Praise for *Botanical Bar Craft*

"*Botanical Bar Craft* is a deeply thorough, well-informed, and tremendously inspired guide to creating herbal beverages for professionals and anyone interested in infusing their imbibing with a bit more nature. From comprehensive herbal-ingredient profiles to recipes that push and blend the boundaries between cocktails and mocktails, this book will be well used and much beloved by its readers!"

—**Rachelle Robinett**, RH (AHG);
writer, artist, and naturalist; author of *Naturally*

"*Botanical Bar Craft* captures something unique among cocktail books—it helps readers reconnect their creative selves with the natural environment and healing plants. This isn't just your average book about building cocktails. Cassandra Sears invites you to use nature as your muse and equips you with the proper bar techniques to harness the power and fleeting beauty of your surroundings. Wild and expansive yet thought-provoking and educational!"

—**Brian Catapang**, bar director and co-owner,
Magnus on Water, Biddeford, Maine

"Ceremonial elixirs and wild plant beverages can be sacred additions to the ritual of socializing. Cassandra unites her bartending background with inspiration from nature in her valuable guidebook, *Botanical Bar Craft*, creating wild and magical cocktails with nature's wisdom woven into the blends."

—**Katrina Blair**, author of *The Wild Wisdom of Weeds*

"In this beautiful and creative book, Cassandra weaves together the time-honored art of making cocktails with a fresh approach to incorporating botanicals for drinks that build wellness and taste delicious! A feast for the senses, her recipes include a deep dive into seasonal elixirs and herbal tonics as well as the foundational practices of mixology. Whether you are new to bar craft or a seasoned mixologist, there is something in this book for everyone. Raising a glass in celebration for *Botanical Bar Craft*—can't wait to try all these fabulous recipes!"

—**Jeff and Melanie Carpenter**, authors of *The Organic Medicinal Herb Farmer*; owners, Zack Woods Herb Farm

"As a Black woman herbalist and herb farmer, I experience the connection between nature and nourishment as more than just a profession—it's a legacy. Cassandra Elizabeth Sears's *Botanical Bar Craft* is a beautiful reminder that plants are not only a source of sustenance but also of creativity, community, and healing. This book reclaims our ancestral relationship with herbs, blending the artistry of mixology with the deep wisdom of the land. Each recipe feels like a celebration of our power to heal and thrive through the gifts of the earth. For those who understand that growing herbs is an act of resistance and resilience, *Botanical Bar Craft* is a vibrant affirmation of our roots, both in the ground and in our hearts."

— **Clarenda "Farmer Cee" Stanley**, herb farmer; founder, Green Heffa Farms

"Cassandra Sears is one of those herbalists who can confidently say, 'Plants chose me.' Her work beautifully captures the seductive intersection of beauty, plants, and playfulness with flavors and botanical effects that come alive in social gatherings. Her plant monographs include both folklore and chemistry and are sure to inspire your creative play with plants, an intention of all great herbalists!"

— **Jane Hawley Stevens**, author of *The Celestial Garden*; founder, Four Elements Organic Herbals

Botanical Bar Craft

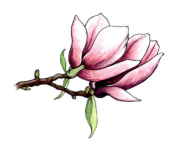

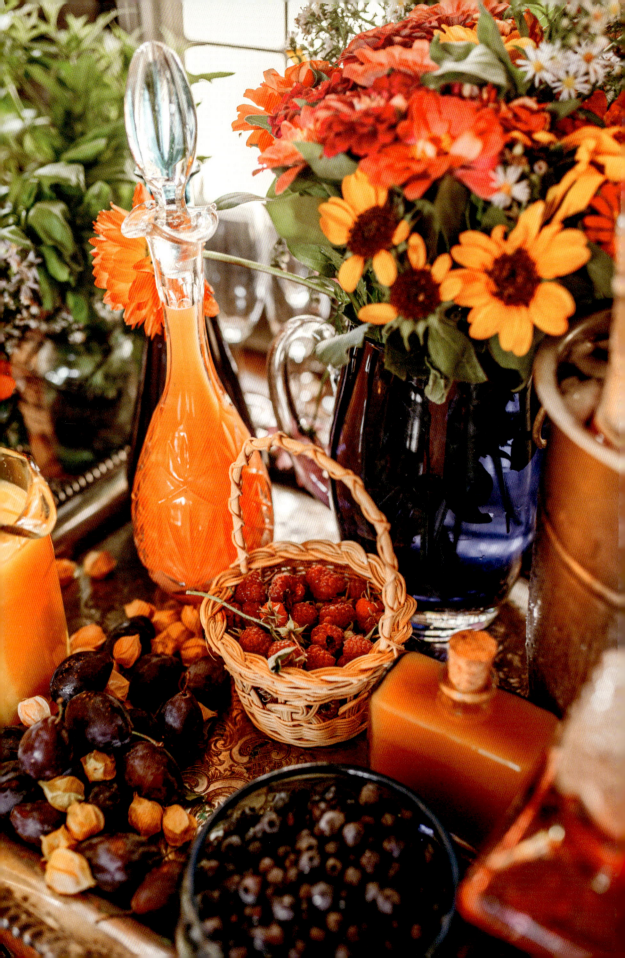

Botanical Bar Craft

A Guide to the Art of Apothecary Cocktails and Herbal Tonic Elixirs

Cassandra Elizabeth Sears

Chelsea Green Publishing
White River Junction, Vermont
London, UK

Copyright © 2024 by Cassandra Elizabeth Sears.
All rights reserved.

Unless otherwise noted, all photographs copyright © 2024 by Cassandra Elizabeth Sears.
Unless otherwise noted, all illustrations copyright © 2024 by Isabella-Zoe Ciolfi.

No part of this book may be transmitted or reproduced in any form by any means without permission in writing from the publisher.

Project Manager: Natalie Wallace
Editor: Fern Marshall Bradley
Copy Editor: Laura Jorstad
Proofreader: Diane Durrett
Indexer: Shana Milkie
Designer: Melissa Jacobson

Printed in the United States of America.
First printing November 2024.
10 9 8 7 6 5 4 3 2 1   24 25 26 27 28

Our Commitment to Green Publishing
Chelsea Green sees publishing as a tool for cultural change and ecological stewardship. We strive to align our book manufacturing practices with our editorial mission and to reduce the impact of our business enterprise in the environment. We print our books using vegetable-based inks whenever possible. This book may cost slightly more because it was printed on paper from responsibly managed forests, and we hope you'll agree that it's worth it. *Botanical Bar Craft* was printed on paper supplied by Versa that is certified by the Forest Stewardship Council.®

Library of Congress Cataloging-in-Publication Data
Names: Sears, Cassandra Elizabeth, author.
Title: Botanical bar craft : a guide to the art of apothecary cocktails and herbal tonic elixirs / Cassandra Elizabeth Sears.
Description: White River Junction, Vermont ; London, UK : Chelsea Green Publishing, [2024] | Includes bibliographical references and index. |
Identifiers: LCCN 2024033584 (print) | LCCN 2024033585 (ebook) | ISBN 9781645022398 (paperback) | ISBN 9781645022404 (ebook)
Subjects: LCSH: Cocktails. | Elixirs. | LCGFT: Cookbooks.
Classification: LCC TX951 .S433 2024 (print) | LCC TX951 (ebook) | DDC 641.87/4—dc23/eng/20240814
LC record available at https://lccn.loc.gov/2024033584
LC ebook record available at https://lccn.loc.gov/2024033585

Chelsea Green Publishing
White River Junction, Vermont, USA
London, UK
www.chelseagreen.com

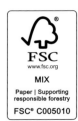

To all of my teachers, especially Jack Pine,
who left a legacy in my heart

To my family and friends:
We are growing together

To the wild & Free

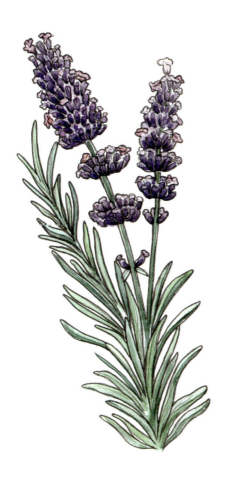

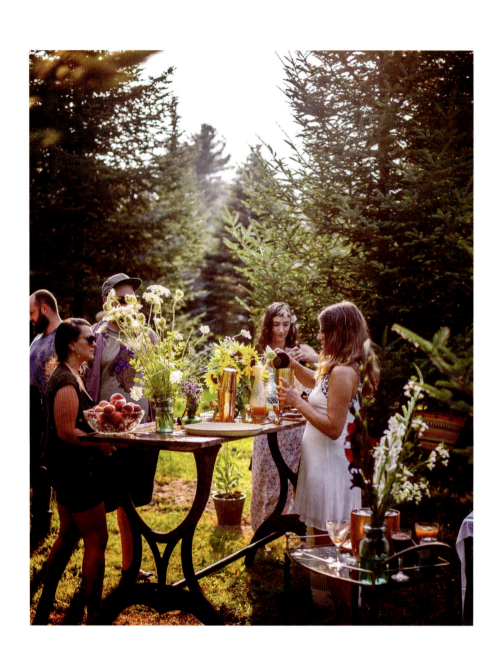

CONTENTS

Introduction: An Inspirited Cocktail Philosophy — 1
1: Ancestral Botanicals in Spirits and Medicine — 11
2: Botanical Bar Craft Essentials — 27
3: Herbal Actions and Tonics — 53
4: The Chemistry of Extraction — 75
5: Distilling Place — 87
6: The Garnish Garden — 107
7: Recipes through the Seasons — 121
8: Plant Monographs — 225
Epilogue: Three Generations at the Bar — 287

Acknowledgments — 289
Resources — 291
Notes — 293
Selected Bibliography — 295
Image Credits — 296
Index — 297

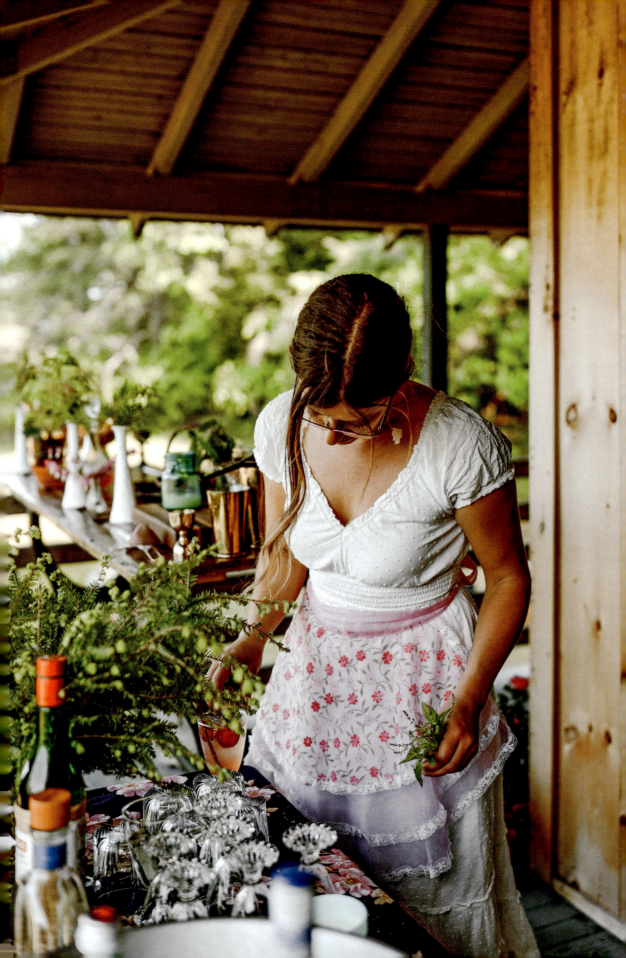

INTRODUCTION

An Inspirited Cocktail Philosophy

The Dandelion Hypothesis compares the resilience of humans with that of plants. It suggests that there is a sweet spot for early exposure to adversity, and that a certain amount of challenge is required to create strength. This concept has become popular in child psychology, especially as a way of evaluating how a person responds to stress in their environment.

Response to stress is largely dependent on an individual's exposure to challenges and the way they must adapt physiologically and psychologically—mind, body, and spirit. If we are to compare people with plants, we might see the difference between the opportunistic, weedy ones and the rare, ephemeral beauties. The example commonly used is the difference between dandelions and orchids. Orchids that require special care and attention are delightfully beautiful but easy to kill if you try to grow them in conditions that don't meet their specific ecological requirements. Dandelions, however, are so strong and resilient, they can bust through concrete. Of course, there can be too much adversity—stresses so great that a living system is unable to overcome them and thrive. This manifests in modern-day culture, where many people face too much challenge in the form of environmental toxins and lifestyle stress. The dandelions among us can survive, but the rest may struggle.

I believe that each one of us has gifts and aptitudes to share in service to the community. Modern society pushes us to act like robots: heartless servants to a monstrous machine. It is easy for an individual's purpose and potential to be stifled by the grind of school and work. It is also easy to focus on our points of disagreement with other people, but what might happen if we focus on the points where we agree and on what we have in common? I think we could all afford a little more live-and-let-live mentality. If somehow you were able to look through everyone's eyes (human, animal, plant, fungi, et cetera), on multiple timelines, before and past death, you might be able to know ultimate truth. But we humans only know what is true based on our own experience, which is highly individual. I don't know why people want to waste their time fighting about who is right when that energy could be a lot more productively channeled. The fact that we cannot possibly know *everything* should be humbling!

My Journey with Plants

Something quite profound that all humans have in common is our dependence on plants. Without plants, we would not be able to exist—we could not breathe, eat, or have shelter. The plant kingdom cares for us deeply, and our DNA has been intrinsically woven together with theirs since the beginning of time.

As a person with a somewhat mystical and literary mind, I often think in symbols and metaphors. One of my English teachers once said, paraphrasing Joseph Campbell, "Change the metaphor, change the world." We are all on our own heroic journey, with gateways to pass through and dragons to tame. My journey began with plants, but how did it lead me to where I am now, serving clients as an herbalist while also working behind a bar and putting on special events? And to write this book?

As a small child, I always found groups of people to be overstimulating. Most of my childhood memories begin with me walking away from a group and end with me sitting in a sticky pine tree for hours, all by myself. Even as a wee person, I knew that nature was the truth. (I would like to thank my mother for letting me sit in the grass and for all the nature walks—and my father for giving me my first herbal remedy.)

For a short time around puberty, I did forget about nature and plants. I was lucky to end up in a small private high school that celebrated free thinking and taught agency to young people. I was a deeply rebellious spirit saved from the fate of inevitable combustion in the public school system. The first class I really loved in school was ecology, and my favorite teacher gifted me a plant press. Poetry was the other subject I connected with deeply. My friends and I were existential teenagers, studying metaphysics and meditation in our free time. The world had made space for us to be ourselves.

Instead of going to a traditional college after high school, I found an apprenticeship at Darthia Farm, an organic farm in Maine. The farmers had been tending their land and crops for thirty years—what an amazing opportunity to learn! Cynthia Thayer saw my interest in plants and put me in charge of the herbal products for the season. I planted, weeded, watched, harvested, dried, processed, and saved my first seeds of *Calendula officinalis*.

I spent most of my twenties working on organic farms or landscaping crews, often learning more about the "weeds" I was pulling out of the ground than the cultivated varieties of vegetables or flowers alongside them. I decided that I wanted to go deeper with herbal medicine than my self-study was taking me. I chose to attend the three-year clinical herbalist program at the

Introduction

Vermont Center for Integrative Herbalism and paid my way by bartending in the evenings and gratefully receiving some help financially from friends and family. A snapshot of a day in the life of twenty-five-year-old Cassandra would include running her dog up a mountain, going to work on an organic medicinal herb farm, jumping into a river to cool off before showing up to bartend in Stowe, and then waking up the next morning to head to class.

After finishing the program at VCIH, I had a strong desire to help people make their lives better through the use of healing plants. I thought I could do this by offering one-to-one consultations, so I rented a room and set up a private practice.

Long story short, that proved a difficult way to make a living. I continued working nights as a bartender in restaurants. For several years I also operated a small edible landscaping business, a one-woman show where I would design and install food and medicine gardens out of my little red pickup truck. Then I decided to start a third business! The Remedy Cocktail Co. embodied the spirit of hospitality and the essential aspects of everything that I loved to do. I had a deep sense of knowing my aptitudes, drives, and passion, but it was a challenge to figure out how to fit it all in. It has taken imagination, guts, and perseverance, as well as many mentors and threshold guardians who gave me gifts, tools, and the keys for getting through the next gate.

Restoring Connections

My vision is to connect people to plants, which inevitably inspires vital health as well as an instinct for environmental stewardship. Healthier people are more mindful and make better decisions. One of the joys of my work with the Remedy Cocktail Co. is journeying to local farms to pick fruit. I take satisfaction knowing it benefits the local agricultural economy and the farmers.

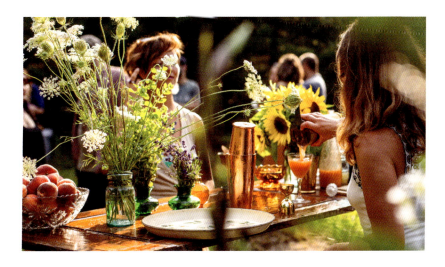

I made a home for my creativity to express and share my gifts, but it benefits the local community as well. I use my platform as a bartender to teach people about the astounding and multiplicitous benefits of plants—and that urge to teach is also ultimately what led me to write *Botanical Bar Craft*.

I chose to include both alcoholic and nonalcoholic tonic recipes in this book because they are equally important. In creating this career that blends my expertise as herbalist and as bartender, I discovered I had to meet the world where it was at. If you want to be of service, it is essential that you perceive and listen! And while I have observed that people want to resensitize and expand their consciousness through sobering up, alcohol continues to have roles to play. As herbalists well know, alcohol is an excellent solvent for extracting many medicinal plant compounds. Alcohol has also had an important role in the development of human consciousness. I am an everyone-is-invited kinda gal!

The hearts and minds of humanity are being called to all that is inherently whole, healthy, and good. The influence of consumer decisions has significant potential in that shift. Voting with your dollar is the most powerful action that you as an individual consumer can take in a capitalist economy. There are also powerful actions you can take in your local communities such as collaborating with other organizations and small businesses that embody shared values, to begin weaving the future together. The consciousness of the importance of quality is rising within many industries, but especially within those that are selling drinks, food, and cosmetics, the things that we put in and on our bodies. Your everyday decisions about what you eat, drink, and wear have an impact. It is important to maintain a holistic view of things when possible, and to always look at the hidden costs of your decisions.

Humans are crying out for connection to each other and to nature. We are not robots. When we build the future together, the transformation can pervade all industries. In some ways we're stepping forward and in others we are stepping back in time, recalling the hand-forged ways of our ancestors. Some folks are worried about artificial intelligence. Could it make humans redundant or unnecessary? Only if humans were posing as robots in the first place! Computer minds do not and cannot possess the knowing or intuition that comes by being a part of the natural world. Emotional intelligence is undervalued, but from the beginning of human existence, wise people have known that vitality and health come from being a part of anima mundi. It is confounding how shortsighted modern people can be. Experience is the foundation of all knowledge and what guides the scientific method. Experience is inherently sensory. Why worry about AI when you can embrace your senses and spiritual intelligence?

Introduction

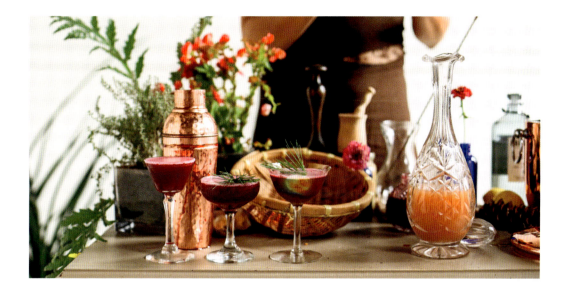

What Is a Tonic?

Sometimes I subconsciously make the mistake of assuming that everyone else knows what I know. But when I share my mission to popularize the use of tonics, people's reactions remind me that they don't really know what a tonic is. When people hear the word, most think of only one thing: the astringent and bitter quinine-laced bubbly mixer called tonic water. This type of tonic water does have medicinal origins, but the essential meaning of the word goes deeper. *Tonic* literally refers to toning; it describes an agent that is toning to the system, that makes it stronger. Tonics are an extension of nutrition and diet, and they can include a diverse world of phytochemicals (natural chemicals found in plants) that gently protect us from the perils of life when we make them a regular part of our diet. It might be argued that in today's modern world, in the face of immeasurable toxicity and stress, there has never been a better time for the knowledgeable use of plants as tonics. Good health is the accumulation of health-promoting choices, like money in the bank.

It is time to say goodbye to sticky-sweet mocktails and a buoyant hello to tonics! We would not be able to eat or breathe without the ubiquitous presence of this green kingdom that we take for granted. Many herbalists, including myself, believe that plants want to help human beings. They mirror us in coevolution. Do we deserve it? Forgive this slip of misanthropy that is a hallmark of my generation. We are evolving together: plant consciousness and human consciousness. Phytochemicals can affect the body in so many ways, including how our genes are expressed. Plants do not speak, but they do communicate. I wonder what they might say if they were talking about us. Do you think they are praising us as good stewards of our home? Perhaps not, but fortunately for humans, it does not seem to be in the nature of the plant world to seek revenge or do harm.

A tonic can be a lifestyle or an activity; it can be a place or a thought. The act of being in nature is inherently tonic and completely necessary. Being dissociated or disconnected makes us sick. We cannot forget that we are a part of the whole wild connection of life's organisms. Health is something that is built over time, and the effects of choices of inputs and experiences is cumulative. As people become healthier, they make better decisions (a fundamental reason to ensure that good nutrition is something available to all).

About This Book

This book is both an herbal medicine book for bartenders and a mixology book for herbalists. My goal as a bartender-herbalist is to use the bar as an engaging platform for teaching about plants. In this book I invite you to step inside the fantastic and magical green realm of the plant kingdom—a colorful place of generous abundance, sparking unlimited curiosity.

Depending on your own experience with making drinks or working with herbs, you will find yourself on familiar ground in some chapters of this book and brand-new territory in others. Embrace it all.

The book begins with my exploration of the ways that herbs and spirits have been part of the practice of medicine from ancient times to the present, as well as reflections on the serious question of whether the risks of alcohol consumption are offset by its benefits. Chapter 2 then turns to the practical essentials of botanical bar craft: basic cocktail-making techniques, the importance of selecting quality ingredients, an inventory of equipment you may want on hand for bar crafting, and an overview of the terminology of classic cocktails.

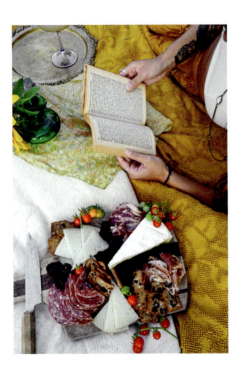

Chapters 3 and 4 introduce the fundamental concepts of herbal actions, energetics, and the chemistry of extraction. Yes, there is some chemistry in this book! But it's all in service to the goal of making tonic drinks that truly embody the healing power of plants—and that tastes *wonderful*.

Chapter 5 is an ode to the art of craft distillation, and a reminder that the creations we make at the bar can only be as good as the quality of the spirits we choose. Mass-market spirits may be popular, but when you learn more about how spirits are made at an industrial level compared with those made by skilled artisans, I believe you will make the commitment to leave mass-market spirits behind.

I love to use flowers, fruit, and herbs fresh from the garden as garnishes for my custom recipes, and one of my goals is to turn more bartenders into gardeners. Toward that end, chapter 6 offers basic instructions for growing herbs and flowers in containers or a garden bed, along with tips for growing some of my favorite garnishes. Gardening is its own journey, and I hope this chapter will help guide some of you to make a start.

I have a great love for the art and process of creating functional tonic beverages and cocktails animated by a close connection to nature. In chapter 7 I share sixty-five of my best original recipes for herbal tonics and apothecary cocktails. The chapter is a tour through the seasons of bar craft, beginning with winter. Recently artisan bartenders and home cocktail enthusiasts have started to extend their high level of craftsmanship to include nonalcoholic libations as well as cocktails. I invite you to walk one step farther into considering the choice of including superfoods and medicinal tonics as daily tonics for your health!

Among the cocktail and mocktail recipes, you'll also find a healthy helping of instructions for making herbal teas, syrups, tinctures, and other extracts, and even a recipe for homemade marshmallows to put in your winter hot chocolate.

In the book's final chapter, a selection of monographs (illustrated plant profiles) provides further knowledge of tonic plants and how to use them behind the bar . . . and anywhere!

Meeting at the Crossroads

Join me at the intersection of herbal medicine and craft cocktails. Both places are inspiring, sensually stimulating, fully alive, and free.

You've let your hair down for the sun to kiss as it swishes across shoulder blades. Balanced at your side is a handwoven basket filled with aromatic plants: resinous pine, a few early seaside roses, apple blossoms, lilacs, and sweet violets. Each harvest is the experience of honoring a moment in time. Each taste has a unique effect on your palate, a palate that you prize for its flexibility and acuity. Each place where you stopped to gather plants affected you differently. The experience was usually therapeutic although not always pleasant. The burning-stinging hairs of the deep green nettle surprised you as you ambled along the sunny side of a river in the spring.

> ### A Prescription to Play
>
> Here is a list of ingredients for an herbal tonic cocktail:
>
> 2 parts artistic rebellion
> 2 parts inspiration directly derived from nature
> 1 part wild-harvested abundance
> 1 part local and seasonally cultivated
> 1 part specific to you in this time and place
>
> *Shake it up, baby!*
> Everything is inspiration and the rest is practice.

On a winding path through mysticism, tradition, and science, I find myself reflecting on how the fate of humanity is inherently woven with the plants. The quest for real and raw sensory experience is part of what it means to be human. Through a shared evolution on planet Earth, we have a deep desire to interact with the wild plants embedded in our consciousness. Our destinies are woven on a biological and fundamental level, from our DNA to our need to breathe, eat, and take shelter, as well as to recover from illness or injury. Humans and plants are interwoven, each requiring the care of the other to thrive.

The quest to be truly alive involves seeking places where nature never left us, or where we have not disassociated from the land. The true heart of science is curiosity. It is not dogmatic. The spirit of science is a continually open-ended question marked by observation, discipline, and experiment. Before modern research, herbal medicine was used effectively for thousands of years. What a wonderful thing that the world seems to be bridging the *tipple* and the *remedy*. The two are intimately linked. From a biochemistry standpoint, alcohol is a strong solvent for many types of medicinal constituents found in plants. And the bar is one of the places that has consistently been infused with plants, even if they're not consistently acknowledged or intentionally engaged with.

Many modern bartenders are intrigued and enchanted by the botanical but lack the deep connection to the elements of their environment or knowledge and practice of using plants functionally. It is my hope that *Botanical Bar Craft* will serve as a guide for those already engaged with bar craft and wanting to expand their knowledge of herbal medicine.

This path is an ode to beauty and creativity—to be a grand host/ess, adorned by, with, and for the plant realm. Happiness is green and flexible, adaptive, and in the flow of all natural things.

Introduction

A party is a wonderful thing. A celebration of the senses. A fostering of connectivity and relationship. An expression of gratitude, a marking of time. Let me say thank you. Let me say Love. Let us laugh and grow together along with the flowers.

Here is my cocktail manifesto: Imagine cocktail hour as a potential ritual for wellness, infusing mindfulness and phytochemistry into a daily tonic. There is no dependence because you are giving your mind-body-spirit what it truly craves: something relaxing, stimulating, hypnotic. Something away from the world—heightened experience, a ritual of self-care or connection.

The drinks I create have a function. They are a way to cultivate health prophylactically and preemptively. It is a daily practice, if you will, to take care of this vessel that we find ourselves in. A ritual creates space for the spirit, mind, and body to talk to one another or provide a healthy escape, a bit of time out of mind. It could be argued that good health begins with motivation, and what better way to be motivated than to be nice to yourself?

The study of plants is a lifelong pursuit of love. The knowledge of plants is key to tying together the creative arts of herbal medicine and craft cocktail making. Whether you are a naturalist, herbalist, gardener, bartender, or some combination thereof, this book will serve as your compass and blueprint for engaging with spirits and flora, the land and its seasons.

As I wrote this book, I found myself answering many of the questions that people ask me when I'm at work behind the bar: What is an herbal tonic? How do I formulate herbs into bar preparations? Is there a mocktail I can make for myself at home—something sensational that hits the spot for relaxation without sedation? This book provides all the answers for those curious readers who have wondered how to make an exceptional drink inspired by and infused with plants. *¡Salud!* To your good health!

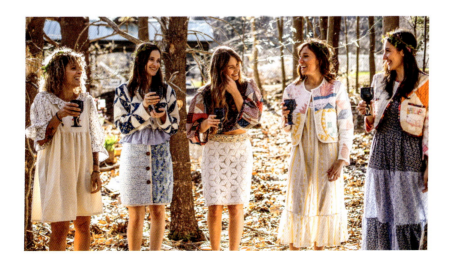

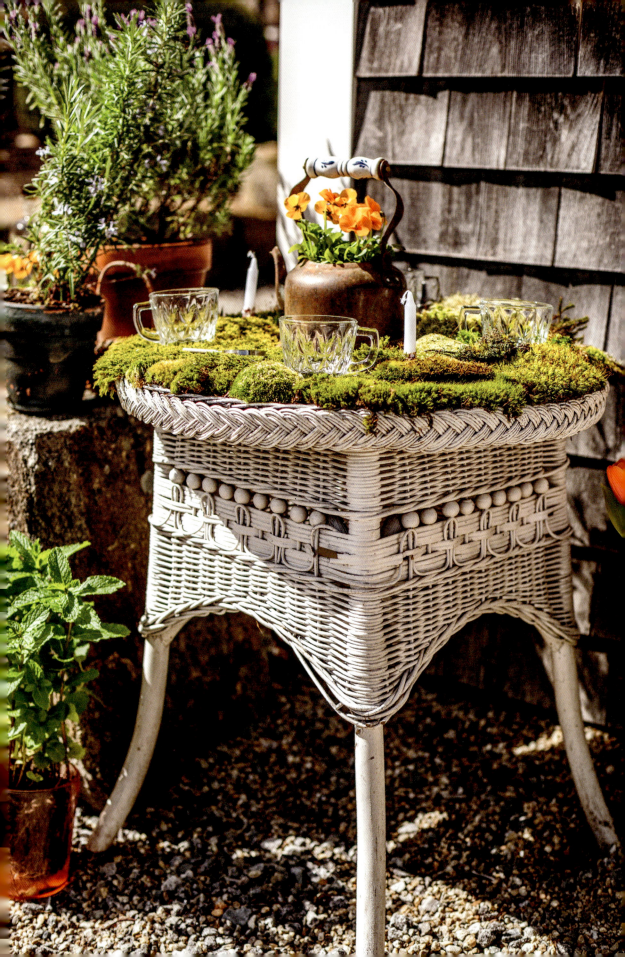

CHAPTER 1

Ancestral Botanicals in Spirits and Medicine

Humans have been evolving their consciousness for thousands of years by stretching and pushing the boundaries of sobriety. Fermented beverages have always been part of our history as *Homo sapiens*. The earliest record of an intentionally made alcoholic beverage is the residue found in a thirteen-thousand-year-old stone jug, and humans were likely brewing even before that. This marks a time often considered the dawn of civilization or the start of the Holocene, the same period when our early ancestors had mastered carving tools out of stone and were beginning to domesticate animals beyond our campfire buddy, the wolf. Humans were transitioning from being nomadic hunter-gatherers to becoming farmers. Some historians believe that it was our desire for drink that drove the discovery and development of agriculture. (If you would like to imagine with me what libations may have tasted like nine thousand years ago, try my Primitivo sangria recipe on page 217.)

Our spiritual origins are deeply tied to plant consciousness, and magical drinks have long helped us reach the outer barriers of our understanding of reality. The mythology and rituals of the great ancient societies were steeped in brew. But what motivates us to alter our consciousness? The urge to transcend reality, although often debased in modern society, is a part of our very nature. This urge has always been integrated fundamentally with a desire to communicate with a higher power. Fermented beverages have been used in ceremonies to achieve elevated states of consciousness that allowed us to speak with the divine. From the libations of ancient Greece to the spit-laced pulque or magic mushroom cacao of the Maya, alcohol was often the carrier for entheogens. Human consciousness evolved through rituals involving drinking in pursuit of spiritual transcendence.

Plants in Ritual and Resurrection

The blue lotus (*Nymphaea caerulea*) flower is depicted in many temple carvings, paintings, and sculptures of ancient Egypt, demonstrating the culture's

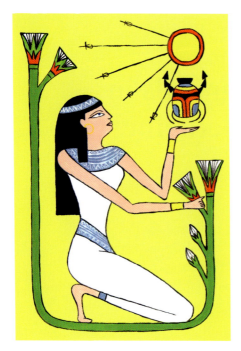

The blue lotus had a deep spiritual significance for ancient Egyptians.

reverence for this beautiful aquatic flower that grew along the banks of the Nile River for millennia preceding the Christian era. The illustrations indicate the use of this plant in ceremony and ritual, as well as its use as an aphrodisiac (including some, ahem, colorful images of very erect pharaohs).

The Egyptians believed this water lily embodied the sun, bridging between day and night, life and death, symbolizing resurrection as well as longevity and immortality. The flower's mention in *The Book of the Dead* confirms this; ancient spells described how to transform yourself into a lotus to assist in fulfilling the quest of resurrection. Perhaps it is in part due to the visionary effects of this narcotic bloom that we can thank the Egyptians for discoveries that continue to influence our lives today, including the very structure of time—the twenty-four-hour day and 365-day year.

The sophistication of ancient cultures is reflected in both their artwork and their rituals. The Mayan Empire extended over what is now Guatemala, Honduras, Mexico, and Belize. There is evidence that cacao played a defining role in the culture. Cacao or *kakawa* was sacred and drunk by all members of Mayan society. Traditional preparations of bitter cacao were used in ritual, connecting the people to their god of maize, Hun Hunahpu.[1] Scientific testing of ceramics that are more than two thousand years old via liquid chromatography and high-pressure mass spectrometry demonstrates the presence of plant-derived compounds such as theobromine, which is found in cacao, thus indicating that the earliest Mayans (600 BCE) drank cacao.[2] Knowing a little bit about the psychoactive chemistry of cacao, I wonder: Did this "food from the gods" contribute to the success of their civilization?

In ancient mythology, Dionysus is the Greek god of winemaking, orchards, fertility, theater, and divine madness. His nickname is the Liberator, and he is depicted with a fennel-stem wand sometimes wrapped in ivy and dripping with honey. This god of wine is defined by freedom. Divine madness is what happens when we partake: Lowered inhibitions lead to full expression and the joy of creation. If you want to summon this god, you may offer Dionysus a libation, which is a ritual pouring of liquid, often wine, accompanied by words of prayer.

The link between alcoholic spirits and spirituality continued in the Christian era. There is a deep tradition of extracting wild herbs into alcohol, preserving them for use and at the same time creating a tasty beverage.

Many orders of monks in Europe made mysterious elixirs—top-secret botanical recipes sometimes known to only one person at a time to ensure that the formula remained confidential. Some popular liqueurs and wines originally (and sometimes still) made by monks include Frangelico, Bénédictine, Dom Pérignon, Amaro Averna, and Mandarine liqueur from Lérins Abbey.

One of the most impressive liqueurs is Chartreuse, a beautiful spirit that has a brilliant verdant color to match its name. It is produced by Carthusian monks in the French Alps, who observe a deeply ascetic lifestyle and have lived in this refuge and sanctuary in the austere Chartreuse Mountains for more than eleven centuries. As the story goes, the monks were given the recipe for an "Elixir of Long Life," but in keeping with the slow, intentional nature of their lifestyle, the first versions of the drink weren't produced by

Blue Lotus Wine Spritzer

1 bottle (750 ml) white wine
1 cup (224 g) dried blue lotus flowers
1 ounce (30 ml) lavender-honey syrup (see the Simple Syrups section on page 37)
4 ounces (120 ml) club soda

Pour the wine into a pot and heat very gently until it is just warm. Put the dried lotus flowers in the empty bottle and then pour the wine back into the bottle. Put a top on the bottle and place it outside in warm sunshine for several hours. Bring it back inside and allow it to continue infusing for about 1 week, and then strain.

Pour 6 ounces (180 ml) of the infused wine over ice in a wineglass, add the lavender-honey syrup and club soda, and stir. Garnish with any type of edible purple flower.

For a nonalcoholic version, brew a strong blue lotus flower tea by pouring 3 cups (720 ml) hot water over 3 tablespoons dried blue lotus flowers. Steep for 30 minutes and strain. Substitute the tea for the wine.

> ### A Chartreuse Trendsetter
>
> First recorded as printed on a 1916 menu at the Detroit Athletic Club, the herbal cocktail called The Last Word was later included in the 1951 cocktail recipe book *Bottoms Up* by Ted Saucier. Absolutely delicious, this trendy, retro, bright-green drink contributed to our renewed obsession with Green Chartreuse during the craft cocktail movement—sometimes referred to as the cocktail renaissance—beginning in the early 2000s.
>
> ¾ ounce (22.5 ml) gin
> ¾ ounce (22.5 ml) fresh-squeezed lime juice
> ¾ ounce (22.5 ml) Luxardo Maraschino Originale cherry liqueur
> ¾ ounce (22.5 ml) Green Chartreuse
>
> Combine all the ingredients in a shaker tin with ice and shake. Strain and serve up in a cocktail glass. Embellish with a lime wheel.

the monastery until more than 150 years later. The lineage persisted, surviving fires, volcanoes, bankruptcy, and eviction.

To this day, only two friars of the Monastery of Grande Chartreuse hold this elusive recipe, which contains 130 kinds of botanicals and spices. The distillery is no longer located at the monastery but is nearby, and the Carthusian monks are the majority shareholders of the company that runs it.

The Deep Roots of Plants in Medicine

Human relationship with plants throughout history is centered in medical as well as ritual and lifestyle uses. The World Health Organization (WHO) estimates that four billion people worldwide rely on herbal medicine as their primary source of healthcare. In the past several decades, herbalists and alternative medicine practitioners have brought new attention to these fundamental natural remedies. And while doing research for this book on the PubMed website, I was pleased to see that the trend is now to refer to herbal medicine as T&C medicine, meaning "traditional and complementary medicine."

How did plant medicine evolve with us? I can't cover the full span of the use of plants in medicine in this chapter, but I can offer some brief glimpses through the lens of doctors, alchemists, and medical philosophers who all shared a belief that good health stems from nature.

Hippocrates of ancient Greece (circa 460 BCE) is a familiar name with the nickname "father of medicine." Hippocrates's work is the beginning of measured rational thought within medical practices: "But conclusions which are merely verbal cannot bear fruit, only those which are based on demonstrated fact."

Hippocrates began the systematic categorization of disease and reliance on the use of clinical observation. Direct observation of a patient's symptoms and behavior remains essential to how effective doctors and herbalists practice today. Hippocrates was also the first to popularize *humoral theory*, no doubt based on the observation of people, their energetics, and disease states in a low-tech world. The four humors were also known as the four temperaments, exemplifying the ability to understand that a person's outward appearance and expression (their "personality") is inseparably related to their *constitution*—the things happening inside the body. This is similar to the energetic categorizations of Traditional Chinese Medicine (TCM) and Ayurvedic medicine. Hippocrates perceived the health of a human as a part of nature and the elements as a whole. The Hippocratic oath begins as a pledge to the gods, demonstrating the connection of health to a larger spiritual context:

Whoever wishes to investigate medicine properly, should proceed thus: in the first place to consider the seasons of the year, and what effects each of them produces (for they are not at all alike, but differ much from themselves in regard to their changes).

Scientific discipline and evidence-based knowledge were bridged with a keen observation and understanding of nature as it presented itself in a human's health. It is the foundation and basis for Western medicine, but at some point along the way, we lost the holistic perspective.

The Hippocratic Corpus, a collection of ancient Greek medical texts, mentions hundreds of species of medicinal plants. And the oldest known medical book, the *Nei Ching*, sets the roots of what is collectively known as Traditional Chinese Medicine, which is a system of holistic health that originated in Tibet, Japan, Vietnam, Korea, and China. The authorship of the *Nei Ching* is attributed to the somewhat mythical Yellow Emperor of China. As described in the *Nei Ching*, TCM sees health as a reflection of the five elements of Wood, Fire, Earth, Metal, and Water, which are also related to the seasons and are mirrored in a person's personality and state of health. (For more description of Five Element Theory, see "Herbal Energetics and Five Element Theory" in chapter 3.)

In Italy in the first century CE, Gaius Plinius Secundus (Pliny the Elder) compiled an ambitious and diverse body of knowledge titled *Natural History*. Pliny wrote about everything in nature, including astronomy, zoology, geology, and medicinal plants. Many scholars relied on this encyclopedia for centuries, even into the Renaissance period (the fifteenth and sixteenth centuries). Much of his work was colored by a Stoic philosophy, which has its roots in Hellenistic Greece, a nature-based school of thought that called for people to maintain *prohairesis*, a will or moral character that is "in accordance with nature." Pliny died on a rescue mission to the active volcano Mount Vesuvius.

Fortune favors the brave.
—Pliny the Elder

Pedanius Dioscorides was of the same era as Pliny but lived in Greece. Their work was similar, but they did not know each other. Dioscorides's *De Materia Medica* includes a five-volume pharmacopeia that served as a reference for more than fifteen hundred years. It eclipsed the work of the Hippocratic Corpus, including a far larger number of medicinal plants, animal products, and minerals.

In the same era, Galen of Pergamon (Aelius Galenus) was a well-educated and well-read doctor, anatomist, and philosopher of classical antiquity. Pergamon was an ancient Greek capital during the reign of the Roman Empire, now placed in modern-day Turkey. Galen's prolific writings reflect his keen logic. He authored hundreds of medical as well as philosophical texts. He was a freethinking intellectual influenced by several schools of thought, not committing to just one. He revolutionized psychology, drawing unique conjectures on the whereabouts of the soul as it relates to the mind and body. He believed there is no sharp distinction between the mental and the physical. Galen posited that reason and experience together ruled knowledge, and this empiricism (the theory that all knowledge is derived from sense experience) drove his individual path of discovery.

A classic medical reference work that includes Islamic theology is *The Canon of Medicine*, a five-volume medical encyclopedia that was used by the Arab world and much of Europe up to the eighteenth century. The encyclopedia's author, Avicenna, was born in 980 CE near the historic capital of the Persian Dynasty in the Islamic golden age. He received basic education but was autodidactic and fueled by his own hunger for knowledge. *The Canon of Medicine* is a synthesis of Greek and Arabic medicine in which Avicenna also imparts his own views on the scientific method and includes his own experience. He added his own resource of Islamic theology to his predecessors: Plato, Aristotle, and Galen. The *materia medica* (a set of treatises on therapeutic properties of plants or other substances) in Avicenna's remarkable work includes eight hundred botanical, animal, and mineral medicines of his time and discusses their energetics, uses, and how to find them in nature.

The contributions of women are often not recognized in the long record of history, but one woman's voice stands out in the record of the uses of plant medicine. Hildegard von Bingen was a Benedictine abbess in Germany during the Middle Ages. Her role offered her the protection to be a mystic, poet, composer, and polymath. She was also confirmed as a prophetic visionary. Her visions were thought to come directly from God and were well regarded and recorded. She wrote two books about medicine: *Physica*, which includes descriptions of the therapeutic attributes of plants, and *Causae Curae*, which concerns matters of the human body and cures for disease. These scientific writings were a result of her work at the monastery's herb garden and infirmary. She was a vitalist who frequently used the word *viriditas*, meaning "greenness" or "lushness," to describe good health. *Viriditas* implies the understanding of vitality as being like a garden, connected to the elements.

Alchemy

The practice of alchemy was the medieval forerunner to modern-day chemistry. Alchemists focused primarily on the transformation of matter to reach sublime perfection. The roots of alchemy trace back to classical antiquity in Greco-Roman Egypt. The alchemists were also concerned about the elements and their qualities, creating highly specialized and methodical processes based on the acute observation of how these materials exist. They fermented and distilled substances, among other complex procedures. It is the alchemists we have to thank for discovering the process for distillation of alcoholic spirits. The alcohol distillations came to be known as *aqua vitae*, water of life. Alchemists thought that aqua vitae embodied the "fifth element" or quintessence—the stuff the stars are made of. For hundreds of years, aqua vitae was believed to be an extraordinary medicine that could cure all ills. Aqua vitae was also called an elixir. Most often this water of life was distilled from grape wine, but the name was used broadly to promote all medicinally intended distillations.

Alchemy is also associated with *hermeticism*, a philosophy arising from the mystical writings of Hermes Trismegistus, supposedly the physical embodiment of the Greek god Hermes and the Egyptian god Thoth. This philosophy combined alchemy, medicine, and astrology with a touch of magic. In modern times people think of *hermetic writing* as a general term for the ancient wisdom of the gods.

Alchemy and its principles of transmutation made their way into the Renaissance period, a time characterized by its massive overhaul of antiquated ideas, spanning all areas of knowledge. The texts of the ancient alchemists were shrouded in secrecy and confounding symbolism, mostly due to opposition from the church. Modern alchemists struggled to interpret and decode. Many elements of alchemical tradition were crystallized during this period, and new works were published during this heyday of alchemy. Alchemists were practicing herbal medicine in the form of spagyrics, which involved transmuting plant matter through various processes of "purification" (such as fire). The etymology combines the Greek *spao*, meaning "I collect," and *ageiro*, "I extract."

Paracelsus, a hermetic physician of the 1500s, coined terms including *calcination*, *projection*, and *sublimation* for methods that embodied the philosophy and tradition of alchemy. The three essential principles, the *prima materia* of the four elements water, earth, air, and fire, are represented as sulfur, salt, and mercury (the soul, spirit, and body). The techniques were intended to essentialize these elements to create the most potent medicine. Spagyric tinctures are still made by herbalists today. The work of Paracelsus, who was living on the bridge of the old and new worlds, carried the mystic thread of alchemy and hermeticism into modern chemistry.

> *Magic is natural, for nature itself is magic.*
> *—Paracelsus*

The Shift to Modern Medicine

The Renaissance was a period of scientific revolution. It was the time of Copernicus, Isaac Newton, Galileo, and Descartes. It was also a cultural and scholarly movement marked by the rediscovery and application of ideas from classical antiquity that had been shrouded in the preceding Dark Ages.

The humoral theory of medicine, which had been the unifying system of thought among physicians for two thousand years, began to be pushed aside by the seventeenth century. Even though it was falling out of favor, certain aspects or practices, such as bloodletting to "purge the bad humors," persisted up until the nineteenth century.

English botanist Nicholas Culpeper was a critic of the unnatural medical practices used by some doctors of the time. Culpeper authored two great works on plant medicine, *The English Physician* (1652) and *Complete Herbal* (1653). He had an affinity for attributing plants to planets (this is the discipline called medical astrology), and his scholarship made a great contribution to the collective knowledge of herbal pharmacology. His work is still highly regarded by herbalists.

The Enlightenment, also known as the Age of Reason, followed the Renaissance, and with it, the magic of the old ways began to fade. The Enlightenment was marked by the rejection of religion as well as superstition and the coveting of intellectual independence. The scientific method and reductionism became the new gods. This had obvious effects on medicine: Traditional ways were suppressed in the pursuit of new truths. But as I mentioned at the start of this chapter, traditional herbal medicine practices persisted and continue to remain the primary means of healthcare in many parts of the world.

In the 1700s and 1800s, as Europeans claimed land and established themselves in many parts of the United States, doctors among them learned from indigenous healers about North American native healing plants. In particular, a group of physicians known as the Eclectics adopted this knowledge, not always crediting those who taught them. The Eclectics also learned herbal healing practices from African healers among enslaved peoples. They were rebel doctors, holding on to the roots of medicine as connected to nature.

Technological advances during the Industrial Revolution played a role in the invention of synthetic pharmaceuticals. The plant medicines commonly available at pharmacies began to be replaced by these human-made drugs. Concurrently, leaning on the deep history of alcohol being medicine, pharmacies and unscrupulous traveling salesmen peddled snake oil and many extracts of dubious value.

In the United States there was no regulation for medicinal substances until 1906. To this day, *snake-oil salesman* is a term used for a so-called quack doctor selling illegitimate medicine. And over the course of the twentieth century, with the advent of the Food and Drug Administration (FDA), the United States has developed an extensive regulatory framework for the practice of medicine, which also relates to herbal medicine. This regulatory framework had some unfortunate results as well. For example, it led to a decline in the teaching of Eclectic medicine; the last Eclectic medical school closed in 1939.

The old magic did find its way into the twentieth century despite the overall heavy reliance on logic and the increasingly narrowing perspective of society and modern science. To offer just one example, although there are many, Austrian scientist and philosopher Rudolf Steiner developed anthroposophy, a wide-ranging philosophical approach influenced by Johann Wolfgang von Goethe and Friedrich Nietzsche. The recorded teachings of Steiner, a self-proclaimed seer, include works that have influenced agriculture (the biodynamic method of farming and gardening), schooling (Waldorf education), and medicine. This focus on cosmology sings to the ghosts of the past alchemists.

Modern regulation of pharmaceuticals in the United States includes herbal and vitamin products. For example, no health claim may be made on a product label unless that product has been reviewed by the FDA. The label of all dietary supplements must contain a phrase such as "These statements have not been evaluated by the Food and Drug Administration. This product is not intended to diagnose, treat, cure, or prevent any disease."

Regulation exists so that you, as a consumer, can trust what's in the bottle of vitamins or herbal tincture you select from the store shelf. It is entirely helpful, but the unfortunate side effect of it is the disbelief in accessible and affordable traditional medicine.

I don't blame people for being wary of herbal medicine, especially given the miraculous cure-alls that were sold for centuries before this arena was regulated. The distrust goes beyond plant-laced potions. Some of the medical practices that were considered safe and effective in past times are horrific to us now: bloodletting, mercury, and lobotomies. Science is always trial and error, and good science always ends in a question mark. It is evolutionary.

I'm not saying that healthcare regulations are unnecessary. But when we place the agency for decision making and awareness outside of the self and delegate it to external agencies, it can remove the people's individual responsibility to do their own research and make carefully considered decisions about their healthcare.

I believe the continued suppression of herbal medicine is a shame. Modern living could use a little more authentic healing, rooted in the elements and in the deep integrated understanding that we *are* nature. Modern medicine is very much "disease care" rather than healthcare. Herbalists work with a person as a dynamic living being, helping them create health from the ground up through lifestyle choices, mindset, nutrition, movement, and hydration. Herbs are tonics and superfoods and an extension of the person's diet, wildly available and abundant all around us. It is a very empowering shift in mindset!

The Risks and Benefits of Alcohol Consumption

Undoubtedly, alcohol has played a major role in shaping human consciousness, but the question of whether alcohol is beneficial to the human body remains highly contentious. The crux of the matter is dosage: How much alcohol can be tolerated with possible benefit? How much alcohol is inflammatory and damaging to the body? Another question is philosophical: For folks without addictive tendencies, is alcohol an acceptable aid to mind expansion? At special occasions that might be similar to those of our ancient ancestors, does the celebratory or sanctified experience of "time out of mind" benefit our spiritual and psychological health? I believe the key word is *occasional*, along with the recognition that every person is differently able to tolerate a dose of alcohol and a particular frequency of poison consumption. I would argue that smaller doses can be tonic to the body, fortifying it against challenge.

People's views in the United States about the benefits and risks of alcohol consumption have long been divided. One of the most dramatic

The Scofflaw

A temperance-supporting banker, Delcevare King, held a contest requesting entries from the public for their best derogatory term to describe those who drank illegally during Prohibition. The winner received $200 in gold. A bartender named Jock at New York Bar in Paris had a better idea of how to use the prizewinning word.

Here is my take on the original recipe. The original is slightly drier, but I believe these proportions better suit the modern palate. I use dry curaçao (for its concentrated aromatics) in place of an orange twist. I also like to make my own version of grenadine from pomegranate juice and sugar (1:1 ratio), with a touch of orange flower water and a splash of lime juice.

1½ ounces (45 ml) rye whiskey
½ ounce (15 ml) dry vermouth
¾ ounce (22.5 ml) grenadine
¾ ounce (22.5 ml) fresh lemon juice
Dry curaçao
Cherry, for garnishing

Shake the whiskey, vermouth, grenadine, and lemon juice vigorously and strain up into a coupe glass. Spritz with curaçao. Garnish with a good cherry.

regulatory steps taken by the US government was the outright banning of alcohol during Prohibition (1920 to 1933). One outcome of this was that the sale of booze and remedies entangled. With the sale of alcohol beverages forbidden, bootleggers became pharmacists and distilleries produced "medicinal whiskey," available by prescription only from the family doctor.

Many Americans were happy to sip their French 75s, Gin Rickeys, Bee's Knees, and Last Words illegally in secret underground bars. I imagine the adrenaline rush they felt was like that of a teenager sneaking out of the house while the family slept, although perhaps a touch more dangerous. One of my favorite cocktails from Prohibition is a rye whiskey grenadine-laced sour called the Scofflaw, a name made up to describe these wild party animals who *scoffed* at the *law*. For those rule followers, the way to obtain alcohol legally was a prescription from the pharmacy.

Despite alcohol's longtime use as medicine or as a carrier for medicine (including medicinal compounds from plants) and its strong topical antiseptic properties, most modern scientists balk at the idea of alcohol in and of itself being medicine. The consensus of modern research is that alcohol intake above one or two drinks per day is disastrous to health. But perhaps ironically, partaking in one or two alcoholic drinks a day is considered moderate and associated with a lower risk of heart disease and stroke. In larger amounts alcohol consumption can cause neurodegeneration and cognitive impairment, but recent studies have indicated that smaller amounts may increase cognitive function.

Partaking in strong substances that can provide benefits but also such serious negative impacts requires respect and discipline. Predispositions to alcohol dependence can drastically tip the scales and remove any of the psychosocial benefits, such as increased sociability and the ability to relax, that most of us can enjoy. The discussion of how much alcohol is too much seems likely to continue. Alcohol is a highly addictive substance with a genetic as well as environmental link; it is not surprising the topic is contentious. Culturally we are obsessed with the stuff. It is either the devil incarnate or the gas on the fire of leading fast and furious inflammatory lives that are centered on productivity, to the exclusion of all other matters.

Alcohol floods the brain with dopamine, creating feelings of euphoria. It also inhibits judgment, impulse control, and memory. It affects our neurotransmitters, and frequent consumption can reduce the number of the receptors that regulate the body's natural ability to relax. Alcohol is often used as a coping mechanism to deal with overstimulation and general excess to "take the edge off." When used in this way, the self-medicating is not offered without cost. The consequences are marked neurological changes in nervous system wiring and behavior, irreversible damage to the cardiovascular system, and preoccupation of the liver that is supposed to be performing many other essential processes for detox, assimilation, and efficient hormone function in the body. Frequent abuse can cause fatty liver, which then leads to cirrhosis. The negative effects can also include blood sugar dysregulation; alcoholism also often includes extreme nutritional deficiencies that exacerbate any neuropsychiatric disorders already tangled up in the mix.

Women exhibit a more profound response to alcohol because of their lower natural production of the enzyme that breaks down alcohol, as well as their higher concentration of body fat, which stores rather than disperses. Studies that include the brain scans of alcoholics have also demonstrated that the brains of women are more responsive to alcohol, with enlarged limbic-reward systems but also less brain damage. Scientists have yet to get to the root of why this is, but the larger rewards systems in response to alcohol indicates that alcohol is a more addictive substance for women than men.[3]

The same substance we use moderately for celebration and enhancing social experiences can have long-term neuropsychiatric effects when used

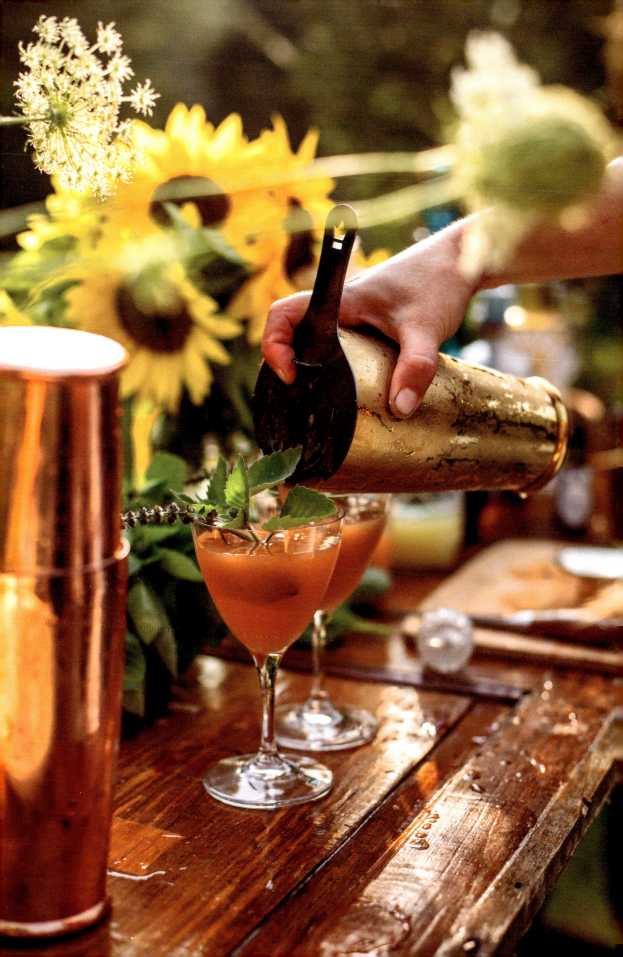

in excess. Excessive drinking also leads to alterations in behavior and associated risks (bad decisions with lack of impulse control) that have been shown to lead to higher incidence of sexually transmitted diseases, violence, and car crashes. Both an acute and a long-term tolerance of alcohol can be accelerated if drinking often takes place in the same environment or is accompanied by the same cues as the brain is set up to "optimize" behavior.

Use of any substance that has powerful effects on the body requires a great deal of discipline. Humanity tends to have trouble with cultivating balanced perspectives, often leaning to one extreme or the other in ideology as well as action. More than one truth can exist along the same continuum. Alcohol is used both to feel and not to feel, to connect and to disconnect.

Even though alcohol use is considered pro-inflammatory, low to moderate use has been shown in studies to have cardiovascular benefits. A lesser-known area of interest is the study of alcohol as a protective substance (dose-dependent) in autoimmune diseases.[4]

Anyone who has engaged in a night of binge drinking knows about alcohol's potential for deleterious effects on the digestive system, but what about small doses? As a circulatory stimulant, there is no doubt that small doses of alcohol get the blood moving, which would in turn affect the digestion and also have stimulating effects on the liver, which plays a prime role in digestion. I believe that, in the absence of any history of abuse or GI inflammation from other sources, like food allergies, small doses of alcohol have the effect of assisting digestion.

What is the root cause of consumption tipping the scales to the side of excess? There are a variety of reasons, but might I suggest looking at cultural implications. Drinking alcohol is often a maladaptive coping mechanism for life in an overstimulated and overworked society. *Maladaptation* is an unsuccessful attempt to fix the problem of being in a bad place. Alcohol may seem to help take the edge off or help you work longer, but as dependence develops, it hurts rather than helps the body. Alcohol is used to help promote an excessive, aggressively empty, go-go society to no effect. We need to respect strong substances and use them accordingly. What creates addictive or maladaptive habits? As distasteful as research on laboratory animals is, we can learn much about our own behavior through the analysis of past research studies, such as the many studies of lab rats. Some of the first addiction-related behavior experiments isolated a single rat in a cage. In the absence of community, the animal would choose to drink drugged water to the point of overdose and death. Is there a parallel to humans who have never lived in a healthy environment? How can they be motivated toward protecting and improving their health? The good news is that alcohol use seems to be downtrending worldwide, as can be seen by the ubiquity of alcohol-free "spirits" on the market.

Something I've noticed through my own experience as a bartender is a positive association between athleticism and alcohol use as well as a link between intelligence and alcohol consumption. Research tells us this is indeed the case. The link with fitness isn't hard to understand—people with sensory-seeking behavior are likely to enjoy exercise, and also likely to enjoy the sensations they experience when drinking their favorite wine or cocktail.[5] The link with IQ is more nuanced. Alcohol use seems to be the behavior anomaly among a group typified by mostly life-affirming behavior.[6] My initial questions about this seeming contradiction shifted as I reflected on the many famous writers who used and abused alcohol. Was it because they were suffering artists, or because of their neurobiology? Some of it seems to be related to the fact that alcohol increases cognitive abilities in the short term. Some scientists believe the positive IQ relationship is simply a socioeconomic one: intelligence-related selection into places in society where frequent drinking is more common.

One thing seems sure to me: There is a fine line on the edge of adaptability, and the only factor protecting you from slipping off the edge is mindfulness. Alcohol is a powerful drug and substance that has played an integral role in our history as human beings. It affects people differently, and choosing whether or not to consume alcohol is dependent on personal sensitivity and preference. Some past cultures were very lubricated, but it seems that this next generation is choosing abstinence more. Perhaps we are at a pivotal juncture in human evolution that requires more acute attention and sobriety. The cultural leaning toward less drinking is no doubt beneficial and is, perhaps, a pendulum swing away from the excesses of past generations. Even if we don't drink alcohol daily, I have no doubt that it will continue to inspire and inform our evolution and continue to be a vehicle for plant medicine as a solvent and carrier for potent phytochemicals.

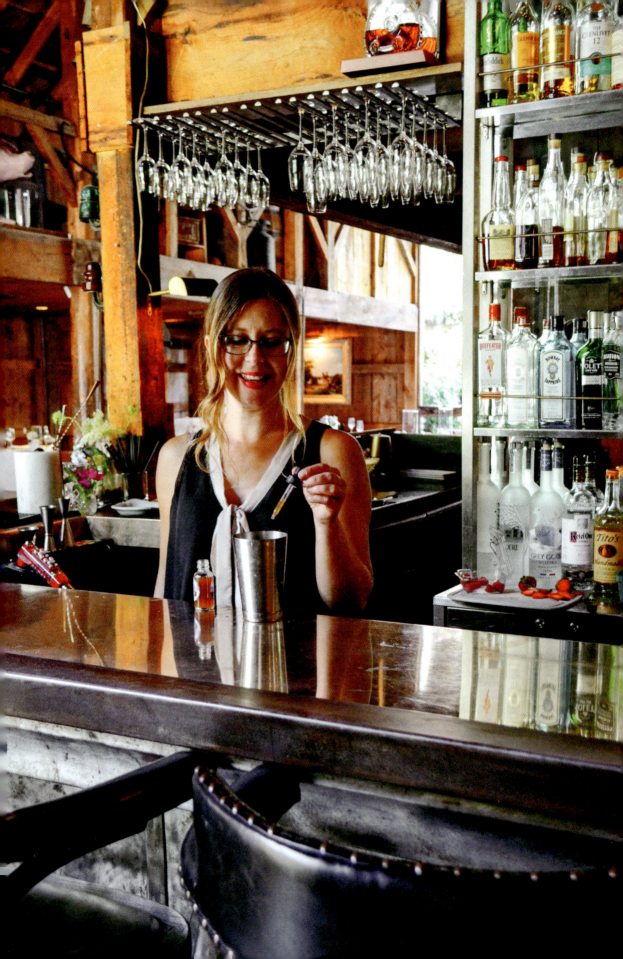

CHAPTER 2

Botanical Bar Craft Essentials

The first step to making an elevated cocktail is to seek ingredients that will inspire you. That might be garnishes you grew in a garden, evergreen tips foraged in springtime, or tart cherries picked at a nearby orchard. Your local farmers market is a wellspring of possibilities. A basket of seasonal fruit and wild herbs becomes the muse for channeling a passion for seasonality into art.

When I am creating signature cocktails for special events, I take many factors into consideration, but the crux of my artistry is capturing the exact taste and feel of a moment in time. This requires mindfulness and being in tune with my environment. It's a call for receptivity. What is nature saying to me right now?

There are other magical threads to capture as well. Who is the imbiber? Do they have favorite colors or tastes? What is the occasion? Is there a story I should weave into this cocktail experience? Are there themes that require the inclusion of certain herbs to encourage a particular effect? Consider metaphysical energetic principles: What is the right remedy for the moment? There is so much we can do with taste, smell, and the combination of the two: flavor. So tell me, what is the flavor of the moment? Feel into it! Indulge in the senses, just like a good chef. Lick the spoon. Feel the sticky resin of calendula blossoms on your fingertips. There are no wrong answers—cocktails are meant to be playful. That is part of the medicine.

Choosing which glass or other type of vessel to use for serving your creation is perhaps an underappreciated aspect of the art form of craft cocktail making. The glass is a significant part of the visual presentation. Sometimes the design of the serving vessel can even inspire the contents! Whenever possible, I like to use fruit and vegetables as a cup, such as half a melon hull.

Be intentional.

One definition of *craft* is "a skilled activity that requires making things by hand." Skill is developed through regular practice, but imagination is

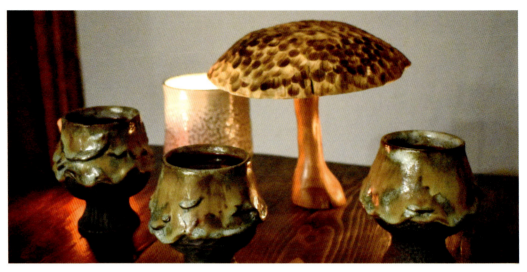

I formulated a special Paloma-esque nonalcoholic fizzy drink called Embrace the Dragon to match these beautiful ceramic cups. (See the recipe on page 155.)

something we can tap into at any time. So embrace the fifth element and enjoy learning a new skill!

The Potential of Fresh Ingredients

When you take a piece of magic grown from the earth into your hands—whether it be fruit or herb—the questions include what to make with it and how to preserve it. Herbalists speak of making *preparations*, which simply means carrying out some type of process to make the herb ready for use as a remedy. In our case, we are making bar preparations—turning raw materials into ingredients we can use in making drinks.

Let's say you have picked a flat of juicy organic strawberries. You could make a variety of preparations from these berries. Perhaps you'll make a complex honey syrup highlighted with herbs, or brew a mead, or dry the berries for later use. The world is your oyster! What grows together often goes together, as the adage goes. When it comes to making functional drinks, however, some types of preparations might be more suitable than others for the best extraction of a plant's potent constituents.

Consider a mineral-rich herb, such as lovely red clover, *Trifolium pratense*. Although its mineral content is not the only boasting benefit of this herb, it is important, and why not benefit from it? Typically to extract minerals from herbs, we add vinegar. So let's make a red clover syrup. The first step is to prepare a strong tea from red clover leaves. Add a tablespoon or so of vinegar to the hot water you pour over the leaves. And to brew a tea that is mineral-rich, it's typical to let it steep for a long time, such as overnight.

Another exceptional method for preserving and capturing the mineral content of red clover or other mineral-rich herbs is to make an *oxymel*—an herbal preparation that consists of 2 parts raw vinegar and 1 part honey—as the menstruum. In turn, *menstruum* is a term for the vehicle for extraction: in other words, your solvent of choice.

I seek out fresh ingredients as often as possible, and I love to make herbal preparations and to preserve handpicked fruits. My recipes in chapter 7 includes many honey tea syrups, tinctures, infusions, and more. The beauty of these preparations is that many of them keep well for months (even years), allowing you to continue including them in your favorite standard drink recipes and in brand-new creations.

I also take care to seek out the very best-quality spirits for the cocktails I make. You may wonder whether there's really any difference between one brand of gin or whiskey and another. Let me tell you, in this exciting era of craft distillation, the differences are very significant. In chapter 5, I dive deep into this topic of the importance and potential of agriculture-driven craft spirits being used for mixing state-of-the-art herbal tonics and apothecary cocktails.

How to Build and When to Shake

Let me introduce some fundamental rules regarding the making of cocktails. How do you *build* a cocktail? By thinking of the cocktail ingredients as your wood, and the cocktail shaker, spoon, and strainer as your hammer and nails. So then, how do you know which ingredients to select first for building a drink? And how do you know which tools to use when?

When bartenders make a cocktail that contains spirits, they typically measure out ingredients in order of the expense, starting with the least costly. Thus, the expensive liquor is measured and poured last into the shaker or other mixing vessel. The choice of vessel depends on whether you ought to stir the ingredients or shake them. That distinction has to do with both the desired degree of dilution and the clarity of the finished drink.

Other techniques for mixing a drink worth mentioning include *rolling* a cocktail and *swizzling*. Rolling requires two shaking vessels. Put the cocktail ingredients in one shaker tin (or Mason jar), add ice, and then pass the ingredients gently between two shakers. This makes sense when the cocktail will be poured over ice to serve and does not require vigorous mixing. To swizzle, stick a cocktail spoon in a cocktail glass filled with some or all the ingredients, and with both hands gently rub the stem of the cocktail spoon to cause the spoon to rotate, which rustles up the ice. Swizzling differs from stirring because when you stir, you move the whole spoon definitively in a clockwise or counterclockwise motion, which moves the all the contents in the glass, not just the ice.

After being shaken, stirred, rolled, or swizzled, many cocktails are poured through a strainer into the serving glass. Traditionally, a julep-style strainer is used with a mixing glass for stirred cocktails and a Hawthorne-style strainer for shaken cocktails. (I describe these types of strainers later in this chapter.)

You may also modify your technique or equipment when you're making a large quantity of drinks rather than just one or two. I have used half-gallon Mason jars for shaking or stirring many servings of a cocktails at once.

The Art of Dilution

Let's explore the topic of dilution. One way to dilute a drink is by adding water, of course. But with cocktails, the dilution often happens while the drink is being prepared, as the maker stirs or shakes the ingredients in a vessel with ice in order to chill it. Shaking typically results in more ice melting—and thus more dilution—than stirring.

Traditionally, spirit-only cocktails that do not contain juices (such as Manhattans or Martinis) are stirred. Drinks that contain fruit juices are usually shaken for a more total mixing of the ingredients (and sometimes more dilution), and clarity of the drink is usually not the goal.

There are good reasons to bend and break these basic rules. For example, I shake Vodka Martinis when the imbiber chooses to omit the vermouth, leaving vodka and ice as the only ingredients. The over-dilution and over-chilling as a result of shaking helps make it easier to drink straight vodka. This is not my personal taste preference, but there are no wrong answers, and everyone's palate is different.

Water is an often overlooked ingredient in a drink, but we use water to create many preparations, from liquor to tea and syrups to the ice used to chill and dilute. Not all water (or ice, for that matter) is created equal. The best water to use is pure, clean-tasting water, such as spring- or well water. If you happen to live in an area that has "medicated" or poor-quality tap water, I recommend either filtration or using bottled spring- or distilled water. Water naturally contains a mixture of minerals from the rock and earth that it is born from, and varying mineral content

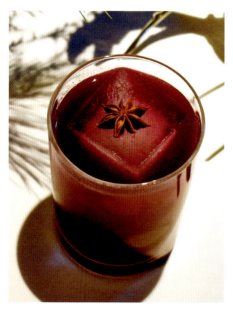

An oversized ice cube can serve as a platform for a creative garnish, like this star anise in a Siren Call (see the recipe on page 212).

can affect the taste. For instance, water that has a strong sulfuric content will make preparations smell and taste faintly of boiled eggs.

This also raises the question: How much ice to use? I usually add enough so that there is just slightly more ice than the amount of liquid, but still plenty of room for the cocktail-in-process to move freely. There's more about the important topic of ice later in this chapter, too.

Botanical Bar Preparations

Plants, of course, are an essential part of botanical bar craft. There are often several appropriate ways to capture the vital essence of freshly picked plant material. Some botanicals lend themselves better to one extraction and preservation method over another to fully capture their essence and the full medicinal value. Here I summarize the preparation methods you will use, including tinctures, teas, and more. These will be key ingredients for building apothecary drinks.

Please refer to the "Quick Reference Extraction Guide" in chapter 4 as well. And in chapter 8 you'll find helpful information about the chemical constituents of specific botanicals, which will help you figure out the best extraction methods for that plant.

"Resources" at the end of this book also includes a listing of reliable companies that make botanical preparations.

Amaro

Amaro means "bitter," and this bittersweet digestif hails from Italy, where there are many, many variations—everyone and their great-grandfather has their own recipe. Amaro does not have an official appellation (region of production) like champagne and some other wines and spirits do. It can be made in a wine or a spirit base. The bitter plants are macerated for several weeks, then strained; the finished product is sweetened. Wine-based aperitifs need to be stored refrigerated and will last one to two months before starting to change flavor. Amaro is often enjoyed neat (plain, without ice) before or after a meal, but it can also be added to digestive-enhancing drinks.

See the Winter Amaro recipe on page 140.

Bitters and Extracts

The definition of bitters varies slightly depending on whether you are an herbalist or a bartender. In the realm of herbology, a bitter is quite simply what it sounds like—something that tastes bitter. Whereas in the bar world, the word *bitters* is synonymous with *extract*, and the method for making bitters and extracts is the same. Typically, an *overproof spirit* is used—a

Extraction Lingo

Herbalists use a few special terms to describe techniques they use while making preparations. Let's quickly define those here:

Extract. In general terms, to extract is to remove something from plant material by using a solvent. When herbalists make an extract, the solvent is often alcohol.

Macerate. When you macerate plant material, you steep or soak it in a liquid until it becomes soft and may even seem to disintegrate.

Menstruum. The menstruum is the chosen solvent for an extraction, such as vinegar in an acetum or alcohol in a tincture.

Infuse. To infuse is to steep in water without boiling.

Decoct. To decoct is to boil down an herb in water to extract its flavor or constituents.

Strain and press. These terms refer to squishing all the liquid out of the herbs and fruit that has been sitting in a menstruum. To strain and press, you can push on the material with a tincture press or the back of a kitchen spoon. Or you can use your (clean) hands to squeeze the material if you're straining through cheesecloth.

---

spirit that is greater than 50 percent alcohol, extending as high as pure ethanol. The exact type of spirit to use depends on what you are extracting. In general, a culinary solvent that is 60 to 75 percent alcohol is sufficient for making aromatic bitters. This higher alcohol proof is better at extracting volatile oils and the terpenes responsible for smell and flavor. If you do not have access to culinary-solvent-grade alcohol, high-quality 100 proof (50 percent alcohol) vodka will suffice.

Many products sold as bitters are aimed at the craft cocktail market—everything from peach bitters to smoke bitters. However, these products may or may not have been made using any bitter-tasting plants! To make true bitters, you formulate a combination of bitter roots and leaves, adding carminative spices. The extraction is most often prepared as a tincture (see "Tinctures" later in this chapter). Alcohol is the usual menstruum, but vinegar may be used instead. Bitters should have a good balance of a clean, strong bitter taste balanced with spice and aroma. I often encourage the patrons who sit at my bar or attend cocktail classes to begin by making their bitters with organic orange or grapefruit peels mixed with fresh rosemary or chamomile and cinnamon or cardamom, because these are all common household kitchen ingredients. Dandelion roots and leaves are another common, free, wild option for the source of a bitter taste.

If you wish to experiment with more complex mixtures of roots and spices, I recommend recording your recipes by using a gram scale to measure out the weights of the various roots and spices you combine.

See these bitter recipes: "Are You a Dreamer?" Bitters, page 128; Rosemary Bitters, page 139; Chocolate Sweetfern Bitters, page 143; Chai-Spice Bitters, page 147; Wormwood Vinegar Bitters, page 159; Black Walnut Bitters, page 223; Cardamom-Orange Bitters, page 223.

Cordials

A cordial is a pleasant-tasting medicine that began as the roots of liqueurs that we know and love today. Cordials are sweetened botanicals extracted in alcohol distillations, implied to have medicinal benefit. They were drunk as daily tonics during the Renaissance, prescribed by European apothecaries to invigorate and revitalize the body.

Edible Flowers and Muddleables

Fresh garnishes add much beauty and aroma to your creatives. These "preparations" involve cultivating the soil in some containers or a garden bed and growing the plants. See chapter 6 for garnish-growing advice, but if you lack the time or desire to garden, farmers markets are a great option for garnish shopping. Strike up a conversation with a farmer, and you may learn about interesting or unusual ingredients on offer if you visit the farm.

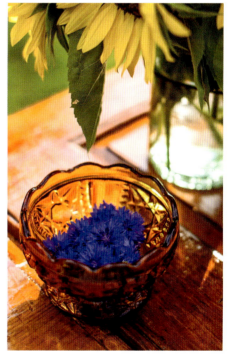

Elixirs

The origin of the elixir reaches back to ancient alchemy, when the word was first used to refer to a mystical substance that could change metals into gold. *Elixir* continues to allude to magic these days. An elixir can be made from any menstruum—a distillation, or a water, alcohol, or vinegar extract—but great attention to the states of matter and consciousness must be applied.

Bachelor buttons waiting to be matched to a cocktail. These and sunflowers are both edible!

Fat Washing

Fat washing is the process of introducing a fat into a spirit for a short period of time (like overnight) in order to change the texture and mouthfeel of the spirit and any cocktails that it might be mixed into. Coconut oil is my favorite fat to infuse or "wash" spirits with for tropical drinks. Olive oil is nice for fat washing vodkas or gin for Martinis. For some drinks, instead of washing the liquor, you can apply drops of oil on the surface of the liquid. One recipe that uses this technique is the Tuscan Garden on page 141.

Ferments

Fermented beverages such as homemade soda, kombucha, water kefir, beer, wine, and mead all make excellent bases if you feel inspired to get down and dirty with making from scratch. It's fine to substitute store-bought fermentations, and there are some lovely products available. The advantage of playing with your own ferments is the ability to create one-of-a-kind seasonal flavor profiles that aren't available anywhere but in your kitchen! Use the concept "what grows together, goes together." Fruits and herbs that are coming into peak expression at the same time often taste incredible paired. Introduce herbs into a ferment of soda, kombucha, or mead at the watery syrup phase.

Flower Essences

An unsuspected cocktail ingredient, flower essences are magical to make and are often used in homeopathic medicines for energetic or psycho-spiritual purposes. Me? I just like the romance. Choose a beautiful day when your chosen flower is at its peak and spend at least ten minutes meditating with the plant. Harvest the flower with clean scissors directly into a small clean bowl filled with water without touching the flower with your hands. Place in the sun for several hours. Mix fifty/fifty with brandy and store in a cool dark place, labeled with the flower, date, and perhaps whatever inspiration you gleaned from sitting with that flower.

See the Hawthorn Flower Essence recipe on page 189.

Glycerites

A *glycerite* is a tincture made using glycerin as the menstruum. Aromatic leaves and flowers such as tulsi, chamomile, and rose tend to preserve well this way. If possible, choose organic, food-grade, non-GMO glycerin, which is poured over fresh material, then blended and allowed to macerate.

See these glycerite recipes: Tulsi Glycerite, page 196; Skullcap Glycerite, page 203; Chamomile Glycerite, page 219.

Hydrosols

Steam distillation is the method for making a *hydrosol*, which is a water-based distillate. Distillation can be done on a stovetop haphazardly, but if you have access to a small still, you'll find it is wonderfully efficient for extracting aromatic compounds as hydrosols. Culinary-grade rose water and orange flower water are two examples of hydrosols that are widely available commercially. Some small cosmetic companies make hydrosols, but avoid buying cosmetic-grade hydrosols commercially because they may be adulterated or made in a non-food-grade facility. If you cannot find a high-quality hydrosol used as an ingredient in the recipes in this book, you can substitute a strongly brewed tea; use twice the volume called for in the recipe.

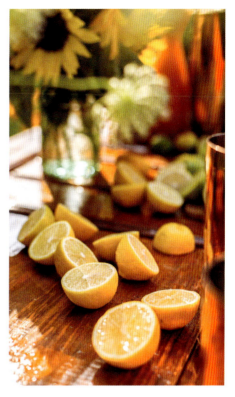

Juicing is a labor of love and absolutely necessary for the best cocktails!

Infusions

A spirit with a flavor imprinted on it is called an *infusion*, and it's made by macerating an ingredient in a base alcohol. Making an infused spirit is an excellent choice for preserving fleeting seasonal tastes and adding complexity and intrigue to your final recipe.

See these infusion recipes: Infused Pisco, page 137; Winter Amaro, page 140; Bitter Orange Cordial, page 148; Hyssop and Teaberry Infused Rye Whiskey, page 149; Cucumber Infused Gin, page 171; Wild Rose Tequila, page 184; Mugwort Infused Gin, page 187; Carol's Elderflower Champagne, page 194; Lovers' Tequila, page 211; Black Trumpet and Butter-Washed Bourbon, page 214; Pear and Cinnamon Stick Infused Calvados, page 223.

Juices

Fresh fruit and vegetable juices can often provide healthy, fresh, and in-season flavor in drinks, capturing the liquid chemistry and nutrition of our most beloved crops, from apples to celery. I often combine juices with herbal teas in nonalcoholic drink recipes. Juicing fresh is a labor of love!

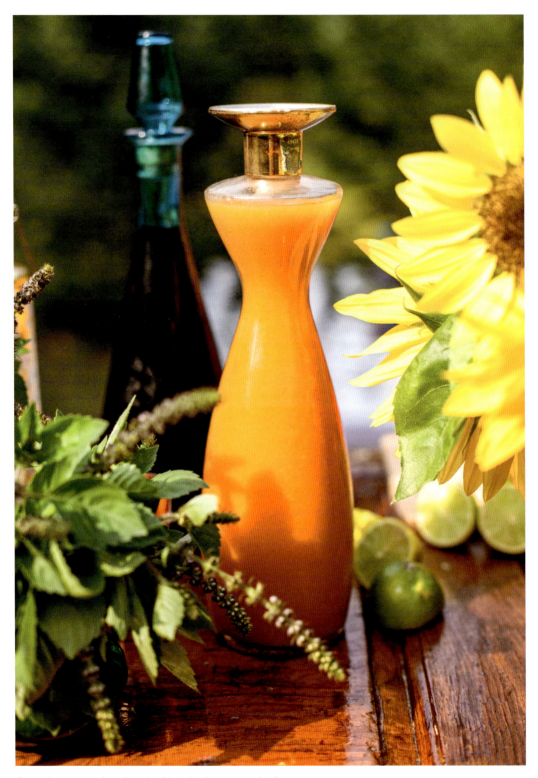

A peach syrup ready to be mixed into high summer drinks.

Powders and Electuaries

Dried herbs and fruit can be ground into powders using a mortar and pestle or a coffee grinder dedicated for this purpose. Herb powders are great for making almost instant herbal lattes. Powdered fruit looks beautiful when applied to the side of a cocktail glass or sprinkled on top of a foamy sour. Note that powdered herbs have a shorter shelf life than whole dried herbs. *Electuaries* are powdered herbs preserved in honey.

Preserves

Preserves can be pickles or jams. Pour a richly spiced syrup over cherries or other fruits to make preserved fruit garnishes. Homemade pickles and other preserves can be stored for several months in the refrigerator, or you can follow guidelines for canning them in a hot-water bath and then store them in a pantry or cupboard.

Shrubs and Oxymels

A *shrub* is usually a mixture of vinegar and sugar in a three-to-one ratio used in the preservation of fresh fruit and sometimes herbs. An *oxymel* has the same ratio of sour to sweet but uses raw unfiltered honey instead of sugar. An oxymel is often employed medicinally. It can contain any type of fruit or herb.

See these oxymel recipes: Spring Tonic Oxymel, page 160; Seafarer's Oxymel, page 213.

Simple Syrups

Simple syrup is sugar and water combined in a one-to-one ratio. You can also make a rich simple syrup with a two-to-one sugar/water ratio. You can substitute all manners of herbal tea in place of water. I often make simple syrups using honey instead of sugar because I like honey's floral taste and its health benefits. I also make what I call honey tea syrups, which are perfect to have on hand for nonalcoholic drinks. Just add one or two other ingredients to a honey tea syrup, and the result will be adequately complex. Honey in a drink also makes it foamy! Generally, it is better to make syrups ahead of time and allow them to cool to room temperature before combining with the other ingredients for a drink. Otherwise, the warm tea may cause too much ice to melt, leading to excessive water and an unbalanced drink.

See these honey tea syrup recipes: Calendula and Gotu Kola Honey Tea Syrup, page 124; Garden Honey Tea Syrup, page 171; Lavender Sage Honey Tea Syrup, page 205.

Sugars and Salts

Mixing herbs with sugar or salt is a time-tested preservation method appropriate for capturing aromatics. This preparation method can also capture the colors of highly pigmented flowers for later use. A food processor is speedy and helpful for preparing herbal sugar or salt; a mortar and pestle will serve for grinding small batches.

Teas and Decoctions

Making teas and decoctions is important for those who do not have ready access to fresh herbs. Many types of tea are available commercially in sachets or loose leaf, and they offer great exploratory ground for exercising

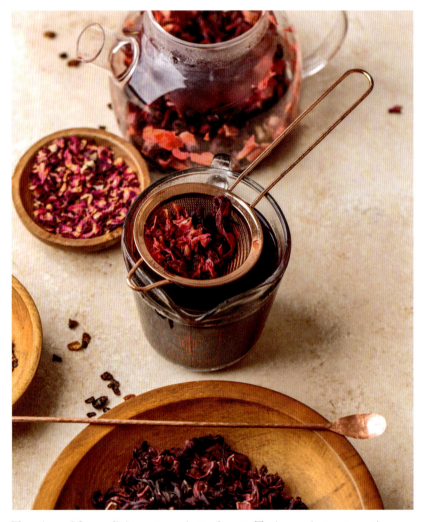

The color and flavor of hibiscus tea make it a favorite. The longer the tea steeps, the more intense the color. Here hibiscus is blended with rose hips and rose petals.

the taste buds. Standard herbal-tea-making instructions are to combine about a tablespoon dried leaves or blossoms (or a sachet) per 8 ounces (240 ml) boiling water and 15 minutes infusing. I often double recommended steeping instructions, although oversteeping some teas, such as green tea, will result in bitterness. Some mineral-rich teas can be infused overnight (with a splash of vinegar). And here is advice I wish I could scream from the rooftops: *Cover your tea!* Put a lid over tea while it infuses. Otherwise all the volatile oils, which are responsible for much of the taste and benefit, will escape into the air.

A *decoction* is a special type of tea prepared by simmering hard or woody ingredients like roots and whole spices in water on the stovetop for varying lengths of time.

See these tea recipes: Aralia Root and Ginger Tea, page 160; Red Raspberry Leaf and Stinging Nettle Tea, page 167; Street Smarts Decoction, page 168; Anise Hyssop and Blueberry Leaf Tea, page 212.

Tinctures

A tincture is an extract made in alcohol or a solvent mix of alcohol and water, which is called a *hydroethanolic extract*. A tincture usually implies medicinal use, but not always. For instance, vanilla extract is a tincture employed for capturing and preserving taste. You can also make a vinegar extract, called an *acetum*. Hydroethanolic extracts typically have a long shelf life, sometimes retaining their efficacy more than ten years if kept in a cool dark place. The length of time an extract remains potent depends on the chemistry of the components extracted. Certain types of molecules such as tannins sometimes fall out of suspension over time, so avoid leaving a tincture preparation sitting too long before straining it.

See these tincture recipes: Street Smarts Tincture, page 168; Reishi Tincture, page 189; Green Coffee Tincture, page 197; Wild Lettuce Tincture, page 201; Milky Oat Tincture, page 203; Schisandra Tincture, page 207.

Vermouth

Many people have no clue what vermouth is, which surprises me. Vermouth is simply aromatized wine. I'm surprised equally that many people (*often Martini drinkers*) think they do not like vermouth. Understanding leads to love. Making vermouth involves gently heating wine and steeping aromatic herbs in it, sometimes with addition of sugar or sherry as a stabilizer. Store vermouth in the fridge and use it up within a couple of months.

See these vermouth recipes: DIY Wild Transforming Vermouth, page 143; DIY Dry Vermouth, page 150.

Botanical Bar Craft

Equipment

The following list of equipment is standard for barware, and I've punctuated the items with recommendations from my own experience. I will say that you can make darn good craft cocktails with almost no special equipment. You can improvise using an ordinary Mason jar and a teaspoon to shake or stir a drink, and a tea strainer works fine for straining cocktails, too.

Shaker Tins

Most cocktail shakers are two- or three-piece types. Boston, French, and cobbler-style shakers are common. The latter is all one piece, so I find it a great choice when camping or on overnight trips (it even has a little strainer built in the top under the cap). Boston glass-on-tin shakers are my personal favorite, but French-style shakers (tin on tin) are the most practical for high-volume service. I like to use a pint glass with a shaker because I like to see the ingredients as I pour them. Stainless shakers have the advantage that they don't corrode or fade. But if your shaker will not see high use, go ahead and indulge in a gold, copper-plated, or hand-painted model.

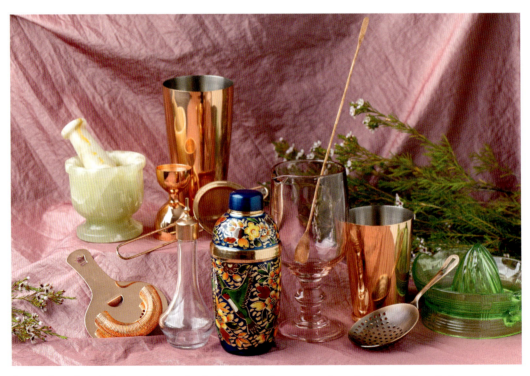

Some of my favorite bar equipment. In the background, mortar and pestle with a bell-style jigger and brass shaker tin. In the foreground, left to right: a Hawthorne-style strainer and a dasher bottle by Cocktail Kingdom, a hand-painted shaker tin, a bar spoon (in a mixing glass) by DMG Designs in Maine, a julep strainer, and an old-fashioned citrus juicer.

Mixing Glasses

A mixing glass is used for stirred cocktails. I have a beautiful footed rose-colored stem glass from Cocktail Kingdom that has held up wonderfully. In theory, you could stir a cocktail in any vessel (such as a Mason jar), but a beautiful mixing glass is appropriate when the mixologist will be on display with the guests watching the process.

Bar Spoons

Bar spoons are taller and slenderer than a dinnerware spoon; the bowl is about the size of a dessert spoon bowl. They're specialized pieces of equipment designed for the optimal stirring of ice. They often are made of high-quality stainless steel and have an extra-long handle with a weighted end. Some bar spoons have a spiral-textured handle, which makes for efficient stirring, particularly if you are stirring two drinks at once. I also love my little copper and brass bar spoons handmade in Maine by DMG Designs.

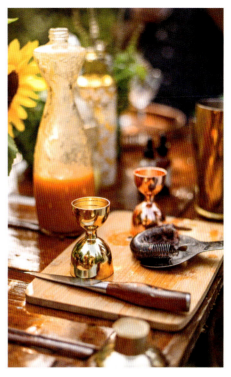

Hourglass-shaped brass bell jiggers like these are my favorite.

Jiggers

Not a person who dances a jig, but a jigger is a simple measuring tool for the bar designed for pouring exact quantities of spirit, juice, or syrup into a mixing vessel. There are two categories. One type is a small hollow metal measuring cup, but the measurements are hard to see in this style. The type more commonly employed is the double jigger, either a bell style or Japanese. The difference between the two is the shape. Each side of a double jigger holds a different amount of liquid. Standard double jiggers come as a 2-ounce / 1-ounce combination or a 1½-ounce / ¾-ounce combination. The 1:2 ratio of the bells is convenient for measuring well-balanced cocktails. Let's dance!

Muddlers

A muddler is a thick wood or stainless stick with a textured bottom end for squishing fruits, sugar cubes, and herbs directly in the shaker. I like my cherrywood muddler because of the way it feels in my hands.

Strainers

Bartenders use just about every type of strainer they can find. Behind the bar, at a minimum you will require a Hawthorne strainer (which has a flat metal disk and a flexible metal spring to help hold the strainer in place) and a small mesh strainer or tea strainer. Sometimes these are used together at the same time for *double-straining* a cocktail, which is important when small bits, such as pieces of an herb like mint, are shaken with the rest of the cocktail's ingredients. For stirred cocktails, a julep strainer (which looks like a spoon with small holes in the bowl) is recommended but not required if your Hawthorne strainer fits in the mixing glass you use. Larger mesh strainers will be necessary when you're making larger batches of herbal syrups, oxymels, mead, and infusions. A *chinois* is a large cone-shaped sieve with a closely woven mesh for straining sauces; it's used in restaurants and commercial kitchens. I use a chinois to strain stewed fruits; a jelly bag works for this purpose, too.

Food Mill

A food mill is not essential, but it's helpful when you're working with fresh fruits and vegetables. If you've ever made homemade applesauce or tomato sauce, chances are you've used a food mill. I like my food mill because it is a non-electrical appliance!

Bottles and Jars

Do you have friends who are herbalists? Then you know that there are never enough glass bottles and jars to satisfy them. The number and types you will require depend on the volume of ingredients you want to process and the range of botanical elixir and cocktail recipes you want to be able to make. I advise a good mix of glass storage for both use and storage: Mason jars, tincture bottles, Grolsch-style (swing-top) bottles, and speed-pour bottles. I like speed-pour bottles from Crew Supply Co., because they come with a cap for storage, for easy use! Swing-top bottles also work well for storage and are especially appropriate for anything fizzy and

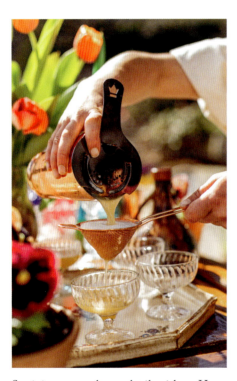

Straining a peachy cocktail with a Hawthorne strainer and brass shaker tin from Cocktail Kingdom.

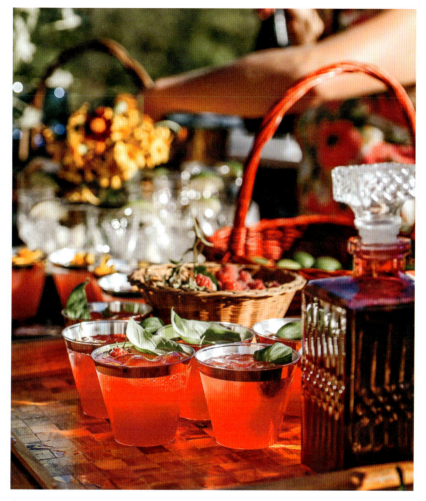

A beautiful glass decanter is the perfect choice for this botanical bar that was set up for a wedding.

fermented like a natural soda, kombucha, or mead. I also wash, sanitize, and reuse store-bought, corked wine bottles for this purpose. Tincture bottles with a dropper cap serve well for bitters. Or you can use dasher bottles, which have a special cap that delivers one dash of liquid at a time. How much is a "dash"? Well, there's no set answer to that question, but some say it's 1/32 of a liquid ounce, or 1/8 of a teaspoon. The volume is dependent on the size of the hole in the dasher bottle top.

Glass decanters and vintage glassware are joyful objects that I love to collect. They can make quite a difference in creative presentation at special events. Happy hunting!

Handblown glassware is lovely to work with. But don't limit yourself to glass. I also look for clay chalices made by local artisans, for example.

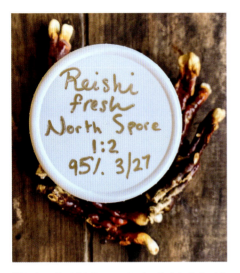

This jar of reishi tincture is clearly labeled with the name of the preparation, the source of the material, the strength of the alcohol used, the ratio of ingredients, and the date prepared.

Blenders

I use my Vitamix high-speed blender for blending tinctures and oxymels prior to maceration. Wand-style hand blenders are also helpful—I use one for blending fruit-based preparations while they are still in the pot.

Labeling Materials

Many preparations must be left to macerate or infuse for a week or longer. Dating each preparation clearly at the time you start it will help you remember when to strain! A good label is also helpful for remembering the story behind the harvest—the place and time. This can inspire and inform the presentation as well as the names of new concoctions.

Microplanes

Microplane is the most popular brand name of rasp-style graters, a tool that was first used in carpentry. Now it is a popular kitchen tool—a long, slender, rasped grater that can be used to zest citrus or grate cheese. A microplane also works well for shaving solid spices to garnish a cocktail. There is even a nutmeg rasp, which is a grater designed specifically for nutmeg!

Atomizer

An aromatic garnish is key for eliciting a positive and multidimensional drinking experience. And don't limit yourself just to flowers or sprigs when

---

Use the Low-Dose Nose

Another fun trick for low-alcohol cocktails is to put spirit into a tincture bottle and use the dropper to drop small amounts on the surface of the drink. This way you get the "nose" and flavor without any of the heavy-hitting effects of the alcohol. This works well for those who are abstaining from alcohol for health and wellness reasons.

Botanical Bar Craft Essentials

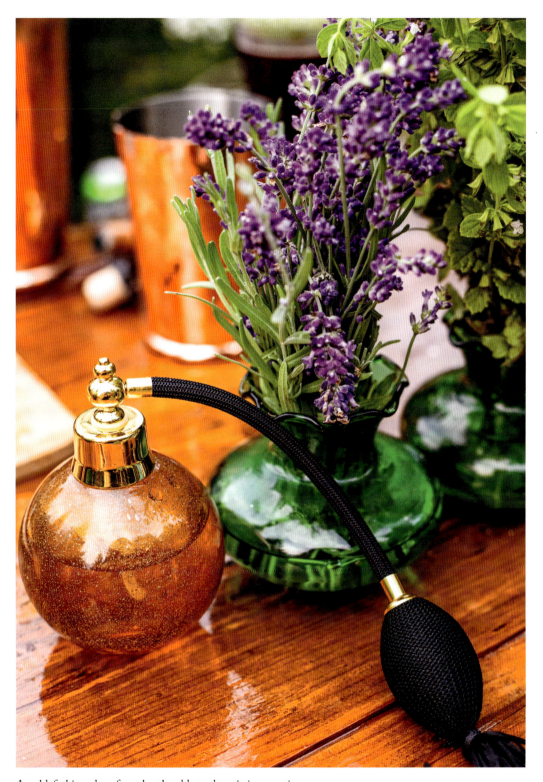

An old-fashioned perfume bottle adds to the misting mystique.

it comes to aromatic garnishes; you can also use an atomizer to mist volatile components over a drink's surface. One good choice for this is dry curaçao, which is made from orange zest, rose water, vanilla extract, and absinthe.

Mortar and Pestle

Although I am guilty of keeping a mortar and pestle on hand primarily as decoration, they are useful for grinding small batches of spices and can also be used for making pastes and powdering dried fruits and herbs.

Spice Grinder

I have always used a high-quality electric coffee grinder as my spice grinder. I keep it separate from the grinder I use for grinding my coffee, though! It is difficult to wash out a grinder fully enough to eliminate all traces of the spice flavors.

Juicers

A high-quality stainless-steel juicer is not a necessity but a beautiful luxury for making fresh vegetable and fruit juices to use as bases and mixers. These machines are capable of juicing almost anything.

Juicing citrus is different, because the bitter peel is usually excluded. There are a variety of methods for juicing lemons, limes, grapefruits, and oranges. A hand reamer is appropriate and quick for juicing small amounts. I like the old-school glass reamers that have a bowl for collecting the juice built into the grooved, pointy appendage. The other option for moderate volumes and made-to-order juices is a mounted citrus juicer. This device has a large handle to press on, which pushes the halved citrus fruit into the reamer. An electric citrus juicer may be the best choice when you need a large volume of juice. Whatever the equipment, I recommend straining citrus juice prior to use to remove the pulp.

Butane Torch

A refillable butane torch is useful for torching herbs or other botanicals to smoke a drinking glass to add flavor. You can also lay a smoldering stem across the glass to add burnt aromatics and intrigue.

Ice Trays and Molds

There is plenty of variety and fun in the world of specialty ice molds: spheres, cylinders, and even roses! Experiment to find what you like best. Some silicone molds make use of a directional freezing method, which creates very clear ice. I like the 1-inch (2.5 cm) square molds—this is a good size for freezing edible flowers in ice cubes. This technique works best when the flower is a little larger than the space in the mold. That way the flower is held in place when the water is added and does not float up and out of the water. It stays in the ice cube, which is where you want it.

Measuring Cups

Jiggers are the go-to measuring device for executing a cocktail recipe behind the bar, but they just won't meet your needs when you're making herbal preparations and drink ingredients at scale. It's good to have both a small (1- or 2-cup) glass measuring cup and a large (4-cup) one on hand in the kitchen.

Building from the Classics

A *classic* cocktail can be defined as one that has been made time and time again, usually spanning a generation or more, and is often reinterpreted and used as the backbone or inspiration for new flavors. As a botanical bartender, you can break down a classic cocktail recipe and craft seasonal tastes into it at every layer. This is a great strategy for a beginning bartender or cocktail enthusiast to learn how to build a well-balanced cocktail and develop their own concept and perception of taste and pairings. Start simple and build from there. See what is happening in nature at an exact moment in time. Often the fruits and vegetative plants that thrive within a particular season will harmonize nicely in a drink. This is in part because they share the energetics of the season they belong to (to learn more about energetics, refer to chapter 3). My advice is to choose one fruit and one herb to add to one of the following classic recipes and gradually build complexity from there.

Ancestrals and Spirit-Forward Cocktails

Ancestral and spirit-forward cocktails are synonymous with the first definition of the word *cocktail*, from the editor of *The Balance, and Colombian Repository*, a New York newspaper, in 1806, as "a stimulating liquor, composed of spirits of any kind, sugar, water, and bitters . . ."

Two stirred, spirit-forward cocktails that fit this description are the Old Fashioned and the Sazerac. Others include Martinis, the Manhattan cocktail, and Negronis as well as the Bijou and Old Pal.

Sours

The category of sours is the most popular modern template, and it contains all the favorites: the Gimlet, Daiquiri, Whiskey Sour, and Gin Sour.

The first sours were the punches and grogs drunk by British sailors in the 1600s.

The golden ratio of cocktailing is 2:1:1—that is, two parts spirit and equal parts sweet and sour. To make any type of sour successfully, use the

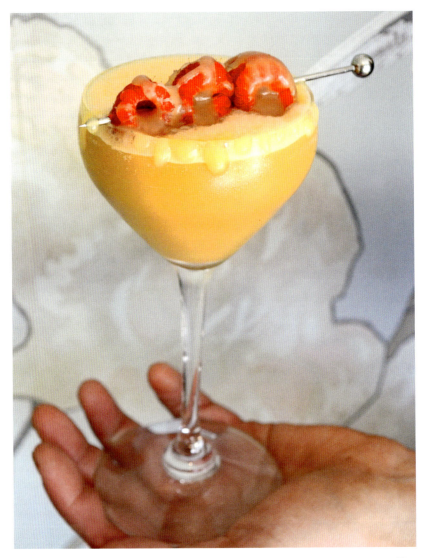

This drink is Euphoria, one of my original recipes, based on an Espresso Martini. (See the recipe on page 211.)

2:1:1 ratio. In the case of nonalcoholic sours, such as a lemonade, the ratio is 1:1, equal parts sweet and sour, to create optimal balance.

Sometimes a single egg white is added to a sour to create foam and enhance mouthfeel. When you're making egg white sours, dry-shake without ice and then shake again with ice, and double-strain.

Fizzes, Collins, Daisies, and Rickeys

There are four subcategories of a classic sour: collins, daisies, rickeys, and fizzes. All are considered predecessors of punch.

Gimlets and fizzes follow the 2:1:1 ratio exactly. A gimlet is sugar and lime in equal proportions made with either vodka or gin. A fizz is a sour that has egg white and club soda added.

A collins is a sour (without egg white) that includes the addition of soda water, served over ice in a tall glass.

A daisy is a sour that also contains a liqueur and a fresh fruit (like Cointreau and a lime in the Margarita), and sometimes also contains club soda. It can be served straight up or on the rocks.

A rickey is classically made with gin or bourbon, lime juice, and soda (no added sugar).

Bucks and Mules

Bucks and mules are bubbly, refreshing drinks made with a spirit topped with ginger ale or ginger beer and citrus. The buck originated as an often whiskey-spiked version of a Horse's Neck, which comprises ginger ale and bitters, with a lemon peel jutting out from the tall glass like the namesake. They are typically built directly in the glass over ice, and swizzled with a spoon or straw prior to serving. A Dark and Stormy fits in this category.

The Moscow Mule (a vodka-spiked buck) is one of the most famous. The name was coined as part of a very successful advertising campaign by Smirnoff Vodka in 1941. The company's branded copper mugs also set the precedent for drinking a Moscow Mule from a mug.

A classic mule is served over ice with a recipe along the lines of 1½ ounces (45 ml) vodka, ½ ounce (15 ml) freshly squeezed lime juice, and 4 ounces (160 ml) ginger beer.

Pousse-Café

A pousse-café is a layered drink. The ingredients have different densities and, when poured very carefully, will sit one atop the other. Translated from the French, the name means "coffee pusher." The first recorded version was in the classic Jerry Thomas book *How to Mix Drinks* published in 1962. These are usually served as cordial-sized or shot servings.

Tropicals and Tikis

Tropicals and tikis are both inspired by *terroir tropicale*, and the names are used interchangeably. These cocktails often have an expressive and colorful flair typified by lots of garnishes. They're made with tropical fruits and spices and often with rum, as that is the most popular spirit distilled in equatorial regions.

Tropical drinks are light and fun, easy to drink and often served with little paper umbrellas: Think Piña Coladas on a Caribbean vacation.

The tiki, on the other hand, originated in New Zealand and Polynesia and emphasizes tropical ingredients but in a more nuanced way, often having layered and complex flavors. The Zombie as well as the classic Mai Tai are examples of classic tiki. The word *tiki* also refers to expressive, sometimes frightening images of faces carved out of stone or wood. The term has a deep cultural and spiritual significance—tikis are talismans and religious artifacts. Thus, a tiki cocktail is a representation of this culture and born from it, but any reference to "tiki culture" is an outsider's perspective and not how Pacific Islanders refer to or see their culture.

Duos and Trios

As you might guess, a duo is a cocktail that has two ingredients (spirit + liqueur); a trio has three (spirit + liqueur + dairy element). Perfect examples are the Black Russian and White Russian, respectively.

Flips, Nogs, and Alexanders

A flip is any cocktail recipe that contains a whole egg or egg yolk as an ingredient. The origin of the classic flip was beer with rum or brandy and an egg, sweetened with molasses and warmed with a hot poker. It was a drink for sailors during the late 1600s. The category has evolved to include all cocktails made with a whole egg. Nowadays a flip is typically served cold and frequently garnished with grated nutmeg.

A nog contains an egg but also a dairy component. Nogs make suitable dessert drinks. And then there are delicious creamy classics like the Brandy Alexander (brandy + cacao + cream), which are shaken with only the white of an egg. A Brandy Alexander recipe was first published in *The Savoy Cocktail Book* by Harry Craddock in 1930, but a previous version made with gin had been drunk during Prohibition.

Juleps, Smashes, and Cobblers

A julep is spirit + sugar + (usually) mint served over shaved ice, traditionally in a metal cup. This cocktail is made by bruising mint and adding it to a mixing glass with 2 ounces (60 ml) whiskey and ¾ ounce (22.5 ml) simple syrup.

The Mint Julep became popular in the Deep South, where it was served in real silver cups that had come to signify achievement. It has been served at the Kentucky Derby since 1875, although the drink's origins likely predate that by a century.

Base spirit, fruit, ice, and an herbal component: Something gets smashed in a "smash"—usually the fruit! A subtype of the julep, the smash has been around since the mid-1800s. With smashes, you can muddle the chosen fruits in your shaker. The template is entirely flexible, but my favorite is what I call a Whiskey Garden Smash. Combine some muddled summer berries with your favorite whiskey, lemon juice, and a sweetener of choice (such as honey syrup). Add ice and shake it up good. Transfer the contents into a collins glass and add a little splash of club soda. (You can also double-strain over clean ice, if you don't like pieces of fruit floating in your drinks.) Garnish with an aromatic garden herb of choice such as basil or mint.

Cobblers, as the name suggests, are also served over crushed ice, but are more often wine- or sherry-based, and the fruit is more emphasized in the garnish. This classic was created around the same era as the drinking straw and the three-piece cocktail (cobbler) shaker. The Sherry Cobbler was a wildly popular drink for most of the nineteenth century.

Marys and Savory Drinks

Spicy tomato, Worcestershire sauce, celery, fresh cracked pepper: The Bloody Mary has paved the way for inviting savory tastes to the cocktail party! Savory drinks are a wonderful way to use fresh juices. Start with vegetable juices such as celery, cucumber, or tomato juice, or explore umami flavors like mushroom and miso combined with herbs and spices. The "savory" is a category, but there is no specific template.

Hot Drinks

Toddies, mulled wine, chai-spiced cider, spiked hot cocoa, Hot Buttered Rum, and Irish Coffee are classic cocktails served hot or warm.

The Hot Toddy is the quintessential warm cocktail consisting of hot water, lemon, honey, and whiskey, sometimes made with additional spices such as cinnamon sticks or a clove-studded orange.

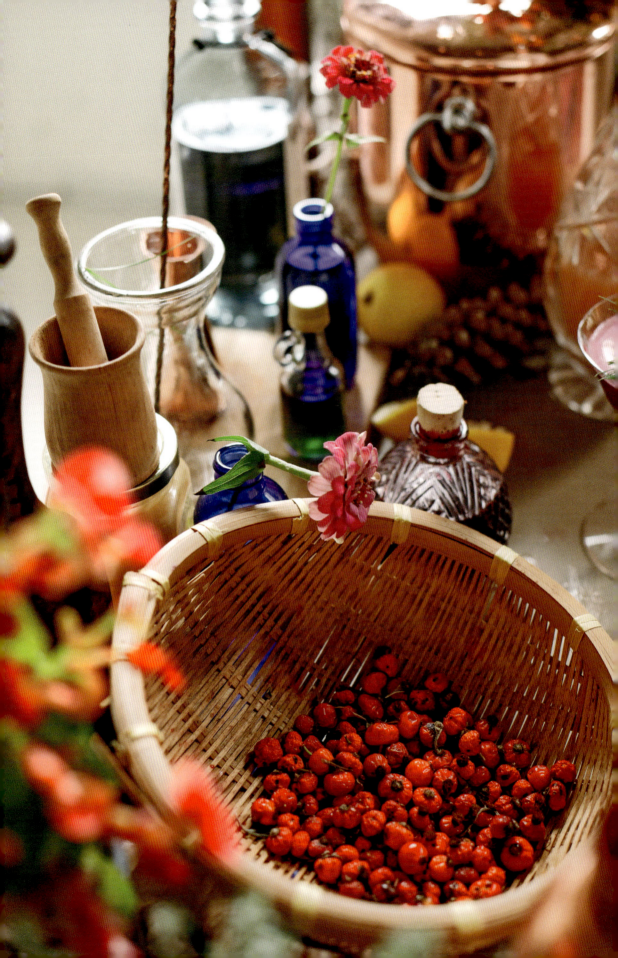

CHAPTER 3
Herbal Actions and Tonics

Herbalists often categorize plants by their actions. Simply put, herbal actions are ways that botanical agents can affect the human body. A familiar example is an anti-inflammatory, which is unfortunately familiar to almost all of us since inflammation is one of the overarching patterns of dis-ease that plague the modern world. Herbal tonics can be part of a healthy lifestyle that helps to prevent and remedy illness and maladaptive states.

It's helpful to learn the terms used to describe herbal actions as a bridge to understanding and remembering key information about botanical allies. This knowledge is a building block to help you appreciate the recipes in chapter 7, which include listings of the herbal actions that each recipe offers. Becoming familiar with herbal actions will also help you work with the information on specific botanicals in chapter 8 as you begin designing your own tonic drinks.

We can also describe the effects of herbs on the body through energetic patterns. Energetic herbalism draws from several healing traditions and focuses less on measurable states of metabolism such as blood pressure or cholesterol levels and more on the overall state of the body—whether the tissues are too moist or too dry, for example. Energetics is a fascinating area of study, and I introduce a very basic description of it at the end of this chapter. It is a subject worthy of a lifetime of study.

What Is an Herbal Action?

In modern herbal medicine, herbal actions are the functions that a medicinal herb can serve. A single species can have many actions. The list of herbal actions is very long, and in this chapter I focus on a limited set of actions (functions) that are applicable to the art of incorporating tonic herbs into beverages. Remember: Tonics work to build and balance health gently over time. They are food-like, meant to be taken daily to achieve desired results, much like daily servings of superfoods help keep our bodies in top shape.

The source of the beneficial effects of many useful tonics rests in the secondary metabolites they contain. *Secondary metabolites* are chemicals produced by plants for their own resilience to protect themselves from

> ## About Plant Names
>
> In day-to-day life we call plants by their common names: Think *parsley*, *sage*, *rosemary*, and *thyme*. But the common names of plants can vary from region to region, and some plants go by several different common names. To be precise, herbalists and gardeners rely on the botanical names (Latin names) of plants. When you are introduced to a new plant friend, learn its full name!
>
> All plants belong to the kingdom Plantae, and from there are subdivided into types and families, such as the rose family (Rosaceae). Plants within the same family often share characteristics. Plant families are further divided into genera and species. Each plant can be identified by its genus name followed by its species name. For example, rosemary is *Rosmarinus officinalis*. The genus name is capitalized, and the species name is lowercase. This system of two-part names is officially called *binomial nomenclature* and it is a key function of the discipline of taxonomy.
>
> If you're not used to associating plants with their botanical names, it may take you a while to get used to binomial nomenclature. But it's a good skill to learn for accuracy in identifying plants as well as safety (making sure you have the right plant). Throughout this book, I include botanical names in plant lists, as well as in any instance where it's helpful to know specifically which herb I'm referring to.

insect or animal damage, and from bacterial, viral, or fungal disease. Secondary metabolites include terpenoids, phenolic compounds, alkaloids, and sulfur-containing compounds. (I describe these categories of secondary metabolites in more detail in chapter 4.)

Adaptogens

Adaptogens are popular, and for good reason! The quintessential "tonics," adaptogens have an overall (not specific) strengthening effect on the body, helping us increase our resilience and adapt to stress, be it physical, psychospiritual, or environmental. Adaptogens interface with the endocrine system, adrenals, immune system, and sometimes other systems, such as the cardiovascular system. Adaptogens can help increase athletic performance, mental acuity, and resistance against disease. There are stimulating adaptogens that can help you run faster from the tiger that is chasing you, while other adaptogens have a regenerative effect—they gently nourish and prevent burnout over time. The phytochemistry of adaptogens typically falls into two large categories of secondary plant metabolites: terpenes and polyphenols (see "Polyphenols" in chapter 4).

HERBAL ADAPTOGENS

American ginseng (*Panax quinquefolius*)
Ashwagandha (*Withania somnifera*)
Astragalus (*Astragalus membranaceus*)
Eleuthero (*Eleutherococcus senticosus*)
Licorice (*Glycyrrhiza glabra*)
Maca (*Lepidium meyenii*)
Reishi mushroom (*Ganoderma lucidum, G. tsugae*)
Rhodiola (*Rhodiola rosea*)
Schisandra (*Schisandra chinensis*)

Alteratives

Alteratives alter the body's processes of metabolism so that tissues can best deal with assimilation of nutrients and excretion of waste. Many herbs that have this action improve the body's ability to eliminate waste through the kidneys, liver (bitters), GI tract, urinary system, skin, and lymphatic system. Alteratives for the urinary system are called *diuretics*; when specifically used for the lymph system, they are called *lymphatics*. Many alteratives work across multiple systems.

HERBAL ALTERATIVES

Burdock (*Arctium lappa*)
Cleavers (*Galium aparine*)
Dandelion (*Taraxacum officinale*)
Nettle (*Urtica dioica*)
Red clover (*Trifolium pratense*)

Anti-Inflammatories

Some botanicals contain compounds that help reduce inflammation in the body. *Anti-inflammatory* is a catchall term; there are many processes in the body that can cause inflammation, and I explore some of them in "Inflammation and the Stress Response" later in this chapter. There are also many means of quelling inflammation. Immunology is a complex subject!

Here are some examples of favorite broad-spectrum anti-inflammatory plants.

HERBAL ANTI-INFLAMMATORIES

Birch (*Betula* spp.)
Ginger (*Zingiber officinale*)
Meadowsweet (*Filipendula ulmaria*)
Turmeric (*Curcuma longa*)
Willow (*Salix* spp.)
Wintergreen (*Gaultheria procumbens*)

Aphrodisiacs

This is an exciting category that includes actions also shown in other groups. The mechanisms that enhance libido and performances differ between the sexes, and aphrodisiacs can affect various metabolic pathways. An aphrodisiac agent might increase blood flow, acting as a circulatory stimulant or cardiovascular tonic. Or it might offer essential nutritional building blocks needed for a healthy libido and sexual activity. Aphrodisiacs may provide a physical energy boost and/or hormone-regulating effects. Among the herbs that improve energy are stimulating adaptogens, nervine stimulants, circulatory stimulants, and nutritive superfoods, depending on the individual(s) involved. Some people need to get in the mood with relaxing nervines rather than stimulants, helping them get out of the sympathetic nervous system state and relax into the parasympathetic, rest-and-digest state of mind and body.

Blueberries, raspberries, blackberries, and some other types of berries are superfood cardiovascular tonics and therefore aphrodisiacs. The act of eating these fruits is also sensually stimulating.

HERBAL APHRODISIACS

Cacao (*Theobroma cacao*)
Cayenne (*Capsicum annuum*)
Damiana (*Turnera diffusa*)
Ginger (*Zingiber officinale*)
Maca (*Lepidium meyenii*)
Pumpkin seed (*Cucurbita maxima*)
Rose (*Rosa* spp.)

Aromatics

I think that aromatics are my favorite plants for cocktails! Aromatics are any herbs that have a strong aroma. Our sense of smell contributes greatly to any sensory experience. The olfactory nerve is closely tied to the memory and pleasure-reward centers in the brain. Burning aromatic plants was an ancient ritual of communicating with and making offerings to the gods, and burning aromatic plants to cleanse a space energetically and physically is still a popular practice.

Many aromatic plants contain beneficial antimicrobial compounds. Essential oils of warming spices are carminatives that enhance digestion. Aromatics also relax the smooth muscles in the body—muscles around our vasculature, heart, lungs, and GI tract. Using an aromatic is perhaps one of the most direct and effective ways to relax the body. Many aromatics also have a stimulating and/or relaxing effect on the nervous system, so they also fit into the category of nervines (see "Nervines" later in this

Aromatics are the spirit of a plant; plants are the spirit of place.

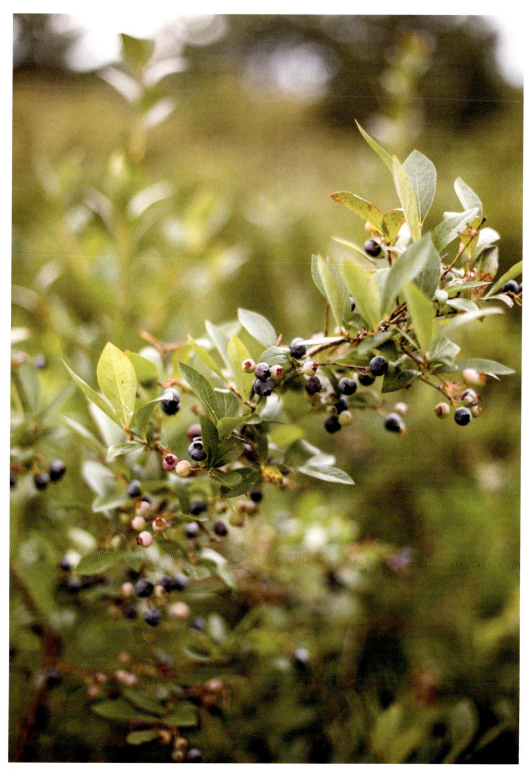
Blueberries are cardiovascular tonics, which improve circulation, creating an aphrodisiac effect.

chapter). Choosing and blending aromatics is especially useful in mocktails to help provide a relaxing experience without alcohol.

AROMATIC HERBS

Anise hyssop (*Agastache foeniculum*)
Bee balm (*Monarda* spp.)
Cardamom (*Elettaria cardamomum*)
Lavender (*Lavandula angustifolia*)
Lemon balm (*Melissa officinalis*)
Peppermint (*Mentha piperita*)
Rosemary (*Rosmarinus officinalis*)
Tulsi (*Ocimum sanctum*)
Vanilla (*Vanilla planifolia*)
Wild chamomile (*Matricaria discoidea*)

Astringents

Astringents have direct tissue-toning effects. Astringents tone by tightening the tissue and therefore can have an acute slightly drying effect that affects mouthfeel.

HERBAL ASTRINGENTS

Green tea and black tea (*Camellia* spp.)
Lady's mantle (*Alchemilla vulgaris*)
Oak (*Quercus* spp.)
Raspberry leaf (*Rubus* spp.)
Rose (*Rosa* spp.)
Yarrow (*Achillea millefolium*)

Bitters

Ah, bitter—perhaps the most underdeveloped taste bud in the Western world, it may also be the most medically useful. When a bitter taste hits our receptors, it stimulates digestion; is hepatoprotective; is often cooling and anti-inflammatory; is grounding; and helps regulate blood sugar levels. Behind the bar, bitter takes the place of salt and seasoning to enhance and balance a recipe. Bitter elixirs are used as aperitifs and digestifs, optimizing digestion before and after a meal. Amaro, from Italy, is perhaps the most popular bittersweet liqueur (and there are many). Bitter drinks are deeply rooted in Italy's food- and nature-loving culture. Many aromatic plants such as rosemary and chamomile are also bitter. Some bitter plants have a more true bitter taste or an earthy bitterness, such as the roots of dandelion or chicory. These taste best when blended with aromatics.

Bitter is a very important action unto itself. If something tastes bitter, then you know it is working! The taste is a medicinal catalyst for multiple processes of the body's digestion, encouraging the liver to make bile, which begins the breakdown of fatty foods, and the pancreas to produce enzymes specialized in helping digest proteins, fats, and carbohydrates. The process starts in the mouth with the first bitter taste receptors that inhabit our tongue. Many of our body's organs—including the lungs and the heart—also have bitter taste receptors! Bitters enhance, balance, and draw out other flavors—in Traditional Chinese Medicine, they are the key taste to balance the Wood Element. In traditional folk medicine and practice as well as in ancient Chinese medicine, bitter has also been used to ground the spirit in the body.

See the Cardamom Bitters and Wormwood Vinegar Bitters recipes on page 159.

HERBAL BITTERS

Angelica (*Angelica archangelica*)
Artichoke (*Cynara cardunculus* var. *scolymus*)
Barberry (*Berberis vulgaris*)
Bitter orange (*Citrus aurantium*)
Blue vervain (*Verbena officinalis*)
Bull thistle (*Cirsium vulgare*)
Dandelion (*Taraxacum officinale*)
Gentian (*Gentiana lutea*)
Grapefruit (*Citrus paradisi*)
Milk thistle (*Silybum marianum*)
Motherwort (*Leonurus cardiaca*)
Mugwort (*Artemisia vulgaris*)
Orange (*Citrus sinensis*)
Wild lettuce (*Lactuca virosa*)

Cardioprotectives

This is a notable category among the system-specific tonics because the vascular system is the body system at highest risk from overconsumption of alcohol as well as from chronic stress. There are many daily tonics we can consume to protect the endothelial lining of our blood vessels as well as our heart. An ounce of prevention is worth a pound of cure here because the damage to blood vessels (atherosclerosis) is permanent and cannot be undone. Aromatics can be included in this category, but the biggest players in protecting the heart's highways are flavonoids.

Flavonoids are some of the most ubiquitous compounds found in plants and include more than eight thousand different types. Many of these are responsible for the varied colors in fruits, flowers, and leaves. For the plant, they function as protection against ultraviolet radiation, feeding damage by animals, and pathogens. Flavonoids often have anti-inflammatory, antiviral, and antibacterial effects in humans as well.

Among the flavonoids with proven antioxidant and cardioprotective effects are anthocyanidins. These active constituents are present in highly pigmented blue and purple fruits, such as blueberries, and often also in leaves (including hawthorn leaves, blueberry leaves, and purple cabbage leaves).

Other types of polyphenols are cardioprotective as well, such as resveratrol in red wine or Japanese knotweed and catechins found in green tea. Any antioxidant will benefit the cardiovascular system, as will anti-inflammatory omega-3 fatty acids and cholesterol-regulating agents.

Not to minimize the value of cardioprotectives, but the most effective choice you can make to protect your heart is to take it easy on refined sugars. Sugar is the number one cause of blood vessel inflammation and damage and the root source of atherosclerosis. High blood sugar can also be caused by stress and tissue damage, or lack of tissue integrity caused by poor nutrition.

SOURCES OF POLYPHENOLS

Blackberry and raspberry (*Rubus* spp.)
Chokeberry (*Aronia melanocarpa*)
Cranberry (*Vaccinium macrocarpon*)
Green tea (*Camellia sinensis*)
Hawthorn (*Crataegus monogyna*)
Japanese knotweed (*Reynoutria japonica*)
Saskatoon berry (*Amelanchier alnifolia*)
Wild blueberry (*Vaccinium angustifolium*)
Wild grape (*Vitus* spp.)

SOURCES OF FATTY ACIDS

Chia seed (*Salvia hispanica*)
Evening primrose (*Oenothera biennis*)
Flax (*Linum usitatissimum*)
Hemp seed (*Cannabis sativa*)
Micro-algae (*Chlorella* spp.)
Purslane (*Portulaca oleracea*)

Demulcents

A demulcent herb is one that changes viscosity. It has a goopy texture and can enhance the mouthfeel of a beverage, making it more full and velvety. Demulcents are used in herbalism to be functionally soothing, hydrating, coating, and healing to the tissues.

HERBAL DEMULCENTS

Ceylon cinnamon (*Cinnamomum verum*)
Chia (*Salvia hispanica*)
Corn (*Zea mays*)
Irish moss seaweed (*Chondrus crispus*)
Marshmallow (*Althaea officinalis*)
Mullein (*Verbascum thapsus*)
Sweet violets (*Viola* spp.)

Nervines

The nervine group contains plants that have an affinity for the nervous system. The category can be further broken down into nervous system stimulants, hypnotics, relaxants (most of which are also antispasmodic), and nutritive restoratives. Together, these herbal tonics are used to address mood-related imbalances (as are nutrition and exercise).

Nervine Stimulants

A nervine stimulant increases the excretion of adrenal fight-or-flight chemicals such as adrenaline, epinephrine/norepinephrine, and pleasure-inducing and excitatory neurotransmitters such as serotonin and dopamine. In a roundabout way, nervine stimulants also increase blood circulation. Caffeine is such a stimulant—it increases the heart rate, resulting in more energy. The effect of many stimulants is the increase of stress hormones like epinephrine from the sympathetic nervous system, causing increased blood flow to muscles and the release of sugar into the bloodstream for energy. This additional energy helps the performance of athletes.

HERBAL NERVINE STIMULANTS

Black tea and green tea (*Camellia sinensis*)
Chocolate (*Theobroma cacao*)
Coca leaf (*Erythroxylum coca*)
Coffee (*Coffea arabica*)
Rhodiola (*Rhodiola rosea*)
Yerba mate (*Ilex paraguariensis*)

Nervine Relaxants

Nervous system relaxants can be antispasmodics, anxiolytics, hypnotics, gabanergics, or some combination thereof. Some relaxants also have a restorative and overall tonic effect on the nervous system.

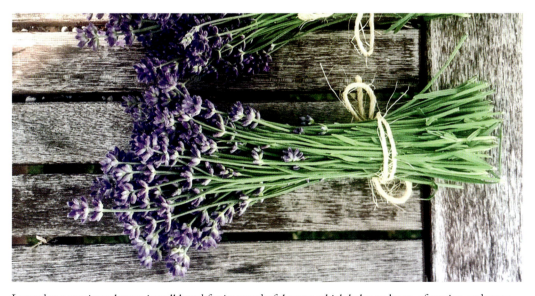

Lavender, a nervine relaxant, is well loved for its wonderful scent, which helps us let go of tension and stress.

GABA is an acronym for "gamma-amino-butyric acid." A gabanergic agent is something that has effect on the GABA system in the body. Within the nervous system there are inhibitory (relaxing) and excitatory (stimulating) receptors. GABA receptors are the body's primary inhibitory transmitters.

HERBAL NERVINE RELAXANTS

California poppy
 (*Eschscholzia californica*)
Chamomile
 (*Matricaria chamomilla*)
Cramp bark (*Viburnum opulus*)
Damiana (*Turnera diffusa*)
Hops (*Humulus lupulus*)
Lavender (*Lavandula angustifolia*)
Nutmeg (*Myristica fragrans*)
Passionflower
 (*Passiflora incarnata*)
Wild lettuce (*Lactuca virosa*)

Nervine Trophorestoratives
A trophorestorative is a nutritive restorative with special affinity to a body system or organ. These strengthen and tonify the integrity of the nervous system without having a marked stimulant or sedating effect.

HERBAL NERVINE TROPHORESTORATIVES

Ashwagandha
 (*Withania somnifera*)
Gotu kola (*Centella asiatica*)
Lion's mane mushroom
 (*Hericium erinaceus*)
Milky oat seed (*Avena sativa*)
Skullcaps (*Scutellaria lateriflora, S. galericulata*)
St. John's wort
 (*Hypericum perforatum*)

Nootropics

Nootropics are plants, nutrients, or drugs that enhance cognitive functions, particularly memory and learning capabilities. In the realm of herbal medicine, nootropics are also often tonics that enhance the nervous system and cardiovascular circulation. Omega-3s and B vitamins are also considered nootropics because of their nourishing and building effect on the nervous system. Note that in addition to boosting these systems, any herb or plant that is anti-inflammatory will have a positive effect on cognition. Leading research studies on cognitive decline indicate that it results from inflammatory diseases. Inflammation is also sometimes caused by deficiency.

HERBAL NOOTROPICS

Bacopa (*Bacopa monnieri*)
Ginkgo (*Ginkgo biloba*)
Gotu kola (*Centella asiatica*)
Green tea (*Camellia sinensis*)
Lion's mane mushroom
 (*Hericium erinaceus*)
Rosemary (*Rosmarinus officinalis*)
Saffron (*Crocus sativus*)

Some Applications of Herbal Actions

There are two major ways that herbs in tonic beverages and apothecary cocktails can promote health. One is by reducing chronic inflammation and chronic stress. The other is by balancing the nervous system, which can be done by protecting the nerves, reducing neuromuscular tension, taking care of the nervous system in the gut, engaging the parasympathetic nervous systems, and encouraging the body's production of endogenous chemicals that produce positive emotions.

Inflammation and the Stress Response

Inflammare is the Latin term meaning "to set fire." Everyone knows that inflammation can cause body tissues to become reddened, swollen, hot, and sometimes painful, but we often fail to look for the underlying cause. Inflammation is a natural response that is meant to heal and repair, but when unresolved or out of balance, it can cause maladaptive illness. Inflammation is the body's *innate immune response*, and it includes changes in basic structural barriers like skin, mucous membrane surfaces, and other inherent features like mucus.

The *stress response* is a cascade of chemical events that unfold as a physiological reaction to perceived stress or actual physical stress. Also known as fight or flight, the stress response is your body's way of protecting you from harm. Adrenals produce and release adrenaline, which causes blood vessels to narrow, increasing blood pressure. Bronchioles dilate, increasing oxygenation. A cascade of precursor hormones mediated by the hypothalamic pituitary adrenal (HPA) axis within the central nervous and endocrine systems causes the release of cortisol, a steroid hormone that in turn calls for the release of glucose from the liver. Chronic exposure of blood vessels to glucose can lead to cardiovascular disease and cholesterol imbalance.

Most of us live in a state of chronic stress, and often we rely on this natural adrenaline-rich response as a way of enhancing productivity and keeping up a fast pace. Our ability to respond to stress defines our strength as individuals and collectively. We find ourselves on a continuum encompassing the trajectory of life and health, a line pointing up- and downhill—uphill is the necessary challenge of adaptability, and downhill is degeneration. You are the fulcrum of balance, your choices and practices tipping the scales. It is much easier and faster to roll downhill than to summon the steady discipline to walk uphill. Genetic predisposition and environmental factors can make that hill steeper. The process of progressive aging due to accumulated inflammation-caused degradation also makes for a harder climb. The temptations of modern life salaciously lure you toward self-destruction.

It is important to consistently move in the upward direction and push your personal edge of capability. But it is just as crucial not to push yourself to a breaking point, because if you fail to adapt and start heading downhill, it is so easy for problems to snowball. Our survival instinct tells us: Adapt or die. The study of epigenetics is proving how important our daily choices are, altering the fate of genetic expression and how our DNA is read in this moment, facts that empower the individual toward agency and responsibility when it comes to their own health. Sickness and health are not random; nor are they due to a victim's bad genetic luck. Someone may have inherited a lot of "bad genes," but the choices they make—including which phytochemicals they put in their body via diet and herbal tonics, as well as nature immersion and exercise—determine how health outcomes play out. Active (intentional) restorative rest when the body requires it is still an active evolutionary step!

Adaptogens are the class of herbs that are indispensable for creating physiological resistance in times of chronic stress. They are nonspecific and nontoxic therapeutics that can promote neuroplasticity (*adaptability*), preventing excess cortisol production and the domino-effect damage that can ensue. These botanicals can prevent endocrine system malfunction such as adrenal insufficiency or burnout and immune deficiencies.

Many of the research studies on adaptogens focus on people's responses in stressful situations, including war scenarios featuring Russian fighter pilots. Adaptogens might be helpful for you if your life feels like an action movie. There is no substituting for the balance of rest, however. Adaptogens are a gift for shorter periods of time to help you get through, but not for long-term use.

Chronic Inflammation

Inflammation in response to injury or infection is an important part of the immune response for healing. But problems arise when there are more inflammatory inputs than the body can handle, and the body never has time to resolve and heal. This is chronic inflammation, which is defined as inflammation that lasts for longer than two weeks and results in tissue damage. Chronic inflammation and stress are interconnected, many times causing each other and both being at the root of many modern disease states.

There are two types of immunity: innate and adaptive. Innate immunity is general, messy, and automatic whereas the adaptive immune response is highly specific, based on a person's immunological memory.

Oxidative stress is a condition in which an excess of free radicals ramble around inside the body. A *free radical* is simply a molecule that has an unpaired electron. Formation of free radicals is a normal part of metabolic processes, but when there are too many free radicals, they can cause damage. Too much of this instability is chaos embodied; it can cause DNA damage and genetic mutations that lead to premature aging as well as heart disease and cancer.

Inflammation and Our Moods
There is an intimate link between mood and inflammation, particularly in those with anxiety and depression. People living in a chronic state of inflammation may experience problems with impulse control, making risky decisions. The gut plays a key role in regulating moods because the majority of serotonin is made in the gut. (More about this in "Gut Feelings and the Enteric Brain," later in this chapter.)

Lifestyle choices that are pro-inflammatory include less-than-adequate sleep, excess alcohol consumption, dehydration, smoking, inactivity, eating food that is not food, and excessive physical labor or exercise that does not allow for periods of recovery.

Generally, antioxidant-rich plants reduce inflammation. In the face of pain due to inflammation, many people rely on nonsteroidal anti-inflammatory drugs such as aspirin and ibuprofen that block the production of prostaglandins, which are hormone-like chemicals responsible for inflammation and pain as well as swelling. Some plants have a high content of salicylates, which are a key ingredient of aspirin. Some medicinal mushrooms contain beta-glucans, which help move the body from a hot inflammatory state relying on innate immunity to a more intelligent adaptive (immunomodulating) response. Additionally, demulcent herbs that are rich in polysaccharides are directly soothing to tissue. They promote the *terrain* necessary for the body to facilitate repair. Terrain is a metaphor used by herbalist practitioners to speak about the holistic health of living tissue.

Vehicle of Consciousness

Electrical wires branching like trees—seeing, transmitting, synthesizing. Your spirit riding on electrical currents. The nervous system is an essential, foundational, and intricate interface that relies on our adaptability. A healthy nervous system is like a finely tuned instrument. We are sensitive beings that can become desensitized to too many stimuli, weakening our intelligence and awareness.

Sometimes we can become monsters due to maladaptive behavior (a neuropsychiatric disorder). But are all behaviors maladaptive? Consider mania, for example. I would argue that while it's perhaps not adaptive, an

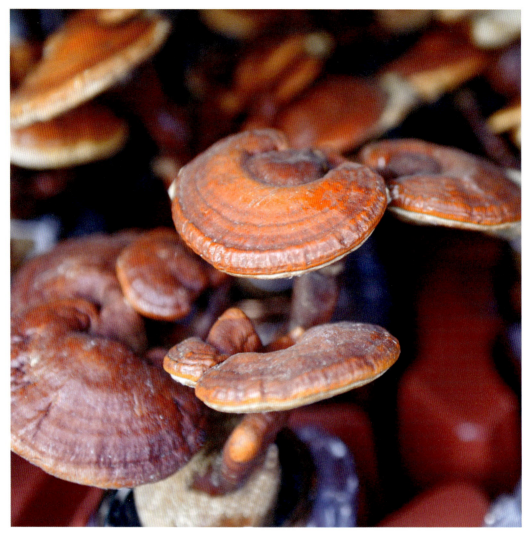

Extracting beta-glucans from reishi mushrooms into a tincture is a way to capture the mushrooms' anti-inflammatory effect. See page 189 for a Reishi Tincture recipe.

abundance of excitation is certainly a reasonable response in some contexts. We live in a world where an overwhelming fountain of information is constantly bombarding us. Desensitization and eventually neurodegeneration leads to the lack of an adequate response. Other events and substances also negatively affect the nerves, but the ridiculous excess of modern Western culture is a very relevant example.

Full-Fat Foods as Building Blocks
The nervous system is electrical, and fat is the insulator on the outside of the cells to help transmit messages. Nerve conduction velocity ranges from

2 to 275 miles per hour (3 to 443 kph) (which is much slower than electricity but faster than blood flow). Our bodies require an abundance of healthy fats to keep our senses plush. Have you ever heard the expression *raw nerves*? I picture this as some nutritionally depleted nerves out in the cold without their comfy blanket of fat—full of fear and quite vulnerable. This is a depleted state that is the picture of neurasthenia.

Essential fatty acids, which we must obtain through diet, include omega-3s and omega-6s, which are two types of unsaturated fats. "Healthy fat" consumption has to do with the ratio of consumption of these omega fatty acids. Taking in more omega-3s than omega-6s is important for preventing inflammation. Fatty and cholesterol-rich foods get a bad rap, partially because they are thought to contain imbalanced ratios of these omegas, and in part because cholesterol tends to stick to damaged blood vessels, causing constriction that can lead to cardiovascular disease. Cholesterol, however, is not the culprit. In fact, sugar (and the hyper-glucose states caused by stress) is the agent responsible for nicking the inside walls of vessels, which the cholesterol sticks to. Over time, high blood sugar can *damage blood vessels as well as the nerves that control your heart.* Everything is connected!

Neuromuscular Tension
Tense nerves and tense muscles tend to go hand in hand. Unhealthy nerves can cause muscle weakness and vice versa. Very active people, such as athletes and people who do physical labor for a living, have a high degree of muscular tension. They are too "tight," and that tension can impede nerves as well as adequate blood flow.

Gut Feelings and the Enteric Brain
Looking to rationalize away that gut feeling or overcome the butterflies in your belly? It might be impossible. Tucked in the walls of the digestive system is a complex interplay of more than one hundred million nerve cells known as the enteric nervous system. This "brain in your gut" is the link between digestion and mood and can even impact the way you think. Serotonin is a neurotransmitter with the nickname "the happiness chemical," as it plays a key role in mood regulation. The gut manufactures 95 percent of the total serotonin made and used in the body, and this neurotransmitter plays a big role in mood as well as important biological processes including vasoconstriction, wound healing, cognition, memory, and learning.

In the gastrointestinal system, inflammation can "leak out" and cause a cascade of inflammation all over the body, particularly in joints or the cardiovascular system. In the case of chronic GI inflammation, serotonin synthesis is interrupted, as are digestion and nutrient assimilation, the very building blocks for tissue integrity throughout the body. In these cases, we may see cases of deficiency, inflammation, and neuropsychiatric disorders all playing the same ball game.

The Vagus Nerve and Heart Rate Variability
The vagus nerve is the longest cranial nerve in the body, extending from the brain to the large intestine. It is responsible for many functions of the parasympathetic mode of the nervous system, letting your body know when it is okay to relax, rest, and digest. It affects heart rate and heart rate variability (HRV), blood pressure, breathing, and digestion. The more the peripheral nervous system is engaged, the more responsive the nervous system will be; this is a reflection of good health and adaptability. High HRV indicates good vagal tone and is a good thing; low indicates an overstressed (and less responsive) state. This is where aromatic compounds do their magic.

Addicted to Love: The Limbic System
The limbic system is a group of structures present in the brains of most animals and positioned just above the brain stem or "reptilian brain." The reward pathways and circuits of the limbic system involve emotions (such as love), the sense of smell, and memory and are responsible for much of our behavior, including libido, addiction, motivation, and will. This system is also essential for maintaining homeostasis in the body. This is where your personality lives. At the biochemical level, love is just a collection of neurotransmitters and sex hormones. Smell and memory are very closely tied, which is the reason aromatherapy is so effective for retraining the mind and recovering from trauma.

The Endocannabinoid System
There has been a rising fascination with cannabis (which is a medicine or drug, not a tonic) and its effects in recent years, which has led to the discovery of a subcategory of the nervous system. Endocannabinoids are a type of neurotransmitter, and the endocannabinoid system (ECS) contributes to central nervous system development, synaptic plasticity, and response to environmental insults. It is a complex network that plays a role in homeostasis as well as overarching nervous system effects from emotion, learning, and pain to immunity, appetite, body temperature, and sleep.[1] The specific actions of these receptors is still a place of active scientific discovery. There are many plants that affect these sites; humans also produce endogenous cannabinoids.

Care for a natural high? The most studied endogenous cannabinoid is anandamide, also known as the bliss chemical (from the Sanskrit term *Ananda*). It is one of the catalysts responsible for runner's high, along with endorphins.

Your body's own cannabinoids act as messengers that play a role in inflammation (particularly in the GI tract), pain, perception, depression, appetite, memory, and fertility. The ECS affects much of our moment-to-moment functioning, and although it has been proven to be essential, it is still mysterious. Plants and mushrooms that have been studied for their positive interactivity with the endocannabinoid system include cacao, echinacea, spilanthes, truffle, chaga, turkey tail mushroom, kava, turmeric, tea, hops, magnolia, black pepper, certain sunflowers, maca, and even carrots! Spilanthes contains spilanthol, which activates a receptor demonstrated to play a role with immune function. Echinacea also contains alkamides, chemicals that are structurally similar to our endogenous cannabinoids such as anandamide.

Natural Performance-Enhancing Highs

Exercise is one of the best means for obtaining a natural high. The transient state of euphoria known as runner's high floods your body with good feelings in the form of natural opiates (endorphins), stimulants (phenylethylamine), and anandamide (a cannabinoid). Myriad botanical allies can assist in enhancing performance. Adaptogens can assist in endurance.

Lying on the Earth

There is a scientific explanation for why it feels good to lie on the beach or breathe while sitting next to a waterfall: negatively charged ions. In simple terms, movement in nature (particularly that of air and water) creates ionic activity—the addition and removal of electrons to and from air and water molecules. Ions are present in the environment around us, and they seem to have positive effects on the human body, possibly boosting serotonin levels (and thus our mood) and enhancing immune system function. I do not feel the need to have researchers prove the obvious healing effect of lying on the ground, but I am impressed that scientists are studying the effects of grounding (also called earthing) on inflammation, the immune response, wound healing, and treatment of diseases.

Nervine stimulants can spark motivation. Circulatory stimulants help get the blood moving, and yin tonic herbs and inflammation-resolving agents can help with recovery. The mindful and skilled combination of these plants will keep you high on life! The tonic categories that boost physical performance and recovery are circulatory stimulants, adaptogens, nerve trophorestoratives, yin tonics, and demulcents. Hydrating ingredients such as electrolytes (calcium, magnesium, potassium) also serve this function.

A *yin tonic* is a moistening agent that prevents the dryness that can be caused by overactivity (yang). The concepts of yin and yang create an easy way to understand the balance of polar energies. Rest can also be considered yin. In the case of exercise, a suitable amount of yin is necessary for rebuilding (and remoistening the muscles).

Herbal Energetics and Five Element Theory

The Latin root *constitutus* means "to enter into the formation of as a necessary part." It is the root of the word *constituents* and also the word *constitution*. Everyone has a unique natural constitution. In discussing the concept of constitution, the emphasis is mostly on the body but also includes personality. Thought affects form, and mind, body, and spirit are intrinsically interwoven. Cultures across the world have developed systems for measuring constitutional energetics of both plants and people. The details of these systems vary, but they all measure degrees of temperature, moisture, and tension as they relate to the human body—scales of hot to cold, dry to moist, and tense to lax. The concept underlying constitutional energetics is that every person has a body type that leans one way or another on these scales. The characterization of these types helps us to observe and identify patterns of balance and imbalance. It provides a framework for observing the energetic architecture of plants—does this plant have a taste or action that is warm and dry, or cool and moist? This kind of observation is simple, but it does take a bit of practice to understand the implications.

Energetics also apply to the seasons and the characterization of basic elements within an individual person. Traditional Chinese Medicine is a beautiful ancient practice that outlines each season with an element and each element with a personality and temperament. I am in love with these methodologies, particularly TCM, because it acknowledges that we, too, are fluctuating, dynamic parts of nature. Other traditional energetic models include ancient Ayurveda from India and the four humors, the ancient Greek model discovered by Hippocrates and further developed by Galen. These systems, despite their diverse origins, share similar and overlapping features. Having a grasp on energetics is a very empowering thing because it is a pattern-based understanding of the world and our health. Through observation of patterns, we can help balance the body.

Different traditions measure energetics differently, but there is often overlap as these effects are based on observation. I have a personal love and preference for the five phases of Traditional Chinese Medicine because I feel it most closely resembles my own experience of life with the elements. In the descriptions that follow, I mention each of the five elements—Water, Wood, Fire, Earth, and Metal—with its corresponding season. It's important to note that each cycle includes associated Organs (using the term *Organs* as understood by the ancients of the East, not by modern Western medicine), but I do not delve into that here. TCM is a complex system of medicine, but I appreciate Five Element Theory (as well as the theory of yin and yang) for its accessibility. Most people can intuitively grasp the concept of the five elements rotating with the seasons, especially as they tune into their own senses. This cycle is viewed as inherently transformative. A personality can have a tendency toward one element type or other, and the keys to unlocking health can often start from that simple observation.

> *The Sages follow the laws of Nature and therefore their bodies are free from strange diseases. They do not lose any of their natural functions and their spirit of life is never exhausted.*
> —*The Yellow Emperor's Inner Classic*

Salty, Winter, Water Element, Fear

Salt has a softening and dispersive quality. It is a yin (receptive, feminine) energy, moving energy downward and inward, like winter. It is hydrating and moistening in smaller amounts, dissolving lumps and masses (think of what happens when you sprinkle salt on vegetables). It can improve digestion and assimilation as well as detox. Salt detoxifies inside and out. Think Epsom salt baths as well as their use as a laxative. Sodium is an essential mineral in the body as well as an electrolyte; it keeps your blood moving, muscles contracting, and fluids balanced. In plants, a salty taste often indicates a high mineral content.

Sour, Spring, Wood Element, Anger

Sour is yin, cooling, and astringent, the quintessential tonic taste, toning or tightening to the tissues, improving elasticity and tissue function. I believe this category can also enhance focus, as it gathers everything together. You know how in the summer it can be "too hot to think" because everything is so relaxed? Sour is a friend to the liver, which helps with the breakdown of fat and protein-rich foods. This is why digestive bitters made with vinegar are extra-digestive-enhancing tonics. A great way to understand the effects of the sour taste is to picture the effects of acidic ashes and masks on sagging facial skin. This same effect can be applied to all tissues and organs in the body. In *Healing with Whole Foods*, Paul Pitchford asserts, "Sour flavors collect and hold together the dispersed, capriciously changing personality."

Bitter, Summer, Fire Element, Joy

Bitter has contracting, cooling, and grounding effects, and often detoxifying or cleansing effects as well. It promotes various pathways of elimination and reduces stagnation, particularly in the liver. It generally reduces excess and is drying to tissues.

In the West the bitter taste is the least developed, but I am eager to witness this change with the prevalence of amaros, cocktail culture, herbal medicine, and general health awareness.

Sweet, Late Summer, Earth Element, Worry

The taste of sweetness indicates nourishment and is building and soothing as well as balancing. In TCM, the Earth element is at the center—each season and transition requires a return to the structural integrity of Earth.

The addiction to sugar in modern culture likely may relate to the place of the sweet taste as the most essential building block of vibrancy. It is important to note that the kind of sweetness under discussion here is natural and unrefined, as in, for instance, sweet, starchy vegetables and grains. I usually advise those with a sweet tooth to incorporate more of these kinds of foods in their diet to help get at the root of the craving.

Spicy, Autumn, Metal Element, Grief

Considered a yang flavor, also known as pungent, this category creates movement, expansion, and dispersion, promoting circulation and digestion. This category includes aromatic plants as well as anything hot, spicy, or acrid. Often pungent plants are warming, but this is not always the case. There are cooling pungents—think peppermint. This taste moves energy upward and out, often causing the release of tension and/or perspiration. Improving blood flow improves the function of all tissues and particularly the heart (cardiotonic). Because it is a blood mover, alcohol falls into this category, but not when used to excess. Too much alcohol leads to cell death rather than movement.

Some of the very warming pungent ingredients have a very hot effect but because of diaphoresis (sweating), the ultimate result is cooling (which may explain why people who live in hot climates tend to eat very spicy foods). This flavor clears any dampness and mucus from the body.

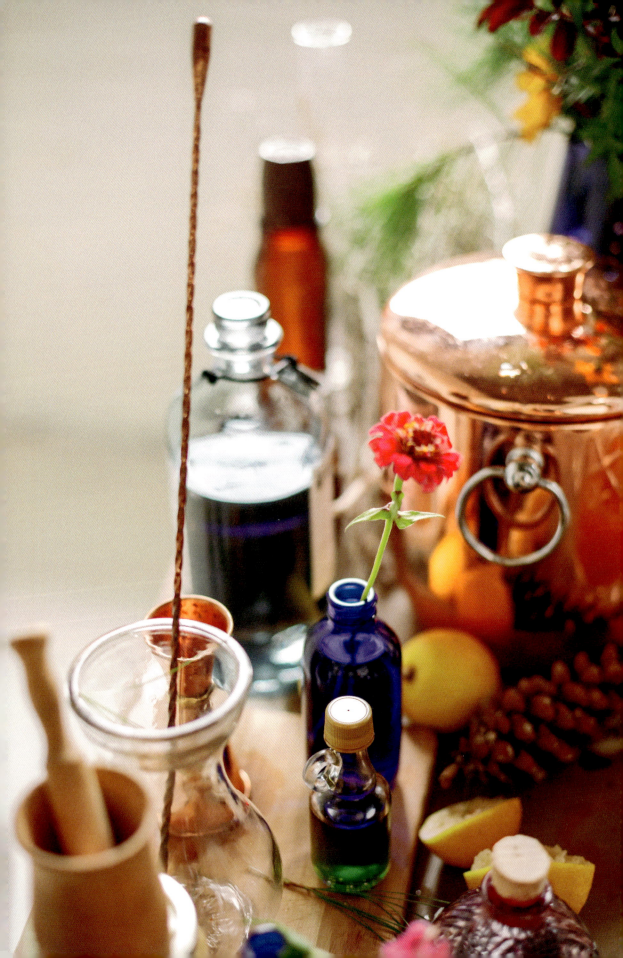

CHAPTER 4

The Chemistry of Extraction

Although you can buy premade herbal extracts and tinctures, one of the joys of creative mixology is experimenting with making your own herbal preparations. As we've learned, the purpose of making preparations is to extract particular chemical compounds from the plants. But to carry out extractions effectively, it's helpful to first learn about principles of phytochemistry. This may sound intimidating, but don't worry. If I could learn this chemistry stuff, you can, too!

Here's how the *Oxford English Dictionary* defines *chemistry*: "the branch of science that deals with the identification of the substances of which matter is composed; the investigation of their properties and how they interact, combine, and change; and the use of these processes to form new substances." Phytochemistry is where botany and chemistry intersect: investigating the matter that plants are composed of and the nature of the interactions of plant matter with the human body. Chemistry is both the solid state and the action. A plant's color, taste, aroma, and effect on its environment and on other organisms all arise from its chemistry. Once you learn a plant's chemistry, the stage is set for you to effectively extract the various compounds it contains.

Chemistry as Cocktail

The decomposition of plants creates fertile ground for all of life. We breathe out and the trees breathe in. It should be no surprise then that our bodies are reflections of this coevolution, and that many of the systems and much of the chemical signaling that happens in the human body is in response to phytochemicals. Many times the secondary metabolites manufactured by plants have actions in human bodies similar to those they have in plants. We often advocate for stewardship of nature by humans, but a concept that is less realized is that plants are stewards of us!

Chemicals in living organisms are in a constant state of flux: complexing, reducing, and oxidizing. Chemistry is often a *cocktail*, the whole greater than the sum of its parts. It is also important to note that plant compounds function differently when within a matrix of other chemicals than they do

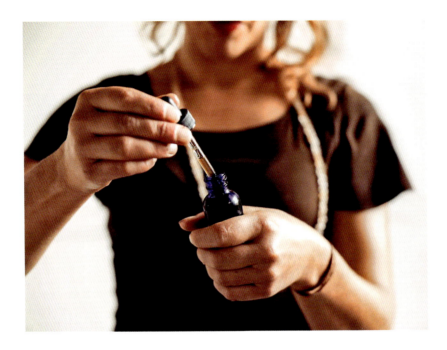

as isolated entities. Often various components will synergize—this is something many of us know in the realm of nutritional chemistry (whole foods versus vitamins). A particular set of constituents may behave quite differently from a seemingly similar combination. This is important when working with isolated molecules extracted from plants, as happens in the making of pharmaceuticals or even natural "herb" supplements—for example, curcumin that has been isolated from turmeric.

Chemistry informs my inspiration of how to process an herb that I've gathered from the garden, whether that is through a tincture, oxymel, glycerite, tea, or hydrosol. Let's say I just harvested some fresh rose petals and want to maintain their aroma. First, I carefully dry said flowers to concentrate their volatile oils; then I store them in a cool dark place in a sealed jar for making aromatic teas and syrups. When I make the tea, I make sure to cover the cup or teapot, because I know these compounds are volatile—in other words, they can escape into steam and be lost from the preparation! There are usually several appropriate preparations suitable for a particular herb. For my beloved rose, I may also make a fresh petal glycerite, a menstruum known for its ability to capture and store aromatic compounds. Or, if I'm tincturing in alcohol, I know that a higher proof will do the trick. When you craft herbal bar preparations at home, the principles of *solubility* and *polarity* will guide the extraction process. Knowing whether the components of a particular species are water-soluble or oil-soluble will lead you to mixer mastery and more potent potions.

The polarity of a compound has to do with its balance of negative and positive ions. Think back to the classic model of an atom: electrons revolving around a nucleus. Those electrons carry a negative charge, and electronegative compounds have a tendency to attract electrons from other nearby sources. Highly "polar" molecules are those that have the most uneven distribution in electrical charge, and thus they are the most chemically active. Water (H_2O) is a highly polarized molecule.

Polyphenols

Phenolic compounds are a large and diverse class of superfood and antioxidant molecules produced by plants to support their own growth and as a chemical defense against pests. I find it somewhat romantic that these superhero molecules have such beneficial effects on our bodies as well. Do plants consider us a predator? When I think about the larger ecological context in which birds and larger animals serve as vehicles for seed dispersal, I reckon probably not!

This class of secondary metabolites includes many tonic groups of phytochemicals, including chalcones, flavonoids, lignans, phenolic acids, and stilbenes. Flavonoids are blue, red, and purple pigments that can be classified in various subgroups, including anthocyanidins and anthocyanins, flavonols and flavanonols, flavones and isoflavonoids (also called phytoestrogens). Chemistry can be the most confusing thing!

Coumarins are a type of polyphenolic compound ubiquitous in plants. A characteristic cut grass–vanilla smell indicates their presence. They are biologically active and have been used in various cancer therapies, but high doses of certain types of coumarins are known to be hepatotoxic, although their toxicity is largely exaggerated and dose-dependent. Coumarins are present in many common foods such as strawberries, cinnamon, carrots, olives, and nuts. See the Cinnamon entry on page 239 for more about coumarin content of cinnamon.

Certain essential oils also contain phenols such as carvacrol (found in thyme, oregano, and bee balm) or rosmarinol, which is found in the essential oils of many members of the mint family (Lamiaceae). These are examples of *monophenols*.

Flavonolignans, curcuminoids, and tannins also fall within the category of phenol.

How to extract: Solubility of these compounds varies. In general, they are solvent in water and alcohol. Prepare plants that contain polyphenols using hydroethanolic extracts (tinctures) with differing percentages of alcohol depending on each type of compound. Water-based preparations such as teas and syrups are also appropriate.

Alkaloids

Alkaloids tip the scales a little more toward poison than superhero, because this category includes some of our favorite daily drugs, as well as some of the most common addictive substances: caffeine, theobromine, nicotine, cocaine, and morphine. Almost all these substances in plants exhibit a bitter taste, which often indicates poison. There are many categories of alkaloids, but all alkaloids share the characteristics of having a basic pH and containing at least one nitrogen atom.

How to extract: Vinegar is a good solvent for alkaloids.

Terpenoids

Terpenoids are a broad class that includes carotenoids (carotenes) and xanthophylls, which are orange and yellow pigments, as well as terpenes and sesquiterpene lactones. Terpenoids are the main bioactive compounds of essential oils and are typically volatile.

Iridoids are bitter-tasting monoterpenes that plants produce as defense against infection by virus or microorganism and to aid in repairing damaged plant tissue.

Saponins are a subclass of terpenoids also referred to as triterpene glycosides. They are bitter tasting and have a foamy quality when added to water. Plants such as horse chestnut (*Aesculus hippocastanum*) and green tea (*Camellia sinensis*) that are high in saponins are being studied for their potential cholesterol-regulating effects. It is thought that these soap-like agents work by binding to free-ranging cholesterol in the bloodstream, which also may have a positive effect on preventing atherosclerosis.

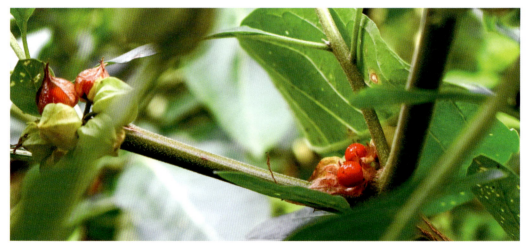

These red berries are ashwagandha (*Withania somnifera*), an herbal adaptogen in the Solanaceae family. The roots contain withanolides and other alkaloids.

The Chemistry of Extraction

The Poison King

Mithridates was the king of Pontus in Anatolia (modern-day Turkey) during the first century BCE, and his poison-laced paranoia has kept his name famous. The term *mithridatism* refers to the king's practice of strengthening his body against poison through the continual ingestion of small doses. Some of the antidotes he relied on were thought to contain the blood of Pontic ducks, which consumed poisonous plants such as hemlock and hellebore. His primary toxic obsession was arsenic, the poison that had killed his father. He reigned during a time wrought by war and anxiety, and his self-poisoning was the eventual cause of his death.

This concept and practice of the dose-response relationship, in which low doses of certain agents are tonic while larger doses are toxic, is called *hormesis*. As Paracelsus said, "All things are poison, and nothing is without poison; the dosage alone makes it so a thing is not a poison."

A modern example is the hermetic effect of alcohol in the prevention of stroke. The concept of hormesis also plays a role in the idea that challenge or stress in the appropriate amount is strengthening on every biological level.

Triterpenoid saponins can mimic the effect of adrenocorticotropic hormone (ACTH), which signals the adrenal glands to release cortisol in the body. These saponins also have all-encompassing anti-inflammatory benefits and often regulate the immune system as well as protecting the liver.

How to extract: Saponins are both water- and fat-soluble. Tea is typically an appropriate method for extraction as well as adding a bit of fat (see the instructions for Matcha Latte on page 248) or consuming these tonics with a fatty meal.

Sulfur-Containing Compounds

Sulfur is needed by all tissues in the human body. It is known as the beauty mineral because it is stored in the skin, hair, and nails and is responsible for the production of collagen, which provides strength and structure to skin and joints. Sulfur is a key component in the building of amino acids and genetic expression as well as DNA repair and protection from pathogens. Sulfur-containing compounds alter the progression of many pathologies by decreasing and slowing the cascade of inflammatory mediators.

Glucosinolates are sulfurous compounds found in plants that convert into bioactive components called isothiocyanates as they break down in the body. Isothiocyanates have beneficial effects in the prevention of cardiometabolic and neurological diseases, musculoskeletal conditions, and certain cancers. Glucosinolates are found almost exclusively in veggies from the cabbage or mustard family (Brassicaceae). This family includes mustard greens, arugula, bok choy, broccoli, brussels sprouts, cabbage, cauliflower, collard greens, daikon, horseradish, kale, kohlrabi, radish, turnips, wasabi, and watercress. Over 130 different types of glucosinolates have been identified and categorized. Some cabbage family crops can be used to help prevent plant pest problems through a technique called biofumigation. The crop is not

The Nutritional Chemistry of Honey

Honey is full of antioxidants including flavonoids and polyphenols, and it contains trace vitamins, eighteen amino acids, and enzymes. This potent, sweet superfood is a concentrated, energizing, balanced sugar source. Honey has been used as medicine since time immemorial for the dressing of wounds and burns, helping to heal tissue. Antibacterial and anti-inflammatory, it also has traditionally been used to promote glowing skin health and treat ulcers, eye disease, throat infections, hepatitis, constipation, eczema, thirst, and fatigue! It is an indispensable home remedy for soothing the common cough and cold, especially when combined with herbs. Bee pollen, also a superfood and medicinal substance, is a mix of seasonally variable flower pollen, nectar, enzymes, honey, wax, and bee secretions—nutrients, amino acids, vitamins, and lipids. It is considered beneficial for alleviating allergies (an immune hypersensitivity), especially if consumed from your local terroir. Bee pollen can be employed as a hepatoprotective agent, protecting and repairing the liver, and as a general immune boost, an antioxidant, and a nutritional supplement.

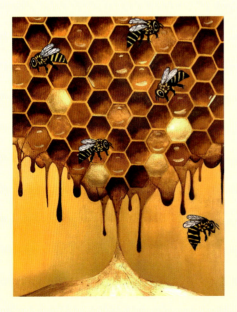

The Chemistry of Extraction

harvested for eating, but instead is turned into the soil. As it decays, it releases sulfurous compounds that are toxic to nematodes, bacteria, and fungi.

How to extract: Glucosinolates are typically extracted through digestion (acid, bile, water, enzymes, et cetera), but in the laboratory they have been shown to be both alcohol- and water-soluble.

Minerals

Minerals are considered inorganic substances because they lack a carbon atom. Scientists have identified thirty-eight hundred types of minerals, yet only nineteen of those are known to be required for healthy functioning of the human body. (There is evidence, however, that more than nineteen are essential, and research is ongoing.[1]) On a body mass basis, humans are only about 4 percent minerals, but that small percentage is essential for life. Minerals regulate heartbeat, help our muscles relax and contract, and play a role in transportation of elements, growth, nervous system function, and the very architecture of the body: our bones.

In the body, minerals are often in the form of electrolytes that conduct electrical charges to keep your blood moving, muscles contracting, and fluids balanced. The minerals required in the largest quantities are calcium, chloride, magnesium, phosphorus, potassium, and sodium. Boron, chromium, cobalt, copper, iodine, iron, manganese, molybdenum, selenium, and zinc are required in smaller amounts.

Most plants contain an array of minerals, and herbalists use plants with exceptionally high content, such as horsetail or stinging nettle, as nutritive tonics or supplements.

Minerals are also considered metals when they are found in the earth, have a positive charge, and can conduct electricity and heat. Not all minerals are metals, but all natural metals are minerals.

How to extract: Minerals are typically absorbed in acidic solvents, such as vinegar. (This is why good bone broth recipes include vinegar.)

Lipids

This category includes oils and their constituents: fatty acids, alkamides, triglycerides, and phospholipids. These are often the remedies that affect cholesterol balance favorably.

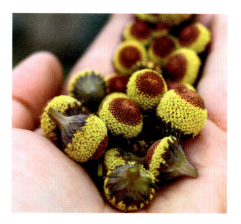

Spilanthes oleracea buds, or buzz buttons, contain alkylamide, which causes tingling sensations in the mouth and has a wide variety of therapeutic effects. Alkylamides from plants are usually lipophilic substances.

How to extract: Lipids have low polarity and are best extracted in other oily substances. Think infused oil or creamy drinks.

Polysaccharides

Polysaccharides are starchy long-chained carbohydrates. These are the molecules responsible for causing characteristic demulcency in herbs such as marshmallow and slippery elm as well as aloe, plantain, and flaxseed. These mucilage-containing plants soothe tissues externally as well as internally, are anti-inflammatory, and are sometimes used as prebiotics and/or aperients (mild laxatives). Mucilage is recognized by its slippery or goopy texture when wet.

The polysaccharides when extracted become viscous and sometimes even gelatinous.

How to extract: Polysaccharides have high polarity and extract the best in water, particularly cold-water teas and infusions. They do not extract in oil and will precipitate out of solution in alcohol extracts.

Tannins

Tannins are a type of polyphenol. Tannin-rich botanicals cause a marked astringent sensation in the mouth. Think tea and red wine. In the beverage industry, the characteristic oakiness in whiskey and wine is due to the tannins they contain. Tannins bind to protein and tone tissue, and they have styptic qualities (can help stop bleeding in wounds). The astringency of green tea is due to high amounts of tannins, which if overconsumed can inhibit the absorption of iron and other nutrients.

How to extract: Typically, tannins are water-soluble, but they can be prepared as tinctures for longer keeping quality. Adding 10 percent glycerin to tinctures to keep the tannins in suspension prevents tannins from binding to alkaloids.

Amino Acids

Amino acids are the building blocks of proteins and peptides (chains of amino acids). The human body requires amino acids for nearly all cellular functions. Proteins are constructed from a set of twenty-one amino acids, some of which are polar, others non-polar.

How to extract: The polarity and thus the solubility of amino acids is variable. The most appropriate way to consume amino acids is in food, as they are the building blocks of protein synthesis. Adding ingredients that are high in digestive enzymes to drink recipes could be a great choice for serving with a protein-rich meal or for your diet in general. Honey is a great example of an enzyme-rich ingredient, as are pineapple, fig, kiwi, and yogurt.

Phytosterols

Phytosterols, also called plant sterols, are the equivalent of cholesterol in animal cells. Phytosterols can have a favorable effect on cholesterol balance.

How to extract: Phytosterols are oil-soluble compounds and therefore lipophilic. They are best extracted in oil or eaten with a fatty meal. Many plants that contain phytosterols are part of a healthy diet, so we don't need to make extractions of them.

Quick Reference Extraction Guide

A basket of fresh herbs is teeming with active constituents. We know that each plant contains its own chemical cocktail, and that these varying compounds respond differently to the common solvents used for extracting them. If you want the daily tonics that you make and drink to be maximally effective, it is helpful to know which extraction technique will work best for which types of constituents.

Table 4.1. Common Culinary Solvents

Solvent	Polar or Non-Polar	Solubility and Storage	Useful For
Water	Highly polarized	Temperature is important when extracting.	Extracts well: tannins, mucilage, acids, starches, gums, pectin, glycosides, mineral salts, and pigments.
Alcohol	High polarity	Different constituents require different alcohol percentages; very long shelf life.	Good solvent for hydrophobic constituents such as volatile oils, alkaloids, and resins.
Glycerin	Food-grade vegetable glycerin is mostly polar	Less shelf-stable than hydroethanolic extracts.	Useful solvent for aromatics. It is usually used for keeping tannins in suspension (10% in tinctures). Can also prevent tannins from binding alkaloids.
Vinegar	Polar	Acetums (vinegar tinctures) ought to be strained within 4 to 6 weeks. Once strained, the shelf life is about 1 year.	Extracts minerals; useful as a proportion of an extract for extracting alkaloids. Sour activates the liver and therefore makes it a beneficial menstruum for carrying remedies there.
Oil	Non-polar, hydrophobic	Dry herbs with high moisture content prior to infusing in oil, or the infusion can become rancid. Strained infused oils last about 6 months stored in a cool, dry place.	Good for extracting fat-like molecules such as sterols and cannabinoids. Aromatics can also be fixed in oil.

Extracting herbs involves immersing them in a menstruum, the chosen solvent: alcohol, water, vinegar, glycerin. When referring to kitchen science, a solvent is a liquid. (Other materials you might use, such as salt or honey, would be functioning as a preservative and not a solvent because no dissolution occurs.) There's a basic rule that like dissolves like, so in essence your method or menstruum for extraction should have the same or similar polarity as the chemical you wish to extract from the plant material. Factors that influence the solubility of a chemical compound include its size or molecular weight, polarity, and structure, as well as what function group it belongs to and who it associates with.

Water, glycerol (glycerin), and ethanol are considered polar solvents, whereas oil has no polarity. Two non-polar substances will mix easily, but if you want to mix polar and non-polar substances (*like oil and water*), it's important to use an *emulsifier*. A true emulsifier is a substance that loves both oil and water and is capable of bonding with both. A mechanical blender can serve the role of an emulsifier, too, but the mix it creates is not a reliable *emulsion* and won't necessarily stay together. Lotion is a good example of a stable emulsion, and lecithin and lanolin are examples of emulsifiers used in natural lotion making.

There are common techniques that increase the efficacy of preparations. The manner in which you process the plant matter affects the end result. The surface area of the plant material, the ratio of material to solvent, the length of extraction time, the energy added during extraction, and the choice of solvent also all have an effect on the outcome of the extraction process. Let's consider each of these in more detail.

Surface Area

The more finely ground an herb is, the more surface area is has, which will allow for maximal extraction. You may purée the material, juice it, or mince it to increase the surface area for more complete extraction. I often process plant material in a high-speed blender prior to tincturing.

Ratio

When making tinctures, it's important to consider the ratio of the quantity (weight) of herbs to the volume of liquid. For instance, a typical ratio might be 1 gram of dried calendula blossoms to 6 milliliters solvent. Standard guidelines for tincture making call for a range of 1:4 or 1:5 when using dried plant material. The ratio may be 1:6 if the material is fluffy, and 1:2 or 1:3 for fresh material (1:4 if not chopped well). Use a simple kitchen-friendly gram scale to weigh herbs. These same ratios can be applied when making bitters, vinegar extracts, and oxymels.

The proportion used when making tea and water-based extractions is typically 1 tablespoon dried herb (or 2 tablespoons fresh) per 8 ounces (240 ml) water.

Time

More or less time equals more or less thoroughness of extraction. Longer is better, though there is a limit to saturation. The length of time also depends on the type of extraction. If you want to make an infused spirit, where the goal is primarily to add flavor, 2 to 7 days is a suitable length of time. To make bitters, allow the extraction to macerate from 2 to 4 weeks. For a tincture, allow 4 to 6 weeks.

A more advanced kitchen chemist might also consider the size of the molecules being extracted. Volatile oils are small, for example, whereas polysaccharides and tannins are large molecules and thus require more time to extract fully.

Energy

Extraction is altered by heat, shaking, rolling, and stirring. "Shake and pray every day" is the rule of thumb to assist diffusion with tinctures.

Heat increases extraction, while cold keeps molecules intact. Mucilaginous constituents, however, must be extracted in cold water because heat damages these molecules. I activate dried herbs by soaking them in hot water before tincturing or placing a jar of infused oil out in the sun or in a Crock-Pot of water on low.

Solvent

Here's a quick summary of which solvent is appropriate for which type of constituents. Remember the general rule that like dissolves like.

- Water is polar. Ethanol is somewhat polar. Triglycerides (oil) are non-polar.
- Oils and waters repel each other chemically because of polarity/charge.
- Less polar equals hydrophobic and more polar equals hydrophilic.
- The type of chemical bonds can affect extraction and bioavailability. Aglycones are less water-soluble than glycosides, which are more water-soluble and therefore more bioavailable.
- The chemical realities inside an extract are variable.
- Chemistry is not stable. It is a dynamic process, and events such as oxidation, polymerization, and precipitation can happen inside an extract.

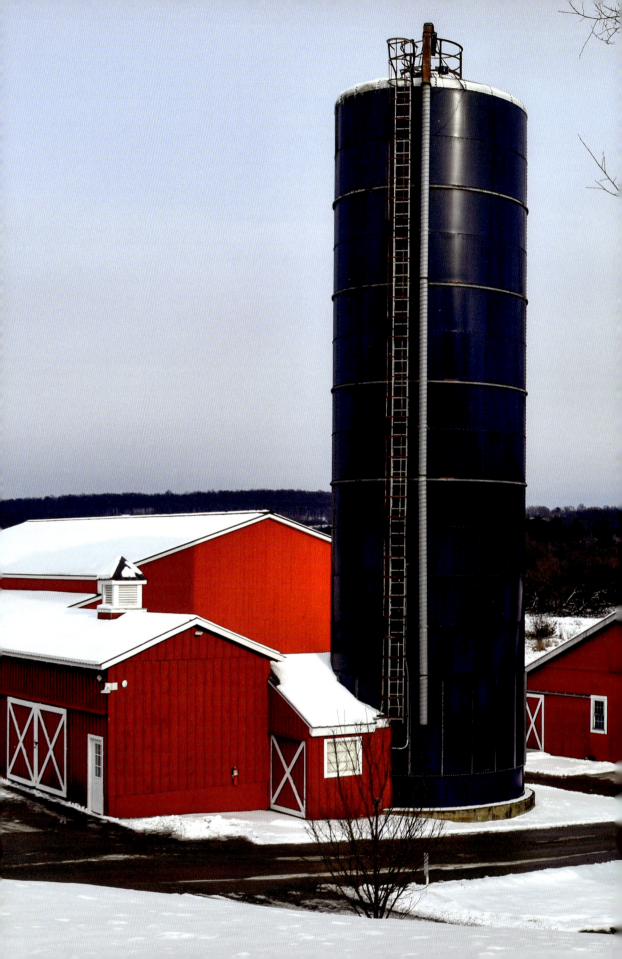

CHAPTER 5
Distilling Place

I love industries that allow individuals to fully develop and express their skills and gifts. It is an invitation to be valuable and be human, and it can be found in the hospitality industry as well as the closely linked world of craft spirits.

Small distilleries that are making spirits from scratch with the crops and botanicals of their local terroir have positive effects on the local economy, supporting farmers and agriculture.

Unfortunately, many brands of spirits masquerade as "craft" or may even include the word *farm* on the label, but those claims are just shiny marketing with no substance behind them. These companies buy grain neutral spirits (GNS) from an industrial mass producer (the neutral spirits are often made using GMO crops) and then rebottle them with their custom label. Their only goal is to maximize the bottom line.

I believe, however, that wealth and success can be measured in more ways than one. One important measure is the health of the fields and the soils. The vibrant community created when small-scale producers collaborate with their neighbors to create a fully local supply chain is another example, keeping money in a dynamic local economic system of relationships. You get to cast multiple votes at once: one for your neighbor who taps the maple trees, one for the mom-and-pop restaurant where everyone knows your name, and one for the soil.

Local spirits embody the souls of real people: their passion, their stories, their lineage. Small-batch production offers the opportunity for the distiller to provide more focused attention to details. These details translate to a positive impact on the local economy, a smaller ecological footprint, and the creation of a better-tasting final product. This is a difference that can be sensed by both the palate and the community. It is like tasting a tomato grown by industrialized agriculture versus from a small garden, lovingly tended.

Also, I'll be frank. As an entrepreneur, seeking out distillers who are creating unusual new types of spirits is a part of my business model—I'm known for the unique recipes I create using innovative ingredients. So seeking out craft distillers and creating partnerships with them builds my business as well as theirs. But even for my own personal consumption, I choose to support these brands, and I encourage you to do so also, whether you're an herbalist, a bartender, or a cocktail enthusiast.

As I was planning this book, I realized that the best way to present the reasons for supporting craft distillers would be to tell the stories of some of the amazing distilleries whose spirits have inspired some of my recipes. So I went behind the scenes to take distillery tours, participate in classes, and talk with the distillers about how their businesses began and what motivates them to make craft spirits. Because I live in Maine, the businesses I profile in this chapter are all based in the Northeast. But no matter where you live, you can find craft distillers making wonderful products.

What Is Distillation?

The Encyclopedia Britannica describes *distillation* as

> *A process involving the conversion of a liquid into vapour that is subsequently condensed back to liquid form. It is exemplified at its simplest when steam from a kettle becomes deposited as drops of distilled water on a cold surface. Distillation is used to separate liquids from nonvolatile solids, as in the separation of alcoholic liquors from fermented materials, or in the separation of two or more liquids having different boiling points, as in the separation of gasoline, kerosene, and lubricating oil from crude oil.*

The entire process of distillation can be achieved because different elements (in this case alcohol and water) have different boiling points. Through the manipulation of temperature, we can separate the two. With the production of alcohol, the liquid is run through a still one or more times to purify it. There is sometimes a "stripping run"—the first run where all of the alcohol is stripped from the wash. Subsequent runs are for removing heads and tails: the more toxic and worse-tasting alcohols and substances. Different chemicals come through the distillation process at different temperatures.

Many unseen factors influence the end results of craft distillation: the way crops are cultivated and harvested, the way the harvested grain is sprouted (the *malting* of that crop) to make the sugar more available, the method of controlled fermentation, and finally the management of the distillation, which often involves multiple runs in stills, of which there are many different types, many of which are custom-made for a distillery depending on its specific needs. In small production the distiller tastes the alcohol for the heads and tails cuts during the process, whereas in large operations, they are automated.

The craft distillation process requires a whole systems approach and the perfect balance between a mechanical mind and a creative one. A good distiller is like a mad scientist in a laboratory. The active, constant creative experimentation requires the maker to be a master of the systems being used. They must be present in the moment so they can rely on their perception of taste and smell to yield to new ideas.

Blue Barren Distillery, Camden, Maine

"We decided to start the distillery one night after discussing the decline of blueberry prices over the last several decades," says Jeremy Howard. Jeremy is a ninth-generation blueberry farmer who embarked on this innovative journey with his friend and now business partner, Andrew Stewart, to ferment and distill blueberries from his family farm Brodis Blueberries in the coastal hills of Hope, Maine.

On a morning in March, I followed the tree-lined dirt driveway leading to Blue Barren's hilltop barn. Beyond the trees I could see blueberry fields lined with classic New England rock walls. The day was cloudy, misty, moody. Bucolic.

Jeremy has a farmer's demeanor—down to earth, kind, and humbled by the elements. His eyes light up when he talks about his family's lineage; one of his ancestors walked up this hill with a land grant in the 1760s. Wild blueberries are everywhere, inviting a path of land stewardship. Jeremy is now teaching the tenth generation to care for 900 acres (364 ha), a living legacy.

In the summertime Blue Barren hosts a daily cocktail hour for guests, serving cocktails garnished entirely with ingredients from an on-site garden. Nearby, in touristy Camden, they run a restaurant and tasting room that features all twenty-three of their products, inspired by the local terroir.

I talked with Andrew Stewart about how some of Blue Barren's spirits are made, including some of their blueberry products and a sugar kelp vodka. The farm crew hand-rakes wild Maine blueberries from the rocky edges of the blueberry fields that cannot be machine-harvested. The berries are fermented traditionally and very slowly with champagne yeast to produce a blueberry wine that is then double-distilled to produce blueberry eau de vie. It is aged for a year in glass before bottling. "It is as close to traditional eau de vie as we can make," Andrew said. "We do not add sugar to the fermentation." Instead they rely on the natural low level of sugar from the fruit to drive the process. One 375 ml bottle of eau de vie requires 33 pounds (15 kg) of blueberries. "It is truly a labor of love!" Andrew remarked. They also blend the eau de vie with blueberry juice and age it in new oak barrels for three years to produce an aperitif they have named

Myrteau in honor of the French *pommeau* it is modeled after. They also infuse vodka with their blueberries during distillation to make a subtly flavored and delicate blueberry vodka.

Blue Barren partners with Atlantic Sea Farms to use sugar kelp, a type of marine algae harvested along the Maine coast. The kelp is infused in vodka for several months before a final distillation. The result is vodka with a uniquely briny flavor. "It's perfect for pairing with seafood of all types but especially oysters," Andrew said, noting that Blue Barren is proud to support the Maine aquaculture industry and local fishermen.

Wiggly Bridge Distillery, York, Maine

The story of Wiggly Bridge Distillery in York, Maine, begins with the vision David Woods Sr. and David Woods Jr., a father-and-son team driven by a shared love for spirits and a desire to create something truly special. Their journey began with a dream of producing high-quality artisanal liquors that would stand out in an increasingly crowded market. Inspired by the rich history of distilling and scenic beauty of their surroundings, the Woods family set out to build a legacy grounded in craftsmanship. Their products include small-batch bourbon and handcrafted gin.

I learned the nitty-gritty of the distillation process at Wiggly Bridge in their Distiller for a Day class. I fell in love with this family operation and brand because of their holistic approach and the heart behind the products they make.

Although I understood the basic theory and process of distillation before I visited Wiggly Bridge, getting my hands into the whole process from grain to glass was a deeply informative experience. The class consisted of "a day in the life" with Dave Sr. and Jr. The amount of information shared in this day is incredibly generous. The seven hours start with learning about the raw corn and rye and end with setting up a barrel in the rickhouse, where whiskey gets stored to age and develop character over time. First we cooked the grain, which was then fermented in mash bins. The fermented grain was channeled into the stripping still and then the pot still for further refinement. Dave weaves his big-picture philosophy into every aspect of his teaching.

Dave and Dave buy all of their grain from a local farmer, who dropped by on the day of the class to learn more about the distilling process. And to extend the network of local connections, the distillery gives its spent grain to another neighboring farmer, who feeds the nutritious material to her prizewinning dairy cows. The distillery's chef-bartender set up a smoker behind the tasting room bar so that he could make bacon-washed whiskey for use in craft cocktails. My classmates and I signed our barrel (barrel

Distilling Place

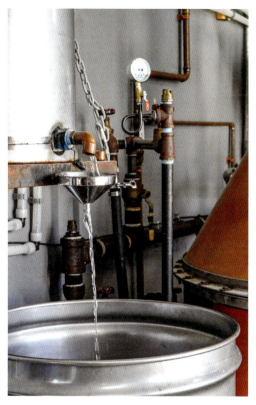 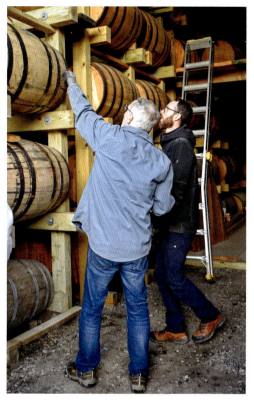

As the distilling process proceeds at Wiggly Bridge, the undesirable parts of the heads and tails are cut to improve the quality of the final product.

The father-and-son team at Wiggly Bridge Distillery choose a place for the new barrel of whiskey in the rickhouse.

1789); anyone who has attended this class can return to the distillery (with a little advance notice) to taste the contents of their barrel.

Dave Woods Sr. explained that their philosophy is to work with nature. "There are lots of moving parts in distilling, and we monitor and constantly observe everything, thus allowing us to maintain a healthy system and process in the creation of our award-winning spirits."

What sets Wiggly Bridge Distillery apart is its commitment to the traditional methods of distillation. One example of this is making heads and tails cuts with their own taste buds versus using an automated system that may result in adding bad-tasting heads and tails into the finished product. Heads and tails are different types of alcohols, oils, and chemicals that also end up being separated out during the distilling process. Heads typically consist of less-desirable alcohols, such as toxic methanol and sometimes acetone, depending on what is being fermented. The tails contain the unpleasant taste and aroma of fusel alcohols. Tails are typically a larger cut than the heads, and at the very end of them some desirable aromatics come

> ### Bad Liquor
>
> The word *fusel* is German for "bad liquor." Fusel alcohol, sometimes called fusel oil, is a mixture of stronger, more toxic alcohols such as amyl alcohol that distill faster. If these bad liquors aren't fully cut, it can lead to off-tasting spirits and possibly worse hangovers for those who consume such spirits.

through again. The product left after the cuts are taken is the heart of the spirit. Wiggly Bridge embraces the nuanced art of crafting spirits in limited quantities. Every step of the process is infused with care and expertise, from selecting grains to meticulously tasting and blending each barrel.

Visitors to the Wiggly Bridge Distillery are welcomed into a world where tradition meets innovation. Father and son embody the spirit of hospitality in their manner, guiding guests on tours to share their passion and hosting regular events and community-building strategies such as a bartender cocktail competition that I recently took part in. This personal connection fosters a sense of community and loyalty among patrons who appreciate the authenticity behind the brand.

New England Distilling, Portland, Maine

It was a short trip for me to visit New England Distilling in Portland. Distiller and owner Ned Wight gave me a tour of their old-school pot stills insulated with bricks from a recycled patio. The extra insulation allows them to reduce their fuel use by 30 percent, Ned said, and it was just one example of the importance he places on efficiency and the ecological footprint of his business. The thing about efficiency is that it often benefits both the environment and the wallet! They use natural cork for their bottling and non-GMO grains.

The direct fire under the pot stills differentiates their spirits. The high temperatures allow for Maillard processes and caramelization, creating a more richly flavored whiskey. Maillard is a complex chemical reaction—also referred to as non-enzymatic browning—that transforms proteins and sugars through heat. It's responsible for toasty, malted flavors. The heating technique most used in the distilling industry reaches temps of 350°F (177°C), whereas the direct fire used here gets up to 1000°F (538°C)—holy hot! Later in the process, the heads and tails are put in a thumper, a centuries-old apparatus that helps to recapture some of the more desirable flavors. We inhaled the aromas of the different stages in cuts. The most

Distilling Place

Mash Bills

A *mash bill* is the recipe that beer and whiskey producers use to indicate how much of which kind of grain is used to create the wort. *Mashing* is the process of combining and heating ground grains with water to catalyze available sugars with yeast and kick-start the natural fermentation process. The wort is the liquid that becomes beer or whiskey. Maltose and maltotriose are fermented by brewer's yeast to produce alcohol.

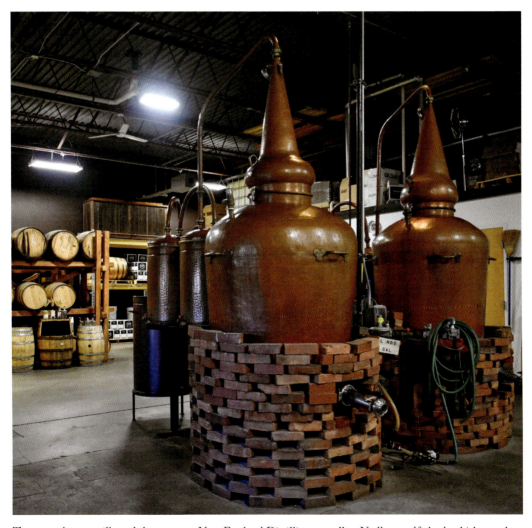

These are the pot stills and thumpers at New England Distilling as well as Ned's grandfather's whiskey rack.

delicious smell was the very end of the tails. Ned explained that the tails are more floral and volatile as we noticed the difference between the smell about 6 inches (15 cm) away from the jar—freshly baked bread. The scent down inside the jar was honey and tropical fruit.

Ned is a sixth-generation distiller, and much of his inspiration hails from his lineage. "The details are murky, but family lore has it that my great-great-great-grandfather John Jacob Wight took over a failing whiskey distillery in the Hunt Valley, north of Baltimore, Maryland, sometime during the 1850s and began producing Sherwood Rye Whiskey," Ned told me.

Ned describes his distillery as being set up like a brewery: "Our process begins in the brew house where we make a distiller's beer, which is essentially an unhopped beer." Once the beer is fully fermented, they transfer it to the stills to boil. In the stills, the alcohol is separated from most of the water, then refined on subsequent passes. The resulting spirit is stored in barrels to mature for up to six years. The flagship product is Gunpowder Rye, named after the river in Maryland where the original Sherwood Distillery was located. This spirit embodies a mash bill and process that produces the quintessential Maryland-style rye, which is known to be more floral and herbal than Midwest rye with its peppery, spicy bite. The wooden rack used to hold the barrels filled with this whiskey is the same one Ned's grandfather used.

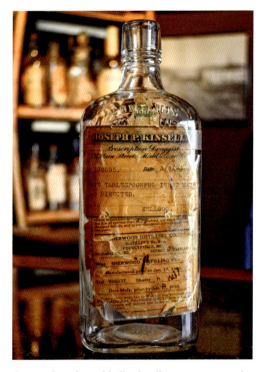

The spirit of collaboration is embodied in their experimental line: Rack 4, for which Ned distills beers from local breweries into whiskey. "I grew up hearing stories of the family's distilling history and dreamed of reentering the family business. My path took me to distilling by way of brewing."

The tasting room is modest but welcoming. Behind the bar is a shelf of memorabilia of his predecessors. I pick up an old whiskey bottle; turning it around I find a prescription on the back. Written during Prohibition, dated March 3, 1923, it called for "1 TB in hot water as recommended."

An artifact from Ned's distilling ancestors who founded Sherwood Distillery and produced medicinal whiskey during Prohibition.

Distilling Place

Matchbook Distilling, Long Island, New York

Matchbook Distilling, a research and design facility located on the North Fork of Long Island, is a brainchild of the inspiring and dedicated Leslie Merinoff-Kwasnieski. This business is deeply aligned with regenerative agriculture and creates imaginative spirits based on what is available from local farms. Everything is scratch-made and organic. Leslie told me, "We think healthy, live soil produces the healthiest ingredients—and the healthiest ingredients produce the best flavor." The Greenport facility infuses and distills many botanicals using grain neutral spirits made from organic New York–grown grains that are milled in-house. They also experiment with landrace varieties to help restore the grainshed of the state.

During my visit, Leslie and I tasted several batches that were in the process of fermenting, infusing, and being proofed down. Everything I tasted blew my mind (and I am not one who surprises easily). This woman is pushing the boundaries of the possible because she is a master of her craft and science. We tasted a wine-based savory vermouth made with tomato, shiso, and olive brine. Leslie invited me to smell the aromatics hovering above the fermenters of a Viognier, but she cautioned me not to stick my head in too far. A blanket of carbon dioxide also forms above the fermenters.

Matchbook also makes wine. Long Island is home to over fifty wineries, and making wine or beer is often the first process prior to the distillation, which separates and concentrates a higher alcohol proof. Grapes are an important part of the North Fork terroir and agri-*culture*.

While looking at their large pot and column stills, Leslie and I discussed the concept of *élevage*, an elegant French word for the idea of "raising" or "bringing up" the peak expression of a crop to its perfect destiny and full potential. She extends this care by further distillation. Leslie explained that "distillation is a process of letting go of what you don't want and keeping what you do want." It seems that slow and intentional is

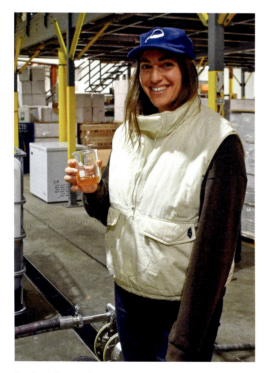

Leslie Merinoff-Kwasnieski, the head distiller and founder of Matchbook Distilling, taste-tests her experimental savory vermouth.

the name of the game of what defines *craft*. The type of distillation varies depending on the desired product, from double pot distillation to using the full column to using only one or two plates, as these perforated sections within the column can also strip some desirable taste.

Attention to detail matters! The barrels they use are cured, not kilned, which preserves some of the organic compounds in the wood, which in turn contributes to the taste of the spirits.

Leslie told me that her mother was an avid biodynamic farmer and farm educator. Leslie majored in political science (but also studied chemistry) and began in the industry as a marketer for Sailor Jerry Rum. She kept asking for a pathway to the production side of the business, but it was never granted. Eventually she quit to follow her distillation dreams.

One of Matchbook's most innovative and surprising spirits is Late Embers, a smoky spirit distilled from sunchokes. Last year, Matchbook roasted twenty-one thousand sunchokes directly over 400°F (204°C) hot coals in a large firepit, a process inspired by local clambakes. The roots are then boiled and crushed, with honey added. The fire helps to begin the process of breaking down sugars through hydrolysis, a process also used for making agave spirits. Like agave, sunchokes contain chains of fructose molecules called inulin. The inulin in the rhizomes converts to sugar, which yeasts then consume, resulting in the production of alcohol.

After two weeks of fermentation, the mash is pumped to the stills. A nearby farm, Rogers Farm, grew the sunchokes used to make Late Embers. As the product gained popularity, Matchbook agreed to purchase a rough quantity at a set price to help the farmer pay for a special piece of harvesting equipment.

I've never tasted anything like Late Embers. The spirit is full, smoky earth, with notes of pepper, pear, and rose. The closest resemblance would be the smoky spirit Mezcal. The nose reminds me of stacking wood and the

Column Stills

In a column or reflux still, the plates create partitions within the column, each section contributing to a cleaner final product. This differs from traditional pot stills, which create flavorful spirits with rich character. Steam is introduced from the bottom of the column. Each plate is cooler than the one beneath it, creating condensation of vapors. This results in the vapors being redistilled, which separates heavier from lighter compounds as they rise up the column.

Distilling Place

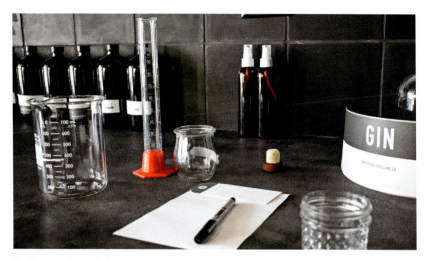

Leslie distills each botanical separately for the "gin apothecary," where Matchbook Distilling guests can create their own custom blend of gin. I made a blend of juniper, orris root, citrus, rose, coriander, bay leaf, and cinnamon.

woodstove smell that clings to our jackets here in the Northeast. I also smell honey and am reminded of a favorite summer activity—sticking my nose into resinous sunflowers and breathing in the aroma. I'm saving some to drink around the first campfires of the season.

In the tasting room at Matchbook, a "gin botanical apothecary" of individually distilled botanicals lines the wall. Visitors can blend their own signature gin from the botanicals. She captures the essence of each plant separately for optimal expression. Florals like jasmine or rose distill low and slow, whereas roots are a hot-and-fast process. Leslie encouraged me to use one of the "stickier" components like bee pollen or orris root, its resinous compounds that help to stretch the palate and change the mouthfeel. I combined several of the distillates, and the result was somewhat of a classic gin with juniper, citrus, orris root, coriander, bay leaf, cinnamon, and rose.

Leslie gifted me with a colorful bottle of amaro called Fieldtrip, which is made from a large, local heirloom squash called the Boston marrow. She also gave me an aperitivo called Elsewhere, made from whole, organic unwaxed blood oranges. The oranges admittedly were not local, but as Leslie said, "When it's not local, it's for a really cool reason."

She purchases from Bhumi Farms, a sustainable broker of citrus. Leslie explained that many small citrus farmers are facing risk of consolidation and having a hard time selling their product. Bhumi helps them find customers and stay afloat.

Each release from Matchbook is unique to a particular moment in time. "We are constantly honing our abilities" to capture "a life-like photo you can drink," Leslie reflected. This is what a research-and-development facility specializes in, celebrating the ephemeral nature of time and constantly evolving with the elements and culture of each season.

Barr Hill, Montpelier, Vermont

I discovered Barr Hill when I was living in Vermont and working at an herb farm in the Northeast Kingdom and also as a beginning bartender. Hands in the dirt during the day and lipstick on at night behind the bar. Barr Hill Gin was the first spirit I could really relate to. This craft spirit was inspired by and named for the place it was grown—the Barr Hill Nature Preserve near Hardwick. Barr Hill began with a relationship between beekeeper Todd Hardie and brewer Ryan Christiansen. The first talented mixologist I worked under, Don Horrigan, introduced me to this brand and the beekeeper. The company has grown exponentially since I first started mixing their raw honey-laced aromatic gin, which is packaged in a gorgeous bottle sealed with real beeswax and marked with a honeybee.

Barr Hill champions land stewardship. Every year the distillery runs a social media campaign called Bee's Knees Week. The Bee's Knees is a delicious sour with a template of 2 parts gin, 0.75 parts honey syrup, and 0.75 parts fresh lemon juice. (Riffs on the original can be quite creative—see the recipe for my version, The Visionkeeper, on page 186.) During Bee's Knees

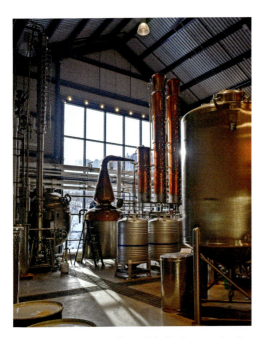

Barr Hill's largest still is "Phyllis," named after Ryan's grandmother.

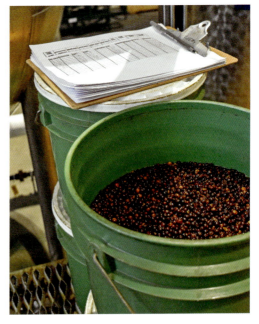

Juniper berries are prepared for the gin distillation in an alcohol solution.

Week, for every photo of a Bee's Knees that is shared online, the Barr Hill team plants 10 square feet (just under 1 sq m) of pollinator sanctuary. In 2023, they planted 220,000 square feet, or 5 acres (2 ha). They have planted over 23 acres (9 ha) since the program began!

Barr Hill's honey comes from family-run apiaries within a 250-mile (402 km) radius, and they use only raw honey that has never been filtered or pasteurized—nothing has been added nor taken away. The honey itself is naturally flavored by the aromatics from the wide range of plants and flowers the bees visit along their pollination journey.

On my visit to Barr Hill, Sam Nellis showed me the production room. First, he lifted off the cap on a 55-gallon drum filled with about 650 pounds (295 kg) of honey. Using a spoon, Sam scraped away some of the waxy parts that had floated to the top. "We've calculated 100 to 150 wildflowers or botanicals found in our raw honey, and this makes up the unique botanical complexity in our spirits," Sam said. "In our opinion, honey is perhaps the most terroir-driven product out there, and we love that our spirits represent the land around us." They use about 200,000 pounds (91,000 kg) of raw honey per year.

In 2019, Barr Hill moved its production facility from the Northeast Kingdom to Vermont's state capital, Montpelier (the only state capital in the United States without a McDonald's). As Sam led me on a tour of the impressive and very busy establishment, he explained that he began here as the opening beverage director and got to help design the bar. Now he has moved into other departments, including sales and marketing, and he's worked closely with Ryan Christiansen, the owner and head distiller, for many years.

Each of the impressive stills is named after one of the production team's grandmothers. Juniper berries were soaking in a green 5-gallon bucket, priming for their inclusion in the gin. To be sold as gin, legally the spirit must include juniper, and at Barr Hill, juniper is the only botanical used; the other nuanced and complex aromatics arise from the raw honey.

Barr Hill is one of very few independent distilleries of its size, Sam said, which allows it to prioritize quality raw ingredients and a minimal-intervention approach to distilling. Many large companies run many distillations as a way to get as much yield out of their product as possible: "they cut corners and disguise their cheap commodity ingredients," Sam explained. Barr Hill never does that. "Our process is simple, and the results speak for themselves. We take a thoughtful-hearts cut and let the flavor of the raw ingredients shine through unhindered. This is what sets our spirits apart in a sea of factory-processed monotony." The distillery's ability to maintain craft-level quality at large scale is impressive: Barr Hill produces more than one hundred thousand six-bottle cases a year; they bottle about twenty-five hundred bottles a day.

Back at the bar, I tasted one of their new ventures: a very special whiskey called Phyllis and the Wide Open Field, a single-barrel rye aged for four years, made with 100 percent Vermont-grown grain. They are releasing only one barrel at a time, and I felt honored to be invited to taste such an expensive pour. I asked Sam what *landcrafted* means—the company has trademarked the term. He replied, "If the land is taken care of, it produces everything we need to make world-class distillates. Our mission at Barr Hill is to reconnect agriculture to cocktail culture." His words are evident in the menu and in the experiences Barr Hill creates for its patrons. I could taste the mission, from the rye nose to the malty finish. "Distillation was always a part of farming," Sam told me. "People have forgotten that. We want to bring folks back to the land with every sip."

Tamworth Distilling, Tamworth, New Hampshire

Founded and owned by liquor brand savant Steven Grasse, Tamworth Distilling focuses on creating one-of-a-kind small-batch spirits that reflect the lush flora and fauna of Tamworth, New Hampshire. Taking a cue from the nineteenth-century Transcendentalists of New England, Tamworth Distilling pulls inspiration and ingredients from the local environment. All ingredients used in the production of spirits are farmed or foraged within 150 miles (241 km) of the distillery, including local grain, pure White Mountain water, herbs and botanicals from the woods and the distillery garden, and local fruits and vegetables.

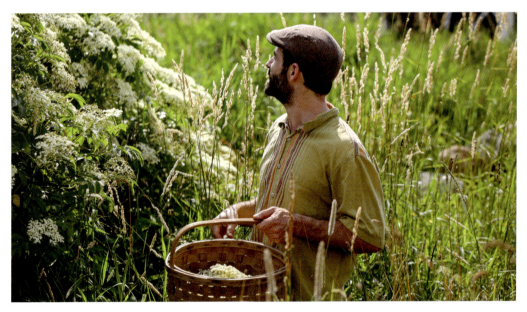

Distiller Matt Power of Tamworth Distilling forages for elderflowers to use in an experimental spirit.

Distilling Place

The distillery was recognized by *Food & Wine* magazine as a 2023 Drinks Innovator of the Year. And for the past several years, Tamworth has hosted my business, Remedy Cocktail Co., to teach botanical-themed, seasonal cocktail classes at the Lyceum, a café-turned-workshop-space down the road from the production and tasting room. These are not ordinary cocktail classes! My favorite has been Foraging for Cocktails, where I lead the group on a wild plant walk around the periphery of the property, identifying springtime herbal tonic green plants and digging up dandelions.

Tamworth's copper still is outfitted with a brandy helmet, whiskey column, gin basket, and rectifying column. These components allow for versatility in producing a variety of spirits, with batches that change seasonally.

Like Matchbook Distilling, Tamworth distills their own neutral grain spirit base, using local organic corn, organic rye, and malt that they mill in-house, on demand, for the freshest flavor.

The town of Tamworth's water comes from the Ossipee Stratified Aquifer, one of the purest sources on the East Coast. More important, the area lies on granite bedrock. Fracking for oil production in granite is not possible, so this pure source is safe from that type of industrial pollution. The distillery test kitchen serves as a hub for creative experiments.

Steven Grasse has been described as the "punk rock prince of small-batch spirits," and is the creative force behind bestselling brands such as Hendrick's Gin and Sailor Jerry Rum. He is an author of several books, including *Brand Mysticism*. I asked Steven about the importance of creativity in craft distilling.

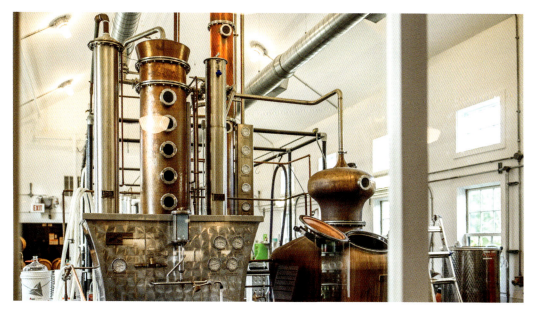

Tamworth Distilling's 250-gallon copper still was custom built by Vendome in Kentucky.

"Creativity is everything," Steven emphasized. "You cannot just create good liquid.... You need to have a great story and great packaging that brings it to life so that it resonates and is intriguing and enchanting to your audience."

Bold experimentation is part of their business plan, and Tamworth Distilling pushes the boundaries of what is possible, producing some weird and wacky spirits such as whiskey distilled from invasive crabs and rye infused with maple syrup tapped from graveside trees. The Deerslayer is a whiskey made with responsibly sourced venison, inspired by James Fenimore Cooper's 1841 novel, *The Deerslayer*. "It is not just liquid, it is story and liquid coming together," Steven told me. "That is what brand mysticism is all about." Tamworth recently released Sylvan Mist, the world's first perfume gin—it is both wearable and drinkable.

In a way, a creative person is a distiller of ideas—taking in lots of information, cooking it down, filtering sensory inputs through their own experience. When pressure is added, new notions rise like vapor into the ether.

Obviously, Steven is a very clever man, but I wanted to know what, from his perspective, makes the Tamworth Distilling brand meaningful, and what, in his opinion, makes a spirits company successful? His reply: "What makes the Tamworth brand meaningful is our never-ending quest for innovation. Our goal is to be the most innovative distillery in the world."

WhistlePig, Shoreham, Vermont

I was guided on a private tour of the WhistlePig Farm in Shoreham, Vermont, on a cold January day with Meghan Ireland, the head whiskey blender. There are thirty employees on this 500-acre (202 ha) farm, along with two kunekune pigs by the names of Orwell and Mortimer Jr. (who is a direct descendant of one of the founding pigs). Their chief purpose is greeting visitors. The farm is open only by invitation to special guests, including members of the barrel program. Restaurants and businesses that purchase a single barrel have the opportunity to stay on the farm for a couple of days, a fully immersive agrotourism-meets-secret-club experience to round out their 53 gallons (*6,784 shots or ounces!*) of craft whiskey.

WhistlePig is known for its rye whiskey, which is spicier than bourbon (a corn-based spirit), and the brand grows much of their own rye on site! Of the 500 acres, 300 (121 ha) are in use. Sustainability is one of its concerns—the farm operates on solar power, and the spent grain is sent to a digester to be repurposed into fuel. WhistlePig also makes barrel-aged maple syrup, in part using sap sourced from sugar maples tapped on their own farm; a partnership with Runamok Maple based in Fairfax, Vermont, makes up the difference. Try making an Old Fashioned with WhistlePig rye and barrel-aged maple syrup.

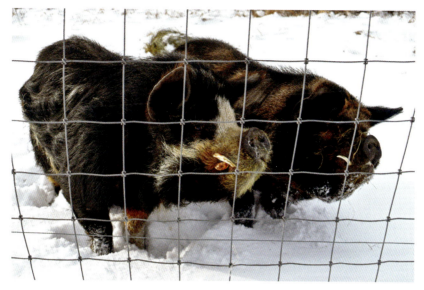

Life is good for these WhistlePigs who live on the land at WhistlePig Farm and Distillery in Vermont.

While talking with Meghan, I learned that she studied chemical engineering. While still in college, she read an article about a woman master distiller who had an engineering degree. She thought that sounded like a fun career path. After college, she got a job with a hard cider company and started to enjoy the blending side of the business.

On an everyday basis, she runs experiments with the whiskey, analyzing the chemistry of different flavors. She can track the amounts of different components within the whiskey. She is also responsible for tasks such as stability testing and filter testing to ensure product quality.

Meghan explained that different woods can impact the whiskeys. "Our Estate Oak Rye Aged 15 Years is finished in Vermont oak, which has a different chemical makeup and offers different flavors to the whiskey, like a nice caramelized sugar note." The Boss Hog X is an example of how WhistlePig is pushing the envelope with never-before-attempted maturation styles. "We finished our whiskey in two barrels," Meghan said, "one of them being a mead and the second one being a whey distilled with the resin frankincense and myrrh that we created. We are trying to create an incredible and unique product."

Wild Sings the Bird, Waitsfield, Vermont

Allison Dellner of Wild Sings the Bird and I attended herb school together at the Vermont Center for Integrative Herbalism. Allison is an herbalist and doula, and she also makes hydrosols (water-based distillates), which I have been buying to blend into nonalcoholic plant spirits that I use in some of my complex, aromatic herbal tonic mocktails.

The art of making hydrosols is ancient and has its roots in perfumery operations. This is the same process as essential oil distillation: The volatile oils concentrate on the surface of water. Essential oils, however, are very concentrated and can be too potent to use internally or undiluted for any purpose. In contrast, aromatic hydrosols are safe and can be used in food and drink. They fully capture the spirit of the plant.

As explained in chapter 3, aromatics are an important part of formulating an effective relaxing nonalcoholic drink. In general, volatile oils are antispasmodic. Also, as essential oils volatilize, they connect us to the greater spirit of all things, carrying our prayers as might be part of a traditional ceremony, like our ancestors.

Most (if not all) of the nonalcoholic spirits on the market are made from hydrosols, but most commercial nonalcoholic spirits also contain less-than-yummy preservatives. There are none added in Allison's hydrosols, because most volatile oils contain their own antimicrobial compounds and are shelf-stable for one to two years in cool, dry, storage-appropriate conditions. These special, small-batch handcrafted hydrosols are like gold. Much of what Allison distills is not available commercially. It is possible to make hydrosols at home with a small still—or in an even smaller way on the stovetop—but good things take time.

I visited Allison this winter in Waitsfield, a quintessentially Vermont small town. We caught up in her apothecary while the copper alembic still was working its magic. She uses an Al-Ambiq traditional copper still that requires making a paste from rye flour each time to seal up the side seams and prevent the steam from escaping. She had also rigged up a pump system in a bin of fresh water for saving the cooling water that's needed for the condenser. The process takes four to six hours. Allison gathered fresh clippings of balsam fir and white pine needles into the water of the still and put it

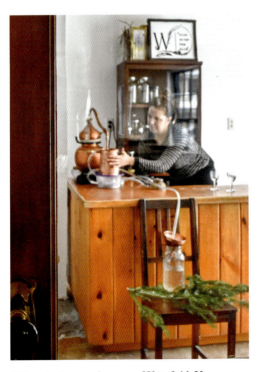

Allison in her apothecary in Waitsfield, Vermont.

Distilling Place

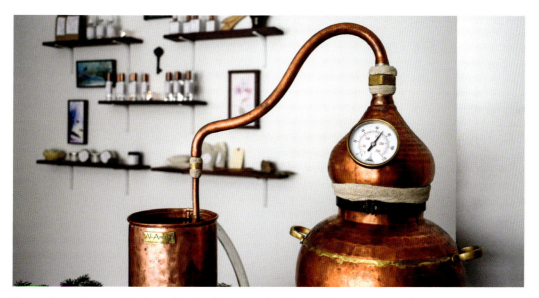

This traditional copper alembic still is hand-hammered in Portugal by the company Al-Ambiq. It is made for steam distillation of essential oils and hydrosols.

on a single burner hot plate in her apothecary. This is what January in Vermont smells and feels like. We are *distilling place*. Last summer Allison and I harvested sea roses together on the coast of Maine in June, which she then distilled in small batches and sent to me! Such a beautiful and romantic way to capture a single moment in time, in a particular place. She offered me a tasting of all the seasons and places she had captured over the past year. We even compared tasting notes of the same botanical and how its hydrosol form tasted different when made from different terroirs.

An herbalist, mother, reader, and lover of wild places, Allison views her work as a combination of practical healing and the magic and art of herbalism. "I preserve plants in the various mediums of oil, spirit, and vinegar for use another day, when these medicines are called upon to help the body adapt to or confront the challenges of illness."

But in addition, Allison explained, each small bottle of hydrosol that she creates is unique to the season of the year, and even to a moment in time. "No process other than distillation really captures this feeling so well," she said. "The ephemeral, unseen, yet liveliest elements of the plants are liberated and preserved in a clear, impossibly fragrant liquid that has the ability to remove your thinking brain from the present moment and bring you back to that rose on the beach, that spruce forest on the mountain. Some remedies that I make are purely to help people remember that they belong to this world; to have a moment of recognition to a flower, a leaf, a root; to see a bit of themselves connected to every living thing."

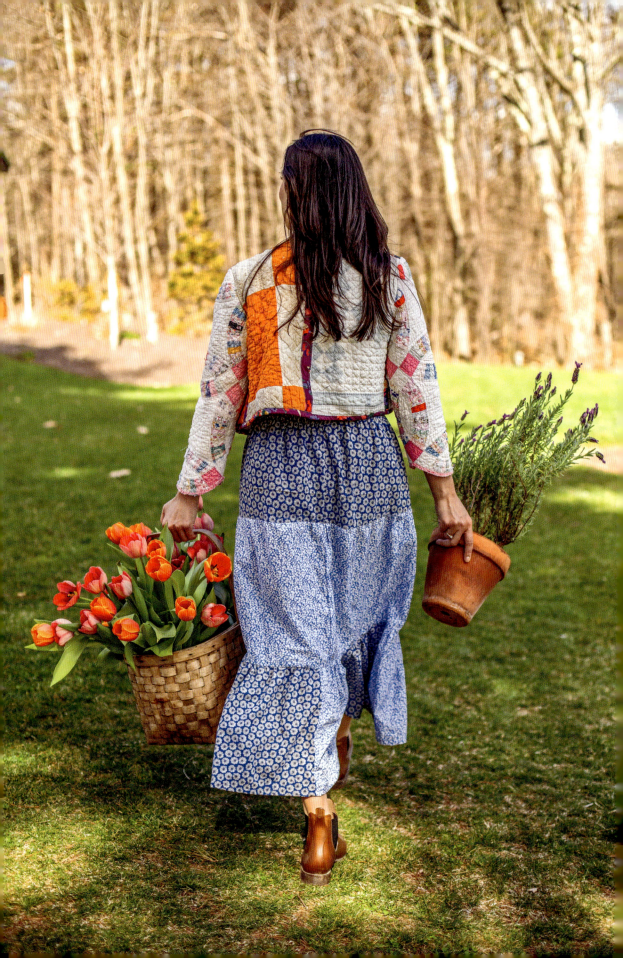

CHAPTER 6

The Garnish Garden

My mission is to connect plants and people, and I hope that everyone who reads this book will try growing some herbs and edible flowers for garnishing your beverage creations—even if you've never grown anything other than a few houseplants or a tomato plant on your patio. Who knows, you may find that your home herb garden can also become your basic herbal medicine chest to use for treating minor wounds, colds, fevers, and pain, as well as providing tonics for daily health.

It's not possible to offer an in-depth gardening guide in this book about botanical bar craft, but in this chapter I walk through the basic steps to planting a first small garden. May it be your introduction to a new lifelong pursuit.

To begin with, here are my guiding principles of ecological gardening:

- The heart of efficient design is observation.
- You are an integral part of nature.
- In a dynamic garden system, everything is connected and in balance.
- Biodiversity is strength, enhancing the lives of all species.
- Be a good steward: Do not poison the ecosystem with pesticides or non-biodegradable household products.

It probably goes without saying, but I am an organic gardener, and I can't stress enough the importance of never using chemicals to control pests or kill weeds in your garden, especially when you are growing plants that you will use as garnishes or ingredients in tonic elixirs and apothecary cocktails!

A garden is a sanctuary. Respect what is already happening there and look for what you can add to provide habitat—perhaps bee houses, birdhouses, and

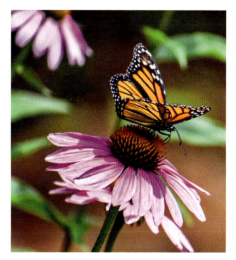

An example of healthy pollinator habitat. A monarch butterfly on an echinacea flower.

even bat houses! Allow leaves to remain covering the ground in some areas—that's habitat, too, as are dead, decaying trees. It may not match your aesthetic of picture-perfect, but gardeners learn that natural is always better.

Step 1: Choose a Garden Site

You may have only one garden site available, but if you have choices, think about sunlight, access to water, and soil quality as you decide which spot is best.

Assessing Sunlight

Plants need sunlight for photosynthesis. In general, a site that gets at least six hours of direct sun per day is ideal for an herb garden. It's important to think about how patterns of sun and shade change with the seasons, too. The sun's trajectory over your landscape is something you can observe directly. Simply stand outside at different times of day and at different times of the year to observe whether your potential garden sites are in sun or shade. Pay attention to tree lines, because often the sun is hidden behind trees in morning and late afternoon during spring or fall, which can effectively shorten your gardening season.

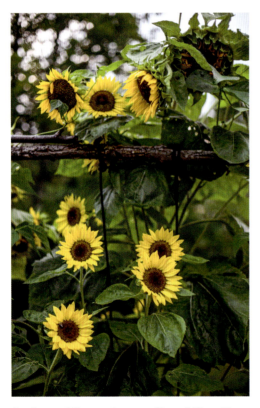

Sunflowers following the sun at Rooted Heart Farm.

Assessing Water

Most garden plants require about 1 inch (2.5 cm) per week, but in high and dry microclimates, more may be needed (for instance, if your garden is on a hill). Is water easily available at your potential garden sites? You'll probably need to water to supplement natural rainfall a few or many times during the season. And how is the drainage on those sites? Many types of plants don't like to have "wet feet" all the time.

Also investigate the quality of the water source. If you are using your household water for watering your garden, you probably have already had it tested for contaminants. But if you plan to use water from a stream or pond to water your garden, you may want to

> ### To Till or Not to Till?
>
> Lots of gardeners own a rotary tiller, but before you decide to borrow or buy one, consider this: Excess tilling is harmful to soil—it makes it harder for the soil to absorb and hold water and nutrients. It also destroys the habitat for millions of beneficial soil organisms.
>
> If you must use a tiller, be sure you add lots of organic matter to make up for the organic matter that will be lost because of tilling. On a garden scale, the broadfork or a simple digging fork are good tools for loosening the soil in preparation for planting.

have it tested. It is not easy to find uncontaminated water in our environmentally stressed world.

I like to include a small water feature in a garden for the pollinating insects to drink from. This can be as simple as a shallow dish of clean water that I change daily. Or it might be a container large enough to include a small solar-powered fountain. Be sure to include spots for insects to perch while they sip.

Assessing Soil Quality

If you have a choice of sites, it makes sense to select the one with the best soil characteristics for gardening. See "Learn about Your Soil" on this page for guidance on how to size up your soil.

Step 2: Gather Tools

There are so many wonderful garden tools! Start with the basics. Here are the five garden tools I recommend for first-time gardeners: hand pruners (I like Felco brand), a hand cultivating tool, a spade, a garden rake, and a trowel or hori-hori knife. If you catch the gardening bug and decide to expand your collection, I find a flat fork or broadfork useful for loosening the earth without tilling, and I like a scuffle hoe for easy stand-up weeding between rows. It's also helpful to have some twine and stakes, 5-gallon buckets, garden shears, and loppers for selective pruning of larger branches. A hose attachment or watering can that dispenses a nice even sprinkle is helpful, too!

Step 3: Learn about Your Soil

Healthy soil is the biological foundation for supporting all life. Soil fertility is the ability to sustain plant growth. The goal is a self-perpetuating closed-loop cycle in which the plant matter decays and provides the organic matter that in turn provides future fertility. How can you assess whether your soil is healthy and fertile? Some simple observations are a good start, and you can also send samples of your soil to a testing lab if you want more detailed information.

Soil texture is one basic characteristic of soil. Soil can be sandy, silty, or clayey. Sandy soil needs watering more often, but it drains well. Clayey soil holds lots of water and sometimes doesn't drain well, but it is abundant in minerals! Silty soil is in between. You can test soil texture simply by wetting a small amount of soil and squeezing it into a ball in your hand. If it makes a very solid ball, it contains much clay. Silt has a silky texture; sand is gritty. Very sandy soil will not hold together—it will fall apart when you squeeze it.

Also examine the handful of soil. What color is it? Dark soil probably contains a good amount of organic matter, which gardeners love because it helps make soil more fertile and better at holding and releasing water. You may see critters in the handful of soil, too: earthworms and millipedes. Critters are also a sign that your soil contains organic matter, because many soil critters feed on organic matter.

Most localities have an organization such as Cooperative Extension that will test samples of your soil and provide a report on characteristics from the nutrient levels to soil pH. They may also offer customized recommendations for what kinds and amounts of soil amendments you should add to your soil.

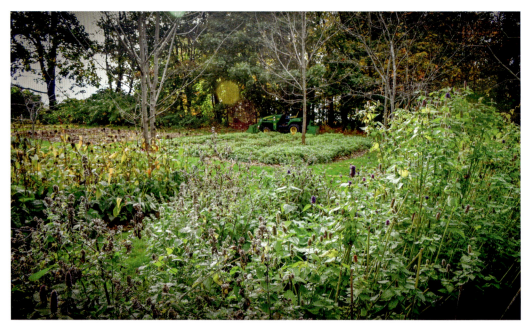

Imagine everything you can't see below the surface of these fall garden beds. The balance and interplay of countless numbers of microbes determine the health and fertility of the soil.

> ### Dirt Is the Best Medicine
>
> If you're a little squeamish about the idea of picking up handfuls of soil, you should know that the best medicine around is the dirt on your hands after you garden. Literally! Beneficial bacteria found in soil help create a balanced microbiome, contributing to immune and nervous system health. Studies done on mice show that a special soil bacteria, *Mycobacterium vaccae*, may increase serotonin release in the brain.[1] Good news for gardening addicts!

If the gardening season is upon you and you haven't had time to test your soil, don't despair! Find a source of high-quality compost and add some to every seed row and planting hole at planting time. Compost, mulch, and careful watering will help most crops succeed, even in less-than-ideal soil.

Step 4: Choosing What to Grow

What are your garden goals? Do you want to visit your garden in search of garnishes for that seasonal libation you have created? Do you want to grow lots of edible flowers? Or would you like to grow a more substantial garden of life-sustaining vegetables and fruits? I recommend beginning with the garnish garden or a small kitchen garden, no bigger than 20 feet by 20 feet (6 by 6 m)—and perhaps as small as 5 feet by 10 feet (1.5 by 3 m). Choose ten to twenty different kinds of herbs and edible flowers, and possibly vegetables, for a first-year garden.

Once you choose what you want to grow, where should you go to buy seeds or young plants? Finding a reputable seed company in your region is the best bet. (Also see "Resources" at the end of this book.) Check to see whether there's a seed swap hosted by a garden group or at your local library. The local farmers market is the place to buy transplants. Avoid big-box stores, because the plants for sale there have probably been treated with chemical fertilizer or toxic pesticides. They are probably water-stressed, too.

When you buy seeds, think about whether those seeds can be sown directly in the garden outdoors, or whether they should be started indoors in small pots or packs. For example, it's easy to plant calendula from seed, but not as easy to grow basil from seed. I recommend that beginners buy seedlings from a reputable source for those that prefer a little head start. But if you decide to start your own seeds indoors, follow the instructions given on the package and any additional growing information available on the seed

Great Garnish Plants for Beginners

Anise hyssop: Full sun; purple flower spikes all summer long are a favorite of pollinators. Grows to about shoulder-high.

Bachelor buttons: Sow seeds directly in the garden in early spring and again in August; knee-high; quick to flower (65 to 70 days); will reseed readily; also called cornflowers.

Borage: Direct-seed; will happily self-seed after that; bears nodding little blue "shooting star" blossoms; mucilaginous and has a mild cucumber flavor; 18 to 30 inches (46–76 cm) tall.

Cherry tomatoes or cocktail tomatoes, which are larger than cherry, but smaller than a full-sized tomato. These like hot, dry conditions; if diseases trouble your tomato plants, try protecting them from moisture with a small, makeshift "greenhouse" to keep off the rain. Use a whole cluster as a garnish.

Cucumbers: Direct-seed under a trellis or plant underneath sunflowers, using their stalks as a trellis; add in nasturtium, gem marigolds, dill, or carrots at the base of the cucumbers. Cucamelon is a fun miniature variety.

Dahlias: All plant parts are edible, from the tubers to the petals. Will not overwinter in cold-winter areas, so dig tubers each fall to replant the following spring. Dahlias taste savory, kind of like a carrot. Heirloom varieties are good bee forage as well as a lovely and flamboyant addition to cocktails. Use the stems as straws, too!

Husk cherry: Heat-loving annuals that will also reseed the following year; husk-encased fruits with unique flavor. Goldenberry (*Physalis peruviana*) has been widely commercialized; it's native to Central America but can grow in cooler climates.

Lemon verbena: Grows eagerly in full sun; cut back the tops and they will continue bushing out. Excellent, versatile aromatic garnish; perennial in Zones 7 through 10; grow as an annual in cooler areas.

Lovage: Leafy, bushy plant that will grow taller than you! Hardy to Zone 4; looks and tastes very similar to celery; the finishing touch on your next Bloody Mary!

Nasturtium: Full sun to part shade; soak seeds before sowing; nice for hanging baskets; spicy-tasting leaves and flowers.

Sunflowers: Look for open-pollinated varieties, which produce pollen that is wonderful sprinkled on top of cocktails. Sow seeds directly in the garden; they will self-sow.

purveyor's catalog or website. Pay attention to how deep the seeds should be planted, and how close together. You will need to buy seed-starting mix (it is also possible to make your own) and clean seedling trays. Lighting is very important, and natural light through a window is usually not sufficient, not even a sunny window. You'll need to set up some type of grow lights, which should be kept on for fourteen to sixteen hours per day.

Some seedlings will need to be thinned out as they develop. Choose only the strongest little seedlings to continue growing; eat or compost the smaller ones that you thin.

These young plants will need to be *hardened off*, a process of gently introducing them to the rougher conditions of light and temperature outdoors. Over the course of a week or two, place the little plants outside for increasing lengths of time each day in a partially shady spot, gradually working up to a day in full sun. Then they'll be ready for planting in the garden (see Step 7).

Step 5: Garden Design and Layout

How do you decide what to plant where on your garden site? A good way to begin is to make a map of the area on graph paper. Set a scale, such as 4 squares equals 1 foot. Draw the outer boundary of the garden space.

Planting a garden in straight rows in rectangular beds is a good way for a novice to begin, but it's not always the most efficient use of space in small gardens. Start by deciding where the beds and paths will be. A good standard is 18-inch (46 cm) wide pathways with 36-inch (91 cm) wide beds (this width allows you to comfortably reach to the center of the bed to plant, weed, and harvest). Think about other features to include, too, like that water

Right Plant, Right Place

Every plant has a preferred ecology, an optimal balance of sun, shade, and rain as well as soil type. Plants are incredibly resilient and often will grow in suboptimal conditions, but there is a greater chance they will be attacked by pests and disease if they're stressed due to poor growing conditions. For plants that are native to your area, observe where the plant likes to grow naturally. What niche is it living in? Each site has microclimates, and sometimes there can be dramatic variability between the microclimate on the north side of a house and that in a sheltered corner on the south side. Keep this in mind if you are planting perennials or shrubs that you won't be planting in your main garden.

feature for the pollinators, or a petite bistro table. Once you've gained some experience, you may want to try a creative bed design such as a keyhole bed.

With your beds mapped out, refer to the list of what you plan to grow. Check spacing requirements for each type of plant as well as height. Where is the solar orientation? You will want to place taller plants on the north or east edges of the garden and shorter ones on the south and west edges. Using pencil at first, begin filling in where the plants will go.

Step 6: Preparing the Garden Beds

If your garden site is covered by lawn grass, you can either remove the sod (which requires some heavy work with spade and shovel) or smother the grass by covering it with cardboard and building the beds on top. I typically employ a hybridized model. I break up the soil and remove the grass, add amendments including compost, then use a broadfork to work the soil to loosen it up—the broadfork is gentler than tilling. If you walk in the pathways and avoid stepping directly in the garden beds, a no-till approach is very easy once you've done the initial bed preparation. Use a garden rake to smooth out the soil surface.

If you till the entire garden site, you can rake up more soil onto the beds so that the beds are somewhat raised. This is advantageous because the raised beds will warm up a little earlier in spring. Mulch the paths with hardwood chips, straw, or leaves, or else they will end up covering themselves with weedy plants that you may or may not want in your garden.

Step 7: Planting

To decide when to plant, it's helpful to know the date of the average last spring frost in your area. Many seed packets recommend planting a certain number of weeks before or after the date of last spring frost. You can find this information easily online or from your local cooperative extension.

String and stakes can be helpful for creating straight planting rows. To make furrows for seeding, use a trowel or the back side of a garden rake. A ruler or yardstick can help ensure that you sow seeds the proper distance apart, but after some time you'll gain a sense of spacings without using a ruler. A fun trick is to use your body. Extend your hand out fully and measure the distance between the tip of your pinkie and the tip of your thumb. For many people, this is about 6 inches (15 cm). Scatter the seeds at the recommended spacing and cover with soil. Tamp down the soil on top of the seeds using either your hand or the back of a metal rake. Water everything well.

When you are planting transplants, be sure to water them well first. Then gently squeeze the bottom of one of the six-pack cells and tip the pack upside down. The plant should slip out. With the plant in your hand,

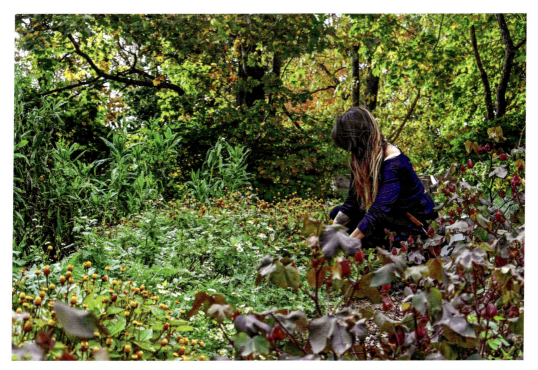

Listen. The land speaks to you. A quiet moment in the garden is a beautiful moment of belonging to a system larger than yourself. (Autumn Gardens at Meeting House Farm.)

tickle the roots and then place the root ball in a small hole dug with the trowel. Cover and press in, ensuring that the base of the plant is even at the level of the ground. If you live in a place that is droughty, you can plant inside a small well.

Step 8: Proactive Pest Prevention

Once your garden is planted and growing, visit it regularly. During those visits, zoom in and look at individual leaves. Is their coloration good, or are they turning yellow or brown? Check for holes or weird patterning. Such patterns or discoloration can indicate fungal or viral diseases. The sooner you spot a problem, the more likely it is that you can take action to help the plant recover.

An important part of a pest protection plan is to plant flowers that attract beneficial insects like ladybugs that eat aphids and mites. Other beneficials include praying mantis, lacewings, ground beetles, predatory wasps, native bees, dragonflies, and damsel bugs, among others! Learn to identify these creatures so you can watch for them on your garden visits.

I have a motto: Anything the bees like, I like. I am a servant to the greater web of Mother Nature. Some of my favorite insectary plants include yarrow,

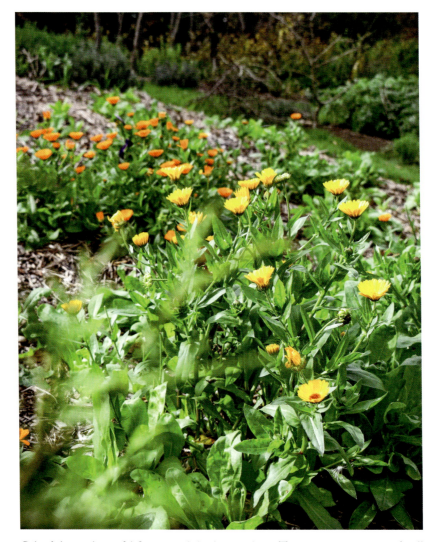

Calendulas are beautiful flowers with healing qualities. They are easy to grow and will attract beneficial insects to your garden, too.

dill, fennel, lemon balm, wild rose, blanketflower, phacelia, bee balm, coriander, and asters. And yes, many of these are plants that you'll want to grow as garnishes—they serve double duty! Maintaining the flowering native plants all around your yard as well as encouraging (and planting more) will attract the good bugs that are already hanging out in your neighborhood.

Step 9: Watering, Mulching, and Weeding

It's helpful to place a rain gauge on a level spot somewhere in your yard, away from trees and roofs, to get an accurate sense of the amount of rainfall in your exact location. Remember that rule of an inch (2.5 cm) of water per week. Newly sprouted seedlings need frequent watering until they establish their roots. New additions to the garden also need extra watering to overcome the shock of transplanting. After they are adjusted, keep an eye on your rain gauge, and be sure you're watering enough to supplement the rain when necessary.

Mulching the garden is a great way to help reduce moisture loss. What is mulch? Typically, it is a drier, carbon-rich material like straw or dried grass clippings. Leaves from hardwood trees like maple work well, too, especially if you can shred them before applying. Applying a layer of mulch on the soil surface around plants prevents soil erosion and keeps moisture in. Avoid mulching very small seedlings or seedbeds until the soil warms up, because mulch also tends to keep soil cool.

Mulching is also part of giving back to the soil, one of the most important tasks for a gardener. Adding finished compost or humus provides organic matter and nutrients that help support the mycological component of soil as well as a range of healthy microorganisms that support soil health and plant growth.

If you are buying compost, keep in mind that not all compost is created equal. Products made with a combination of mineral-rich seaweed, manure, grass clippings, leaves from healthy unsprayed places, and perhaps some stone dust are a good choice.

I consider weeding a meditative task. I imagine that I am symbolically removing the weeds of my mind. However, weeding can seem overwhelming to new gardeners. To avoid turning this simple gardening task into a war, keep the plants around the garden—whether that's grass or some other vegetation—mowed so they don't create seeds that will blow into

Following the Cycles

Every plant has a particular life cycle: annual, biennial, or perennial. Some species are perennials in mild climates but are grown as annuals in cold-winter areas. Some seedlings, such as cilantro and dill, grow quickly and are harvested quickly, so to ensure that you have access to this herb all summer, you will need to seed at intervals. Plant new small patches of seed at least once per month throughout the season. Actually, you do not have to actively remember to do this; all you must do is be present. When the plant finishes its cycle, pull it out and prepare the ground for the next.

the garden beds. Some herbs can grow pretty aggressively and turn into weeds if you allow them to spread or go to seed—they may create an abundance of eager "volunteers" in unwanted places. Volunteers make for great candidates to bring to the next plant swap, though, or to trade with your neighbors. It takes practice to identify very small seedlings as they come up in the garden. Many common garden weeds are edible and nutritious. Working on farms and landscaping crews and learning about the so-called weeds was what first fueled my thirst for knowledge of plants. If you get the knack for identifying plants, you may decide to invite certain "weeds" to stay.

Step 10: Harvesting and Drying

Continual harvest generally encourages the production of more leaves, flowers, beans. The basic rule is to keep it picked. Pinching is different from harvesting: You simply pinch the bud at the tip of the stems of leafy herbs. This encourages the plant to bush out and produce more leaves. When you're harvesting, do not cut at the middle of the stem. Follow the stem to a point where side stems or leaves branch off and clip directly above that point. At the end of the harvest, if there is still some season left, plant or seed another crop in its place, even if it is just a cover crop.

Drying herbs is so easy, everyone should do it. Watch for dry, warm temperatures and time your drying to align. You can make a rudimentary drying rack or buy one, or you can simply unfold a plain paper bag on the kitchen table. Herbs will also dry well and quickly inside paper bags inside a hot car. When I first discovered this, I dried some fresh reishi mushroom in my car, but I do not recommend this because my car smelled like fungus for more than a month afterward!

Aeration is key while herbs are drying: open a window and put on a fan to create a cross breeze. Make sure there are no rodents in the space because their droppings can spoil the outcome (pet hair can, too).

You can dry fruits outside in hot sun by spreading the fruit on a tray and covering it with mesh to keep flies and other bugs away from the fruit. Last resort for drying both herbs and fruit if the weather is not optimal: an electric food dehydrator or an oven at low temperatures.

Aside from drying, I cover many of my favorite preservation techniques—from making infused salts and vinegars to tinctures and oxymels—in chapter 2 and the recipes in chapter 7. So turn the page and start to discover all the wonderful drinks you can make using the harvest from your garnish garden.

The Garnish Garden

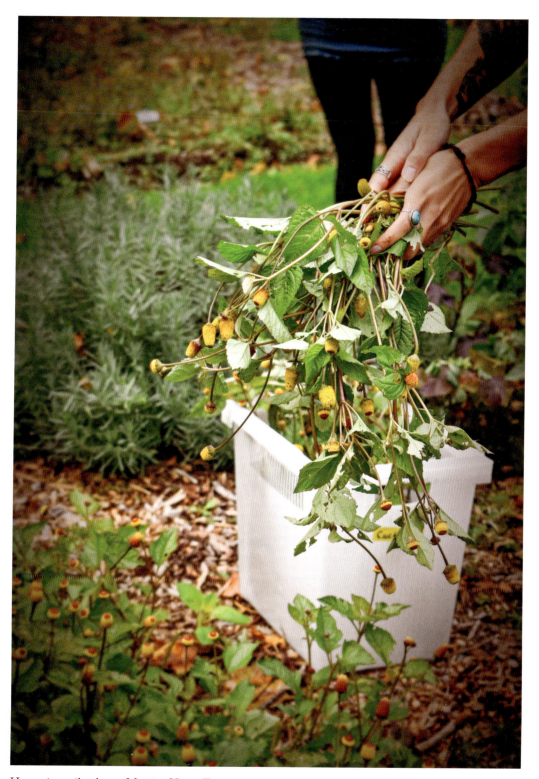

Harvesting spilanthes at Meeting House Farm.

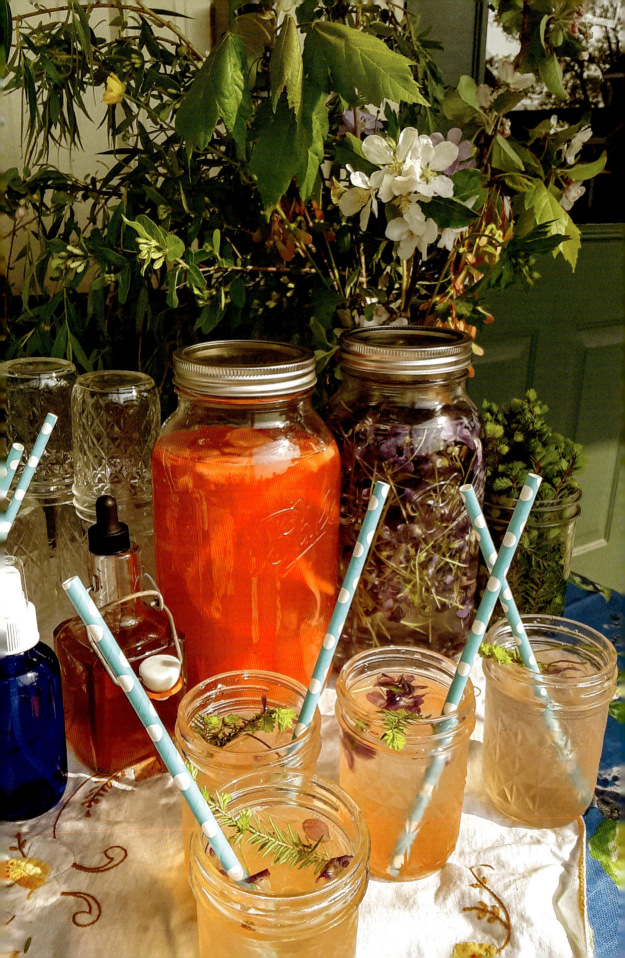

CHAPTER 7

Recipes through the Seasons

My recipes are a form of art inspired by nature. As you look through the pages that follow, you'll notice that the recipe titles center on mystical musings and observations. They are the vivid matter of my dreams and connections made while sitting alongside the brook in the forest near my home. Some of the names are nods to the stories of people and places that inspired the creation of a recipe or the choice of a particular ingredient. Good recipe names are evocative, creating a storyline to tickle the imagination of the imbiber.

I've organized the recipes by season: winter, spring, summer, fall. Within each season, you'll find the nonalcoholic herbal tonics first, followed by the apothecary cocktails that include classic spirits. You'll also find suggestions for making the tonics boozier and for changing the cocktails into no- or low-alcohol tonic elixirs. Essentially, the recipes are reversible, providing the potential for a two-for-one outcome. Some of the nonalcoholic herbal tonics do contain a small amount of alcohol because they include herbal tinctures. If you're abstaining from alcohol for recovery or spiritual reasons, you can simply leave out those tinctures when you make the tonic or substitute a nonalcoholic tincture. There are instances when a nonalcoholic drink contains herbs that are contraindicated in pregnancy. These are noted where applicable. Please be advised to always try a conservative amount of any new herb, because it may result in an individual idiosyncratic allergic reaction.

Some of the preparations may be unfamiliar to you. Refer back to chapter 2 for definitions of extraction methods and instructions for each type of extraction. In some cases you may choose to purchase a tincture rather than making it from scratch. In "Resources" at the end of this book, I provide a list of reputable companies for sourcing raw botanicals as well as tinctures.

Try the recipes as is, or let them be a springboard for your own inspirational flavor pairings. Bend them—they are flexible! Some of the recipes invite you on an adventure to try growing or foraging for herbs and flowers. If that tempts you, revisit chapter 6, "The Garnish Garden," for an introduction to the delightful pastime of planting and harvesting your own cocktail garnishes. The recipes also include some fascinating facts about botanicals, and you can extend that learning by reading the plant monographs in chapter 8.

A list of herbal actions and system effects further illuminates the therapeutic and tonic effects of the botanicals within each recipe. (Revisit chapter 3 to learn more about the meanings of herbal action terms.) It's part of my overall design for this book to help you see the potential of the artful cocktail as an herbal formulation and an invitation to creating functional beverages. Sometimes a new recipe is inspired by the function you wish the drink to serve. Other times a drink comes to life through the energy and flavor of a moment, and its tonic effects are one of the wonderful spontaneous benefits of making and drinking botanical beverages.

Most of these recipes include herbal preparations such as teas, syrups, tinctures, and glycerites that need to be made in advance of mixing the drink or cocktail. For a tea, the brewing and cooling time may only add up to an hour, but tinctures need to be started 2 to 4 weeks in advance to allow for complete extraction of the desired constituents. If a drink recipe catches your eye, be sure to also read the recipes for the related herbal preparations, or you may get caught without an essential ingredient when it's time to shake up and serve.

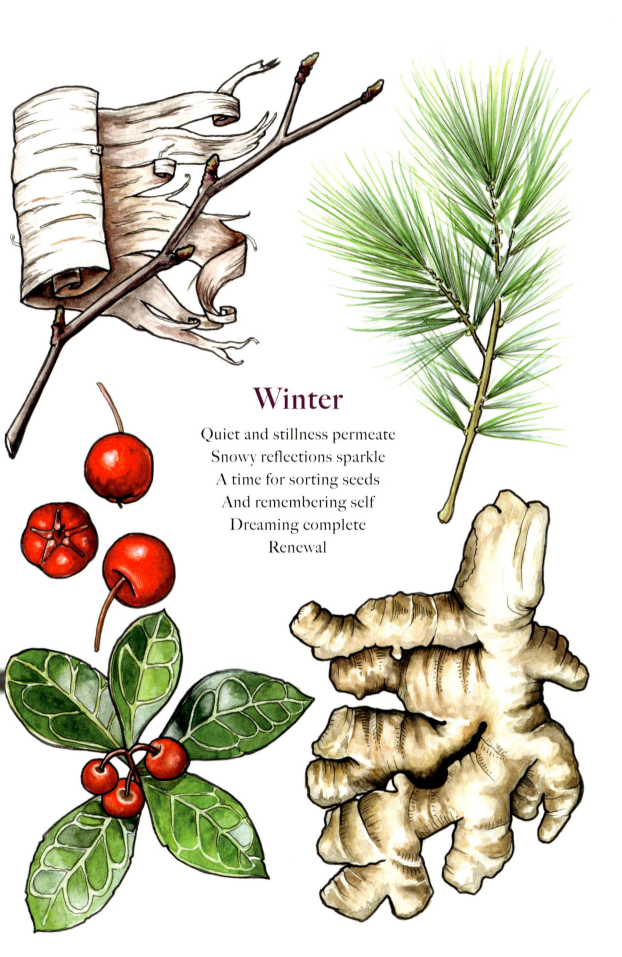

Winter

Quiet and stillness permeate
Snowy reflections sparkle
A time for sorting seeds
And remembering self
Dreaming complete
Renewal

Free the Qi

adaptogen • antidepressant • circulatory stimulant • connective tissue tonic • hepatic • lymphatic • nervine

A mood-boosting tonic that can help free up stagnation in the liver as well as in the circulatory, nervous, and lymph systems to promote the free flow of vital energy (qi) in the body.

Makes 1 drink

1 ounce (30 ml) rosemary hydrosol
3 ounces (90 ml) grapefruit juice
3 ounces (90 ml) fresh blood orange juice
½ ounce (15 ml) ginger juice
1 dropperful Happiness Tonic (made by Anima Mundi Herbals)
1 ounce (30 ml) Calendula and Gotu Kola Honey Tea Syrup (recipe follows)
2 ounces (60 ml) club soda
Lavender hydrosol, for misting
Dried lavender sprigs, for garnish

To build a Free the Qi, fill a glass with ice and add the rosemary hydrosol, grapefruit juice, orange juice, ginger juice, Happiness Tonic, and honey tea syrup. Add the club soda last. Swizzle with a bar spoon. Use an atomizer to mist the lavender hydrosol over the surface of the cocktail and garnish with the lavender.

NOTE

I use rosemary hydrosol from Wild Sings the Bird, but you can make your own. Do not use a commercial lavender hydrosol made for cosmetic use.

Calendula & Gotu Kola Honey Tea Syrup

Makes 1 pint (460 ml)

1 tablespoon dried calendula blossoms
1 tablespoon dried gotu kola (*Centella asiatica*) leaf
12 ounces (360 ml) hot water
12 ounces (360 ml) honey

Add the calendula and gotu kola to the hot water. Steep, covered, for 15 minutes and then strain. Dissolve the honey in the strained tea and allow to cool to room temperature. Store the leftover syrup in an airtight container in the refrigerator and use within 4 weeks.

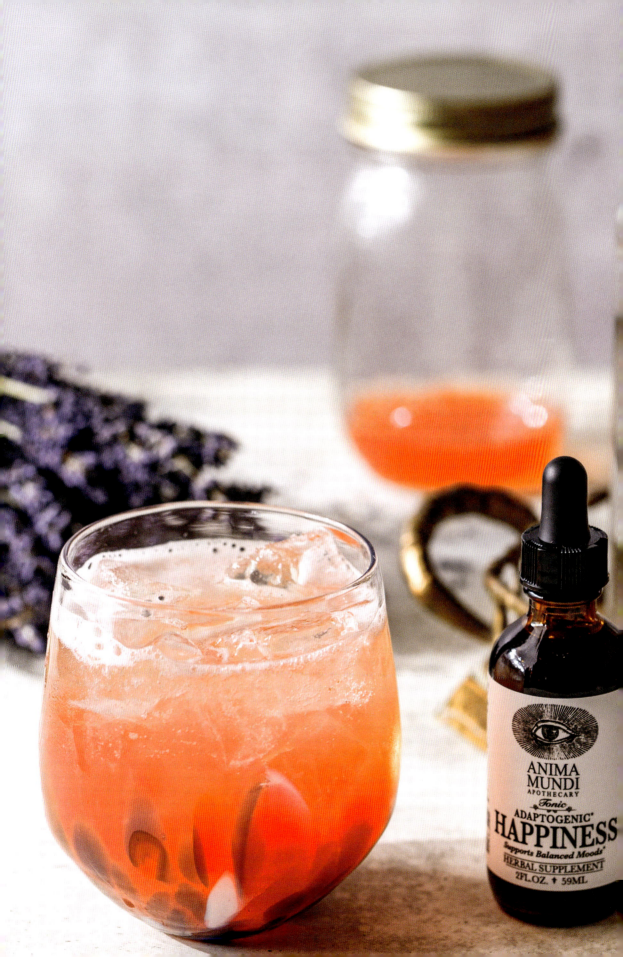

Blueberry Jamboree

antimicrobial • antiviral • cardiovascular tonic • nervine
• nootropic • stimulant • uterine tonic

My impetus for creating this recipe was living in the Northeast, where no local fresh fruit is available in the wintertime, but where I have a pantry stocked with canned jam. This lemony tonic is a simple way to incorporate summer flavors (and antioxidants) into the mix during the cold season. And you can make a delicious jamboree with any kind of fruit jam—try your favorite!

Makes 1 drink

1 ounce (30 ml) strong juniper berry tea or ½ ounce (15 ml) juniper hydrosol
¾ ounce (22.5 ml) lemon juice
¼ cup (77 g) wild blueberry jam
1 dropperful lemon balm tincture
1 egg white
Sparkling apple cider or nonalcoholic champagne (optional)
Loose lavender blossoms, for garnishing

Add the juniper berry tea, lemon juice, wild blueberry jam, lemon balm tincture, and egg white to a cocktail shaker and shake vigorously. Add ice and then shake again. Strain into a coupe glass and top off the glass with the sparkling cider or champagne. Sprinkle with several dried lavender blossoms.

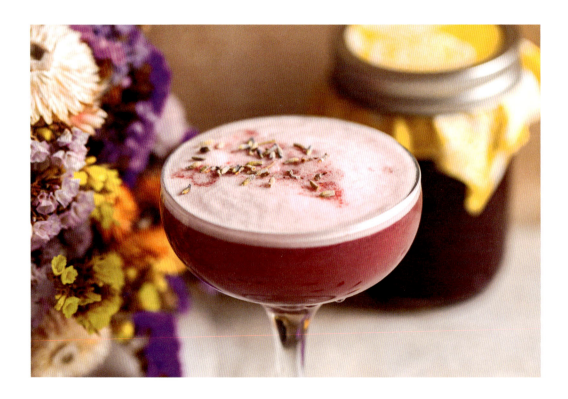

Recipes through the Seasons

Kava Cacao Flip

antidepressant • bitter tonic • carminative • demulcent • immunomodulant
• nervine • neuromuscular relaxant • oneirogen • stimulant

Kava is a neuromuscular relaxant that helps to relieve tension. It is mildly intoxicating and loosens the mind as well as the body. It should not be used excessively or combined with alcohol.

Makes 2 drinks

1 tablespoon marshmallow root powder
8 ounces (240 ml) coconut cream
¼ cup (50 g) chopped cacao paste
2 ounces (60 ml) maple syrup
1 tablespoon kava root powder
1 tablespoon astragalus root powder
1 teaspoon ground cardamom
1 teaspoon ground cinnamon
2 vanilla beans, scraped (see the note)
1 dropperful "Are You a Dreamer?" Bitters (recipe follows)
1 whole egg
Wild rose petals, powdered (see the note)

Let the marshmallow root powder infuse in 8 ounces (240 ml) of cold or room-temperature water in the fridge overnight. This will be added in separately.

In a small saucepan, gently heat the coconut cream with another 8 ounces (240 ml) of water. Dissolve the chopped cacao paste in this warm liquid. Add the maple syrup, and then whisk in the kava root, astragalus root, cardamom, and cinnamon. Remove from the heat. Pour into a jar and add the chilled marshmallow infusion, vanilla seeds, bitters, and whole egg with ice; shake vigorously. Strain into a chalice-style glass and garnish with a sprinkle of the rose powder.

NOTE

The best way to get the good stuff from a vanilla bean is to cut through the pod lengthwise. Then run the blade of a butter knife or metal spoon along the inside of the bean, scraping the aromatic seeds into a container or mixing vessel. The shell can be discarded.

You can purchase powdered rose petals or use a mortar and pestle or electric coffee grinder to grind dried petals.

"Are You a Dreamer?" Bitters

This recipe was inspired by mugwort (*Artemisia vulgaris*), the key aromatic bitter botanical. Mugwort is an oneirogen that inspires vivid dreaming. These bitters are aromatic and floral, excellent in gin cocktails or simply with club soda and a small grapefruit wedge.

Makes 4 ounces (120 ml)

1 tablespoon fresh or dried mugwort
1 teaspoon dried lavender
1 tablespoon dried angelica (*Angelica archangelica*) root
1 tablespoon grapefruit peel, chopped fresh or dry
4 ounces (120 ml) overproof spirit

Add all the ingredients to a 4-ounce Mason jar and cover with an overproof spirit and lid. Let infuse on the counter for 4 weeks prior to straining and bottling.

Hawthorn Honey Syrup

Makes 4 cups (960 ml) syrup

2 tablespoons fresh or dry whole hawthorn (*Crataegus* spp.) berries
2 cups (480 ml) raw unfiltered honey

Simmer the hawthorn berries in 2 cups (480 ml) of water on medium-high heat for 30 minutes, adding up to ½ cup (120 ml) more water if necessary. Use an immersion blender to break up the berries into the water. Strain into a measuring glass and add an equal amount of the honey. Dissolve to complete the syrup. Store in the refrigerate in an airtight container for up to a month.

Pumpkin Seed Milk

Makes 1½ pints (720 ml)

6 tablespoons (66 g) raw organic hull-less pumpkin seeds
2 tablespoons maple syrup
½ teaspoon vanilla extract

Soak the pumpkin seeds in 3 cups (720 ml) of water for 4 hours, then transfer to a blender. Add the maple syrup and vanilla extract and blend on high for 20 seconds. Strain through a fine-mesh strainer. This milk can be stored for 3 to 5 days in the refrigerator.

Vision of Adonis

aphrodisiac • cardiovascular tonic • carminative • circulatory stimulant • demulcent • nervous system trophorestorative • nutritive • superfood • testosterone-boosting • hypoglycemic

Adonis was the epitome of male beauty. The archetypal golden boy of Greek mythology, he was the lover of both Aphrodite (the goddess of love) and Persephone (the goddess of the underworld). He was not a god but rather a mortal who had achieved god-like status. The story of Adonis inspired this aphrodisiac recipe geared toward men.

Makes 2 drinks

12 ounces (360 ml) Pumpkin Seed Milk (page 128)
1 whole egg
1 ounce (30 ml) Hawthorn Honey Syrup (page 128)
1 teaspoon ginger juice or 4 ounces (120 ml) strong ginger decoction
2 dropperfuls nettle root or saw palmetto tincture
2 dropperfuls Milky Oat Tincture (page 203)
1 teaspoon maca root powder
1 teaspoon ground cinnamon
1 teaspoon pine pollen, plus extra for garnish

Put all the ingredients in a blender and pulse on high for about 20 seconds. Fill a rocks glass with ice and pour in the contents of the blender. Garnish by sprinkling the surface with a little more pine pollen.

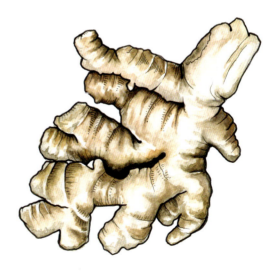

Secret Grove

adaptogen • antioxidant • aperitif • aromatic • carminative
• circulatory stimulant • immune tonic

This festive winter-holiday cocktail is nonalcoholic but surely not missing anything. Dark fruit and spice mingle with the winter woods aromatics. This is a perfect gently stimulating aperitif to sip while sitting around the fireplace with friends and family before an abundant meal.

Makes 1 drink

½ ounce (15 ml) balsam fir and pine hydrosol or 1 ounce (30 ml) strong evergreen tea
2 ounces (60 ml) pomegranate juice
1 dropperful Tulsi Glycerite (page 196)
½ ounce (15 ml) Ginger-Clove Syrup (recipe follows)
Club soda
1 sprig pine or rosemary
Pomegranate arils (seeds)

Build the drink in a collins glass filled with ice, starting with the hydrosol, pomegranate juice, Tulsi Glycerite and Ginger-Clove Syrup. Stir well. Top with the club soda to fill the glass and garnish with a pine or rosemary sprig and a small handful of pomegranate arils.

NOTE
For the hydrosol, I use a Winter Woods blend by Wild Sings the Bird.

Ginger-Clove Syrup

Makes 1 cup (240 ml)

2 tablespoons chopped fresh ginger
1 teaspoon whole cloves
1 cup (200 g) organic sugar

Bring 16 ounces (240 ml) of water to a boil and add the ginger and cloves. Simmer on medium-high for 20 minutes. Strain into a measuring glass. Dissolve an equal volume of sugar into the hot liquid to complete the syrup. Store the syrup in an airtight container in the refrigerator for up to 4 weeks.

Recipes through the Seasons

Opening Doors

antimicrobial • carminative • intuition enhancing • nervine • nootropic • oneirogen • psychotropic

Born from a desire for a nonalcoholic drink that carries the weight and mouthfeel of a "real" drink, this potion looks and sips like a glass of red wine and is formulated with astringent tannins, baking spice, and psychotropic (mind-altering) botanicals that provide a boost to intuition. It's great to have on hand to serve like wine, with dinner.

Makes ½ gallon (1.9 liters)

- 1 tablespoon dried blue lotus (*Nymphaea caerulea*) flowers
- 1 tablespoon dried mugwort (*Artemisia vulgaris*)
- 5 grape leaves, cut up (see the note)
- 1 tablespoon red raspberry leaf
- 1 tablespoon whole allspice
- 1 cinnamon quill, about 5 inches (13 cm) long, broken into small pieces
- 1 teaspoon whole cloves
- 1 teaspoon juniper (*Juniperus communis*) berries
- 1 teaspoon dried lavender flowers
- 1 quart (960 ml) Concord grape juice

Place the lotus flowers, mugwort, grape leaf pieces, raspberry leaf, allspice, cinnamon pieces, cloves, juniper berries, and lavender flowers in a ½-gallon glass vessel or jar. Add boiling water to cover, stir several times, and then cover the vessel with a lid to steep. Strain the tea after 30 minutes to 1 hour. Add the grape juice to the strained tea. Serve in a wineglass, ungarnished. This drink mixture can be stored in the refrigerator for up to 10 days.

NOTE
When I first created this recipe, it was late fall and I used fresh grape leaves, but dried leaves may be used.

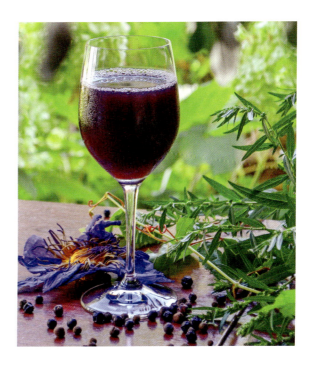

Sexy Hot Chocolate

aphrodisiac • carminative • circulatory stimulant • nervine

Invite heart opening and a sense of connection with this spicy, sultry blood-moving cacao drink. This is the quintessential aphrodisiac.

Makes 2 servings

1 tablespoon damiana leaf
8 ounces (240 ml) coconut cream or raw dairy cream
½ cup (100 g) raw cacao paste, grated or chopped
1 teaspoon ground cinnamon
1 teaspoon gingerroot powder
1 teaspoon cayenne pepper
¼ teaspoon sea salt
1 vanilla bean, scraped (see the note on page 127)
2 dropperfuls Wild Rose Elixir (page 139)
Honey, to taste
Cinnamon Marshmallows (recipe follows), for garnishing

Prepare damiana tea by pouring 8 ounces (240 ml) of boiling water over the damiana leaf. Cover and steep for 15 minutes, and then strain. While the tea steeps, heat the coconut cream over medium heat and add the cacao paste. Stir until melted. Reduce the heat to low. Stir in the strained tea and the cinnamon, ginger, cayenne, sea salt, vanilla, and Wild Rose Elixir. Add honey to taste immediately prior to serving, but do not cook. I love to transfer the hot chocolate to a high-speed blender to blend in the honey because it makes the drink delectably foamy. Garnish with the homemade Cinnamon Marshmallows. If you are spiking this cocoa, Mezcal is the best choice!

NOTE
If you don't have the time or wish to make your own marshmallows, they are available from specialty producers such as Vermont Marshmallow Company.

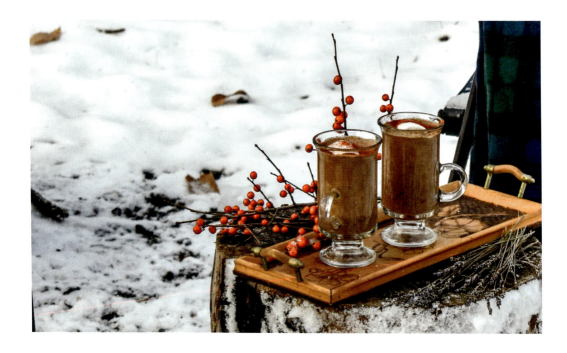

Cinnamon Marshmallows

Makes 30 marshmallows

3 packets unflavored gelatin (7 teaspoons)
2 cups (400 g) granulated sugar
¼ teaspoon salt
⅔ cup (160 ml) light corn syrup (preferably non-GMO)
1½ tablespoons vanilla extract
Confectioners' sugar
Ground cinnamon

Line a 9 x 9 x 2 inch (23 x 23 x 5 cm) or 8 x 8 x 2 inch (20 x 20 x 5 cm) pan with parchment paper and lightly oil it using your fingers, or spray with nonstick cooking spray. Set aside.

In a heatproof, medium-sized mixing bowl, sprinkle the gelatin over ½ cup (120 ml) of cold water and leave it to soak for about 10 minutes.

In a small saucepan, combine the sugar, salt, corn syrup, and ¼ cup (60 ml) water; whisk until the sugar is dissolved. Bring to a rapid boil. As soon as it is boiling, set a timer and allow it to boil hard for 1 minute without stirring. If you have a candy thermometer, check the temperature; it should reach 242 to 245°F (117–118°C) (firm ball stage). Pour the boiling syrup into the soaked gelatin and mix vigorously (an electric mixer is helpful) for 10 to 12 minutes, or until the marshmallow is fluffy and cooled close to room temperature. Add the vanilla extract toward the end of beating. Use a greased rubber spatula to transfer and press the fluffy marshmallow into the greased pan. Press another piece of greased parchment paper lightly on top of the marshmallow, creating a seal. Let set overnight.

Combine confectioners' sugar and cinnamon in a 1:1 ratio. Sprinkle a cutting surface very generously with the mixture. Remove the marshmallow from the pan and lay it on top of the cinnamon sugar. Dust the top surface of the marshmallow generously as well. Use a large, sharp knife to cut into squares. Separate the pieces and toss with the cinnamon sugar. Store leftover marshmallows in an airtight container in a cool, dark place and use within 2 to 4 weeks.

Golden Touch

Golden milk has roots in India as *haldi doodh*, which is warmed cow's milk, ground turmeric, and crushed pepper. The pepper tickles the lining of the GI tract, enhancing the absorption of the active compounds in turmeric. Golden Touch is my rum-spiked take on golden milk, and it is delicious warm or at room temperature. Served in cordial glasses, this warm and cozy recipe is a scrumptious offering at winter-holiday parties. The fat from the cream is deeply satiating. The spices are carminative (enhancing digestion), blood moving, and anti-inflammatory.

Makes approximately 1 quart (960 ml)

¼ cup (35 g) minced turmeric root
2 tablespoons minced fresh gingerroot
1 cup (240 ml) organic raw cream
1 teaspoon powdered turmeric
    (for color)
1 tablespoon ground cinnamon
1 vanilla bean, scraped
    (see the note on page 127)
1 teaspoon cracked black pepper
1 teaspoon ground cloves
1 teaspoon ground cardamom
8 medjool dates, pitted and chopped,
    or ¼ cup (50 g) jaggery
Medium-bodied rum (optional):
    1 ounce (30 ml) per 8 ounces (240 ml)
    Golden Touch
1 whole nutmeg, for garnishing

Bring 1½ quarts (1.4 liters) of water to a boil in a large pot. Add the turmeric and ginger and reduce the heat to medium-high. Simmer for 30 to 45 minutes and then strain. Let cool to lukewarm. Add the decoction to a high-powered blender with the cream, turmeric, cinnamon, vanilla seeds, black pepper, cloves, cardamom, and dates. Blend on high until you can no longer see the date pieces in the mixture. Decant into small glass jars for holiday gifting. If you want to spike the golden milk with rum, be sure to leave enough space in each jar.

Serve in small cordial glasses. Use a rasp grater to grate nutmeg on top of each cordial as a garnish.

NOTE

You can substitute nondairy cream for the dairy cream if desired. If so, also add 2 tablespoons of fat such as coconut oil during the blending process. When I spike this drink, I like to use Bully Boy Rum Cooperative Volume 2.

Recipes through the Seasons

Tonic & Tonic

antimalarial • antimicrobial • antioxidant • antiviral
• immune tonic • nootropic • urinary tonic

This nonalcoholic tonic sips like a classic Gin and Tonic. The recipe is for my winter version 1.0, but this drink can be adapted for any season of the year by using different aromatic hydrosols, juices, and garnishes.

Makes 1 drink

- ¼ ounce (7.5 ml) juniper berry hydrosol or ½ ounce (15 ml) strong juniper tea
- 2 ounces (60 ml) 100 percent unsweetened cranberry juice (see the note)
- 1 dropperful cinchona bark tincture
- 2 teaspoons elderberry syrup
- Club soda
- Skewered cranberries, juniper berries, and edible flowers, for garnishing

Build the drink in a collins glass filled with ice: the juniper berry hydrosol, cranberry juice, cinchona bark tincture, and elderberry syrup. Stir well. Top with club soda and skewered cranberries. Float several juniper berries in the glass. Adding edible flowers is optional, but fun!

NOTE
Often products labeled as cranberry juice aren't real cranberry juice! They're blends of cranberry with other juices or overly sweetened with toxic, unnatural ingredients such as high-fructose corn syrup.

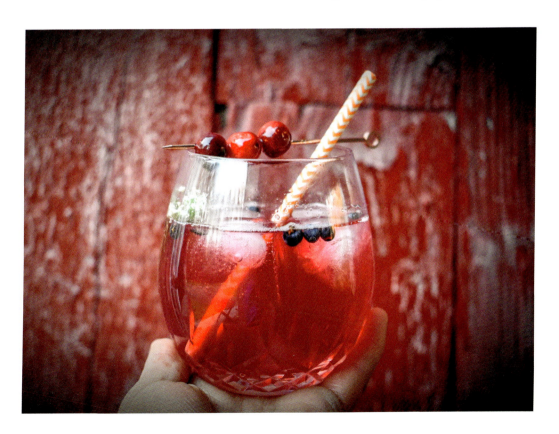

Quantum Entanglement

Quantum entanglement is a concept that describes the phenomenon of two particles affecting each other, even when they are separated by great distances. Subatomically romantic. This cocktail was inspired by the sensuous mouthfeel of a classic Pisco Sour. I enhanced the fruity notes (as well as color) by choosing red açai and raspberry fruits, which are also aphrodisiacs. The trophorestorative Milky Oat Tincture is my encouragement to "seed your wild oats." Maca is deeply nourishing to the endocrine system and production of sex hormones.

Makes 1 drink

- ¼ cup (40 g) chopped dark chocolate or chocolate chips
- 2 ounces (60 ml) Infused Pisco (recipe follows)
- 1½ ounces (45 ml) Maca Chai Syrup (recipe follows)
- ¾ ounce (22.5 ml) lemon juice
- 1 teaspoon ginger juice
- 1 egg white
- 1 dropperful Milky Oat Tincture (page 203)
- Raspberry on a skewer (optional)

To rim a small cocktail glass with chocolate, heat chopped dark chocolate in a double boiler, stirring continuously. To avoid overheating the chocolate, remove it from the pot as soon as it has melted. Allow it to cool for 30 seconds. Upend the glass and dip it into the warm, melted chocolate. Set the glass upright and set aside. Add the pisco, Maca Chai Syrup, lemon juice, ginger juice, egg white, and Milky Oat Tincture to a cocktail shaker and shake vigorously. Add ice and shake again. Double-strain into the chocolate-rimmed cocktail glass. Garnish with fresh raspberries on a skewer if desired (or you can use frozen, freeze-dried, or powdered raspberries—whatever you have available).

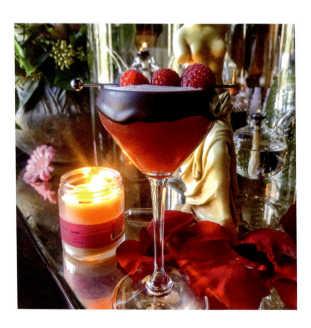

Infused Pisco

Pisco, a fruity and floral spirit, is technically a brandy made in Peru and Chile from distilled grape juice. Seven hundred fifty milliliters is the size of a standard bottle of liquor in the United States.

Makes 750 ml

1 cup (165 g) fresh mixed açai berries and red raspberries
750 ml pisco

Place the berries in a large jar with a lid. Pour the pisco over the berries, ensuring that the liquid completely covers them. Save the empty liquor bottle for storing the strained liquid after infusing. Place the lid on the jar and shake up the contents. Infuse for 3 to 6 days before straining.

NOTE
You can also use frozen berries, but thaw them before adding the pisco.

Maca Chai Syrup

Makes 8 ounces (240 ml)

1 teaspoon chopped gingerroot
1 teaspoon whole cloves
1 teaspoon cardamom pods
1 teaspoon cinnamon chips
1 teaspoon vanilla extract
2 teaspoons maca root powder
1 cup (200 g) organic raw cane sugar

Place the gingerroot, cloves, cardamom, and cinnamon chips in a saucepan with 10 to 12 ounces (300–360 ml) of water and bring to a boil. Reduce the heat to medium-high and simmer for about 30 minutes, adding slightly more water if necessary as it boils off. When finished, the liquid will be reduced to about 1 cup (240 ml). Strain the liquid into a Mason jar. Add the vanilla extract, maca root powder, and sugar. Dissolve. Bottle and store any leftovers in the refrigerator; the syrup will keep there for up to 4 weeks. Double or triple the recipe if you intend on making more than five drinks.

The Gypsy & the Monk

This drink is inspired by the different types of wisdom gleaned from nature and direct experience, sometimes quite mystical.

Makes 1 cocktail

2 ounces (60 ml) potato vodka
¾ ounce (22.5 ml) unsweetened cranberry juice, preferably not from concentrate
¾ ounce (22.5 ml) Cranberry, Rose Hip, and Ginger Syrup (recipe follows)
½ ounce (15 ml) Bénédictine
1 dropperful Rosemary Bitters (recipe follows)
1 dropperful Wild Rose Elixir (recipe follows)

FOR GARNISHING

1 sprig rosemary
1 cranberry, soaked in Bénédictine (optional)
Dry curaçao

Shake all the ingredients with ice, strain, and serve up in a coupe or Martini glass. Garnish with the rosemary sprig and the cranberry, and use an atomizer to mist the surface with dry curaçao.

NOTES

I use Maine Cold River potato vodka.

Dry curaçao is a liqueur flavored with aromatic bitter orange.

You can buy rosemary bitters and wild rose elixir or make your own, following the instructions on the next page.

Cranberry, Rose Hip & Ginger Syrup

Makes 1 pint (480 ml)

1 tablespoon cut ginger slices
1 tablespoon whole cranberries
2 tablespoons dried rose hips
2 cups (400 g) organic cane sugar

Add the ginger slices and whole cranberries to 16 ounces (480 ml) of water in a small pot. Bring to a boil and simmer on high for 20 minutes. Add another 8 ounces (240 ml) of water as it boils off, then blend with an immersion blender. Add the dried rose hips and let steep for 15 minutes. Strain into a measuring glass and then add the organic cane sugar; stir until the sugar dissolves. Store the syrup in an airtight bottle or jar in the refrigerator, and use within 1 month.

Rosemary Bitters

A small glass jar is a suitable container for making bitters. I suggest a ¼-pint-sized Mason jar, which is 4 ounces (120 ml).

Makes about 4 ounces (120 ml)

6 tablespoons chopped fresh rosemary
4 ounces (120 ml) overproof spirit

Fill the jar with the rosemary, up to the first ridge. Cover with the overproof. Make sure the spirit completely covers the herbs. Cover the jar and label it. Shake the jar daily for 2 weeks. Strain into a glass tincture bottle.

Wild Rose Elixir

Harvest fresh rose petals on a bright summer day. I collect petals of *Rosa rugosa*, which grows along the coast of Maine. You can collect petals from any wild rose species or from garden roses (not sprayed with pesticides!). Note, though, that many hybrid garden roses do not have the characteristic rose aroma.

Makes 1 pint (480 ml)

Fresh rose petals, chopped
Food-grade vegetable glycerin

Fill a glass pint jar about three-quarters of the way full with fresh, chopped rose petals. Cover with food-grade vegetable glycerin. Let extract for 4 to 8 weeks prior to straining. Strain into another glass jar or bottle and store in an airtight container in a cool, dark place. Label appropriately. Will keep for 1 to 2 years.

Winter Amaro

I make Winter Amaro with Maine botanicals. I forage for them in late fall and early winter, before the snow covers the ground. It is quite beautiful to find all this local flavor in the forest after the leaves have dropped, but you have to know where to look in the seemingly barren landscape.

Wintergreen (*Gaultheria procumbens*) leaves and "tea" berries
Sweetfern (*Comptonia peregrina*)
Juniper (*Juniperus communis*)
Birch bark (*Betula* spp.), shaved from twigs
White pine (*Pinus strobus*)
Turkey tail mushroom (*Coriolus versicolor*)
Wild rose (*Rosa virginiana*) hips
Wild sarsaparilla (*Aralia nudicaulis* or *A. hispida*)
Overproof spirit
Raw local honey

Gather your botanicals. Have an experienced forager or botanist help if you are unfamiliar with how to identify plants. The aromatic winter botanicals in your area may be different species and types of plants than those I collect in Maine.

Put the botanicals you have gathered in a large jar, about an equal amount of each species. Pack the jar full and cover the plant material with the overproof spirit. I chose rum, because although it's not local here, it maintains its aroma even at a high proof, which I feel contributes to the finished product. If you have a local distiller that makes a high-quality overproof, I suggest you use that.

Leave the plants to steep for at least 6 weeks and then strain into a measuring glass. Add about 1 cup (240 ml) of honey for every 2 cups (480 ml) of strained, infused spirit. Shake to dissolve. Drink as is, adding small amounts of water for palatability.

NOTE
For the overproof, I use Wray and Nephew white overproof rum.

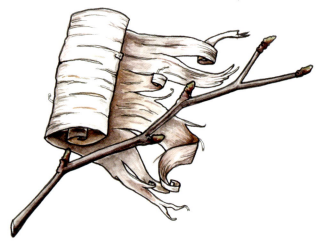

Tuscan Garden

I created this cocktail as I was anticipating my first trip to Italy. The taste reminds me of the experience of meandering through a Mediterranean garden.

Makes 1 drink

1 sprig rosemary
2 ounces Barr Hill Vodka
1 ounce (30 ml) honey syrup (see the note)
¾ ounce (22.5 ml) Meyer lemon juice
¼ ounce (7.5 ml) yuzu juice
3 basil leaves, torn

FOR GARNISHING

Freshly cracked pepper
9 drops Rosemary Infused Olive Oil (recipe follows)
1 pink peppercorn

Torch the rosemary sprig and place the smoldering sprig inside a cocktail glass, then cover. Set aside. Combine the vodka, syrup, lemon juice, yuzu juice, and basil in a cocktail shaker. Add ice and shake vigorously. Strain the liquid into the smoky glass. Add 3 grinds of black pepper, the drops of oil, and a pink peppercorn for garnish. Enjoy!

NOTE

To make honey syrup, dissolve unfiltered local honey in hot water at a 1:1 ratio.

Rosemary Infused Olive Oil

The basic ratio for making this oil is 1 ounce (30 ml) oil for each sprig of rosemary.

Makes 4 ounces (120 ml)

4 ounces (120 ml) high-quality cold-pressed olive oil
3 or 4 sprigs fresh rosemary leaves, chopped

Place the oil and chopped rosemary in the top portion of a double boiler. Bring the water in the lower pot to a boil, then reduce the heat. Put the top portion in place on the pot, cover, and leave on low heat for about an hour. Another option is a low-and-slow method: Put the oil and leaves in a glass jar and cover it tightly with a lid. Place the jar in a slow cooker filled with water. Turn the cooker on low and allow the jar to heat for several hours.

When heating is complete, strain the oil. Funnel into a tincture dropper bottle for easy use. Store in a cool, dark place and use within 1 month.

Botanical Bar Craft

Savant or Savage?

Sometimes we exist on fine lines. Try this foraged-in-Maine Manhattan to channel your inner wild and wise.

Makes 1 cocktail

- 2 ounces (60 ml) bourbon
- ¾ ounce (22.5 ml) DIY Wild Transforming Vermouth (recipe follows)
- ¼ ounce (7.5 ml) Winter Amaro (page 140)
- ¼ teaspoon ginger juice
- 2 ml Chocolate Sweetfern Bitters (recipe follows) or other chocolate bitters
- Preserved cherry, chocolate-dipped cherry, or any canned fruit, for garnishing

Add the bourbon, Wild Transforming Vermouth, Winter Amaro, ginger juice, and bitters to a mixing glass. Add ice. Stir for approximately 40 rotations, more or less depending on the room temperature. Strain into a small cocktail glass. Garnish with a piece of canned fruit or the traditional good cherry.

NOTE
I use Angel's Envy bourbon for this drink, but you can use the bourbon of your choice.

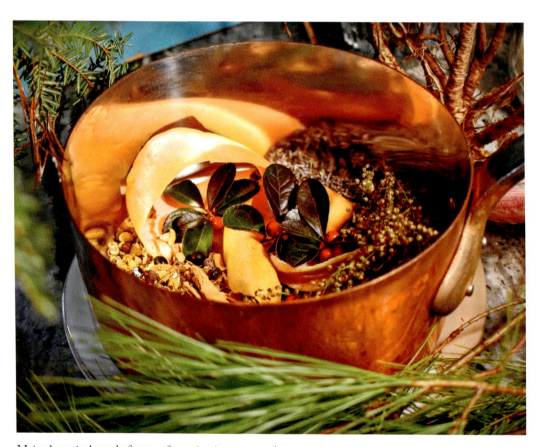

Maine botanicals ready for transformation into vermouth.

DIY Wild Transforming Vermouth

This vermouth is a great capture of a particular transforming microseason.

Makes 1 quart (960 ml)

Several handfuls fresh aromatic plant material
1 bottle dry red wine
Organic cane sugar (optional)
Maple syrup (optional)

Gather some common wild aromatics native to your local terroir. Have an experienced forager or botanist help if you are unfamiliar with how to identify plants. I used a handful each of: wild blueberries, black cherry (*Prunus serotina*) leaves and bark, white pine (*Pinus strobus*) needles, mugwort (*Artemisia vulgaris*) leaves, birch twigs, sweetfern (*Comptonia peregrina*) leaves/buds, and mountain mint (*Pycnanthemum* spp.) leaves. Place in a medium pot and cover with 1 bottle (750 ml) dry red wine. Gently heat with a cover on for 10 minutes. Turn off the heat and steep another 10 minutes. Strain and sweeten. I chose to sweeten with 1 cup (200 g) organic cane sugar and 1 cup (240 ml) maple syrup (because maple is a taste of my landscape). Transfer the finished vermouth into the wine bottle.

Chocolate Sweetfern Bitters

Makes 4 ounces (120 ml)

Chopped sweetfern (*Comptonia peregrina*) leaves/buds
Cacao beans
Overproof spirit

Fill a 4-ounce (120 ml) jar three-quarters of the way full with chopped sweetfern and cacao beans. Cover with overproof spirit. Let set for 4 to 6 weeks. Strain and bottle into a tincture or bitters dasher bottle.

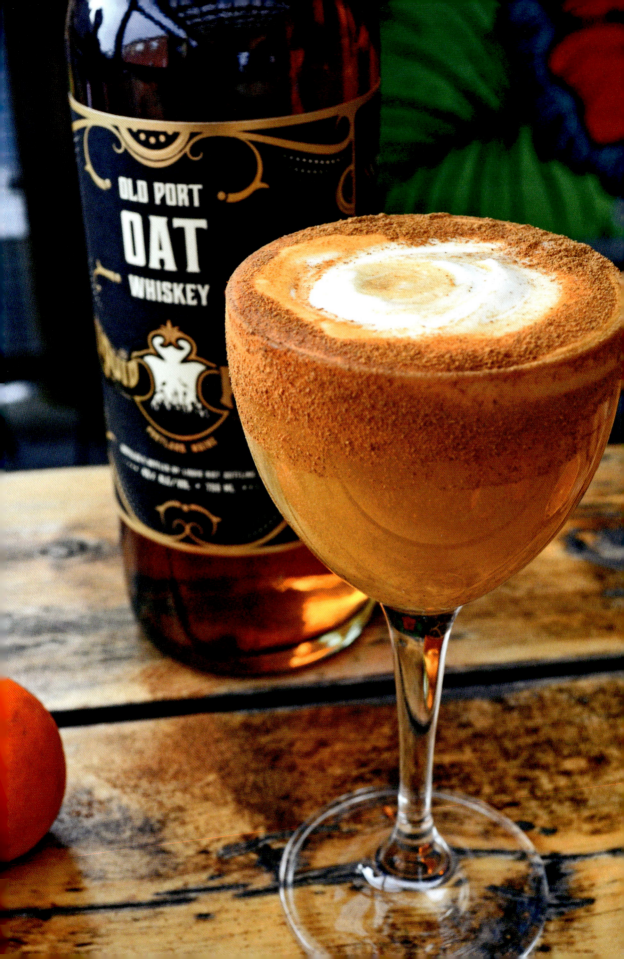

Recipes through the Seasons

Cinnamon Girl

This is a Whiskey Sour bolstered by warming winter spice and foraged botanicals. It is at once cozy and refreshing.

Makes 1 cocktail

1 tablespoon ground cinnamon, for the rim
1½ ounces (45 ml) Liquid Riot Old Port Oat Whiskey
1 ounce (30 ml) Birch Bark Syrup (recipe follows)
¾ ounce (22.5 ml) lemon juice
1 ounce (30 ml) mandarin juice
1 egg
Several dashes Chocolate Sweetfern Bitters (page 143)

Rim a coupe glass with cinnamon: Hold the glass upside down and dip it in water first, then cinnamon. Dry-shake the whiskey, Birch Bark Syrup, lemon juice, Mandarin juice, egg, and bitters in a cocktail shaker. Shake vigorously first without ice, then with. Double-strain into the rimmed coupe glass.

Birch Bark Syrup

Makes 8 ounces (240 ml)

¼ cup (8 g) shaved birch bark (see the note)
2 slices fresh ginger, ¼ inch (6 mm) thick
1 cinnamon stick
1 small birch polypore (*Piptoporus betulinus*)
Peel from 1 organic orange
Maple syrup

Bring 12 ounces (360 ml) of water to a boil in a small pot. Add the birch bark, ginger, cinnamon stick, polypore, and orange peel; cook on medium-high for about 30 minutes, covered. Strain the decoction into a measuring glass and add an equal part maple syrup.

NOTE
You can cut bark from any species of birch. Use sharp pruners to remove twigs or branches, cutting on a diagonal at a node. Use a regular kitchen knife to shave off the bark (or a draw knife for large branches).

Botanical Bar Craft

Wisdom of Old

A medicinal Old Fashioned, this cocktail also works very well as an egg white sour with the addition of lemon juice, whiskey, and syrup in a 2:1:1 ratio. I like to garnish this drink with Maine's state tree, the white pine (*Pinus strobus*), but you can use a pine from your local area.

Makes 1 cocktail

Absinthe, for rinsing
2 ounces (60 ml) tulsi, birch, and hyssop infused bourbon
¾ ounce (22.5 ml) Chai-Spiced Elderberry Syrup (recipe follows)
3 ml Chai-Spice Bitters (recipe follows)
Pine sprig, for garnishing

Rinse a rocks glass with the absinthe. Put the infused bourbon, elderberry syrup, and bitters in a mixing glass and stir. Strain over a large ice cube in the rinsed glass. Garnish with the pine sprig.

NOTE
This recipe features an infused bourbon made by Wiggly Bridge Distillery because I created this recipe to enter in a cocktail contest hosted by Wiggly Bridge.

Chai-Spiced Elderberry Syrup

Makes 1 quart (960 ml)

1 pound (450 g) fresh elderberries or 3 cups (225 g) dried
Several sticks astragalus root
Several turkey tail mushrooms (*Coriolus versicolor*)
1 Ceylon cinnamon stick
¼ cup (35 g) chopped fresh ginger
About 4 cups (960 ml) raw unfiltered honey

Bring 2 quarts (1.9 liters) of water to a roaring boil. Add the elderberries, astragalus, mushrooms, cinnamon stick, and ginger. Simmer on medium-high for 25 minutes. While it's still warm, strain the liquid into a measuring glass, then let it cool. Mix with an equal volume of honey. If you plan to keep this syrup for the duration of winter in the refrigerator, I recommend adding several tablespoons freshly squeezed lemon juice per cup of syrup to extend the shelf life.

Chai-Spice Bitters

Makes 4 ounces (120 ml)

2 tablespoons cinnamon chips
1 tablespoon chopped fresh ginger
1 tablespoon cardamom pods
½ teaspoon whole cloves
½ teaspoon black peppercorns
4 ounces (120 ml) overproof spirits

Place the cinnamon chips, ginger, cardamom pods, cloves, and peppercorns in a 4-ounce (120 ml) Mason jar and cover with overproof spirits. Strain after 2 to 4 weeks. Store tightly covered.

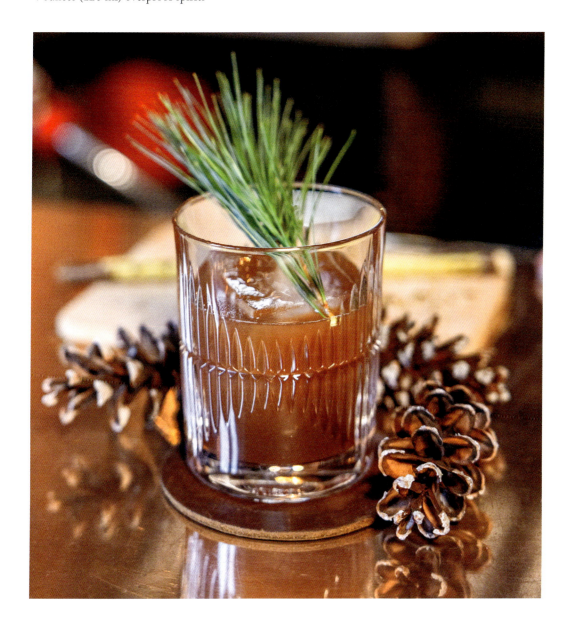

Bitter Orange Cordial

A naturally colored orange aperitivo made with golden beets, aromatic organic orange peels, and bitter tonic botanicals. This recipe can be drunk as is or used as an ingredient in a cocktail.

Makes about 1 quart (960 ml)

½ cup (50 g) chopped fresh orange peel
¼ cup (45 g) chopped kumquats
1 teaspoon gentian root
1 teaspoon cinchona bark
1 teaspoon coriander seeds
16 ounces 100-proof vodka
½ cup (70 g) chopped golden beets
2 cups (400 g) organic sugar

Place the orange peel, kumquats, gentian root, cinchona bark, and coriander in a glass jar. Pour in the vodka and cover the jar tightly with a lid. Leave to macerate for 1 to 2 weeks, shaking occasionally.

When the macerating period is over, strain the vodka into another glass jar and set aside. Prepare a syrup by placing the beets in 12 ounces (360 ml) of water in a small pot and bringing them to a boil. Boil for 10 minutes. Strain the liquid into a glass jar and add the sugar to dissolve. Allow to cool.

Combine the infused vodka and the beet syrup. Store the finished cordial in the refrigerator and use within 6 months.

Doctor's Orders

This drink is delicious and medicinal even without the whiskey. Hyssop is an underrated botanical, perfect for a Hot Toddy!

Makes 1 serving

1 ounce (30 ml) Hyssop and Teaberry Infused Rye Whiskey (recipe follows)
Juice of ½ lemon
1 ounce (30 ml) elderberry syrup
1 dropperful echinacea tincture
2 slices fresh ginger
1 whole licorice root
1 sprig fresh hyssop (*Hyssopus officinalis*) or thyme, for garnishing

Build in a footed glass mug: Add 8 to 10 ounces (240–300 ml) of hot water to the rye whiskey, lemon juice, elderberry syrup, echinacea tincture, and ginger. Use the licorice root to stir gently. The licorice will infuse into the toddy as you stir. Garnish with the fresh herb sprig.

NOTES

You can double or triple this recipe, but do not exceed using one licorice root.

You may use any type of elderberry syrup for this recipe. Store-bought works fine, or you can incorporate my Chai-Spiced Elderberry Syrup recipe (page 146).

Hyssop & Teaberry Infused Rye Whiskey

Makes about 1 quart (960 ml)

Fresh hyssop (*Hyssopus officinalis*) sprigs
20 to 40 teaberries (*Gaultheria procumbens*)
Rye whiskey

When I created this drink, I used a locally produced rye whiskey. Harvest a large handful of fresh hyssop sprigs and collect from 20 to 40 teaberries—the berries are present on the plants at most times of year. (Ask a mentor for help if you're not experienced at identifying teaberry plants.) Crush the berries and place in a quart-sized glass jar with the hyssop sprigs. Pour whiskey over the herbs, ensuring that the liquid covers the plant material completely. Allow to infuse for 3 to 7 days prior to straining and using.

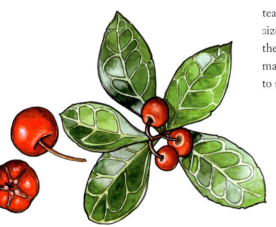

Boles's Dirty Gardener Martini

The friend for whom I created this drink hates weeding but loves pickles! This concept is simple: If you are a Dirty Martini drinker, use your own canned goodies for garnish and the brine for dirtying your spirit of choice. You can use all kinds of colorful pickles that you or your local farmer friends made from last year's bounty.

Makes 1 Martini

- 2 ounces (60 ml) gin
- 1 ounce (30 ml) DIY Dry Vermouth (recipe follows)
- ¼ ounce (7.5 ml) pickle or sauerkraut brine
- Various type of pickles

Fill a Martini glass with ice and cold water to chill. Set aside. Add the gin, DIY Dry Vermouth, and pickle brine into a mixing glass with ice and stir until cold, approximately 30 seconds. Strain into the chilled glass and garnish with all the local pickles.

DIY Dry Vermouth

You can use dry or fresh herbs to make this vermouth. The aromatics are more concentrated when the herbs have been dried properly. Herbs purchased from a mainstream supplier may not have much aromatic punch. The quantities listed below are for dried botanicals. If you're using fresh, double the quantity used.

Makes about 1 quart (960 ml)

- 1 standard bottle (750 ml) dry white wine
- 4 tablespoons coriander seeds
- 2 tablespoons chamomile flowers
- 2 tablespoons fennel seeds
- 2 tablespoons rose petals
- Peel of 1 organic grapefruit
- 1 cup (240 ml) Fino sherry

Gently heat the wine in a pot. When it has been warmed, add the coriander, chamomile, fennel, rose petals, and grapefruit peel; cover. Leave at a low heat for about 20 minutes with the cover on. Proceed to strain and bottle. Add the sherry to fortify (raise alcohol content slightly and improve longevity). Store the vermouth in the refrigerator and use within 1 to 3 months.

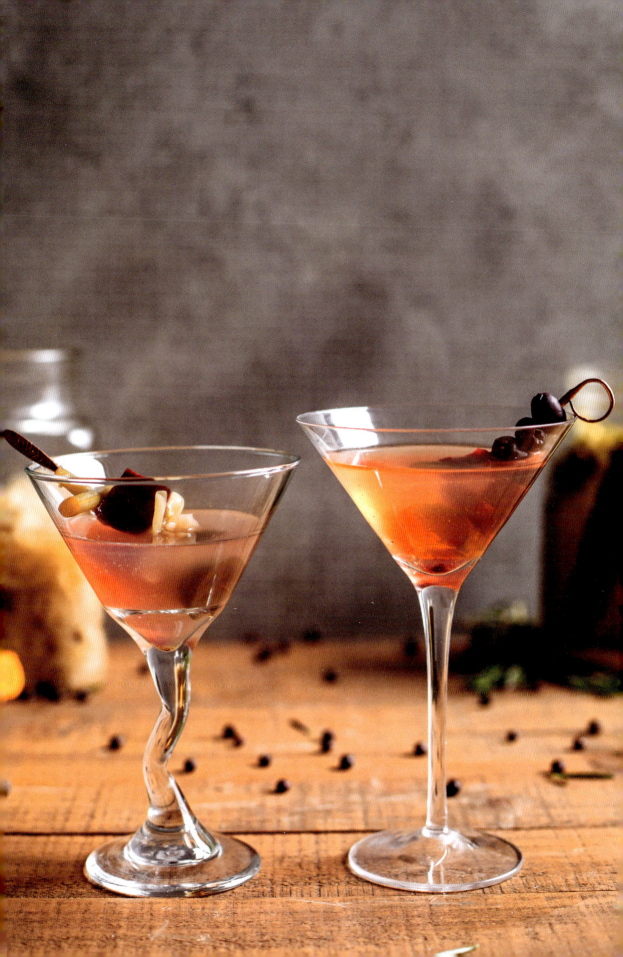

Bloody Botanist

If you have not had a Bloody Mary in the winter made from your very own home-canned heirloom tomatoes, then you have been missing out! This recipe is a treasure for your home pantry.

Makes 1 drink

1½ ounces (45 ml) vodka

6 ounces (180 ml) Bloody Mary mix (preferably homemade; recipe follows)

FOR GARNISHING

Freshly cracked pepper

Pickles of choice

Sprig of fresh rosemary or basil

Fill a collins glass or Mason jar with ice. Add the vodka and proceed to fill the glass with the Bloody Mary mix. Gently toss/roll the liquid between the glass and a cocktail shaker. Garnish with freshly cracked pepper and your choice of pickles. I use pickled burdock and spicy dilly beans. If one is available, add a sprig of an aromatic herb such as rosemary or basil.

NOTES

Basil (greenhouse grown or hydroponically produced) is usually available fresh at grocery stores even during the winter.

If I'm making a virgin Bloody Mary, I've found that I like using the nonalcoholic Ritual brand spirits. Their mock tequila is oaky and spicy and really good in a Bloody!

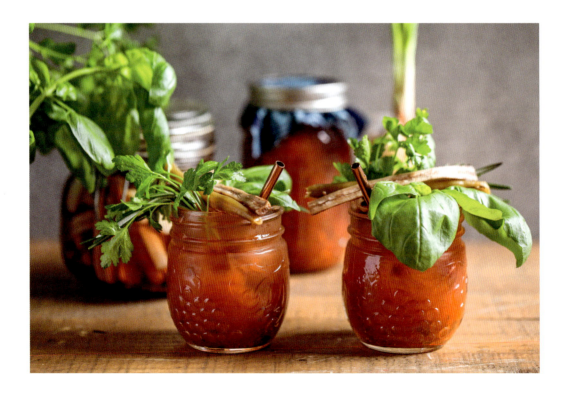

Homemade Bloody Mary Mix

I've listed quantities for the seasonings for this mix, but I recommend adding only half the specified amounts to start, and then tasting the mix as you go. You may want to add more or less of each seasoning than listed here, depending on your palate.

Makes 12 pints (5.7 liters)

- 20 pounds (9 kg) heirloom tomatoes at peak ripeness
- 2 tablespoons horseradish, preferably fresh and grated
- 2 teaspoons cayenne pepper (or 1 to 2 chopped hot peppers from the garden)
- 2 tablespoons oregano
- 2 tablespoons thyme
- 2 tablespoons rosemary
- 2 teaspoons black pepper
- 1 tablespoon smoked sea salt
- 4 tablespoons Worcestershire sauce
- 3 cups (720 ml) lemon juice
- 4 cloves garlic, minced (optional)

Put the tomatoes through a food mill to separate out some of the rougher bits. Transfer the milled tomatoes to a large pot. Heat to boiling and boil for 10 minutes. Reduce the heat to medium and simmer for several hours until very thick, then add the spices to taste. With a gloved hand, gently use an immersion blender to liquefy the tomatoes, being careful not to splatter and burn yourself with the hot tomato mixture.

I use a traditional hot-water canning method to process my homemade mix. If you're not familiar with how to can tomato products, consult a reliable source of information to learn the technique. When you fill sterilized jars with the liquid tomato, add ¼ cup (60 ml) lemon juice per jar to ensure proper acidity. Leave ¼ inch (6 mm) headspace. Wipe the rims before adding the lids back on, finishing the canning process. Store the mix in a cool, dry place such as a traditional pantry, and use or gift it within 2 years.

NOTE
While the quantities of spices are flexible, do not adjust the amount of lemon juice if you plan to process your tomatoes in a hot-water bath. The low pH of the lemon juice is required to acid-adjust the tomatoes, which have varying levels of acidity.

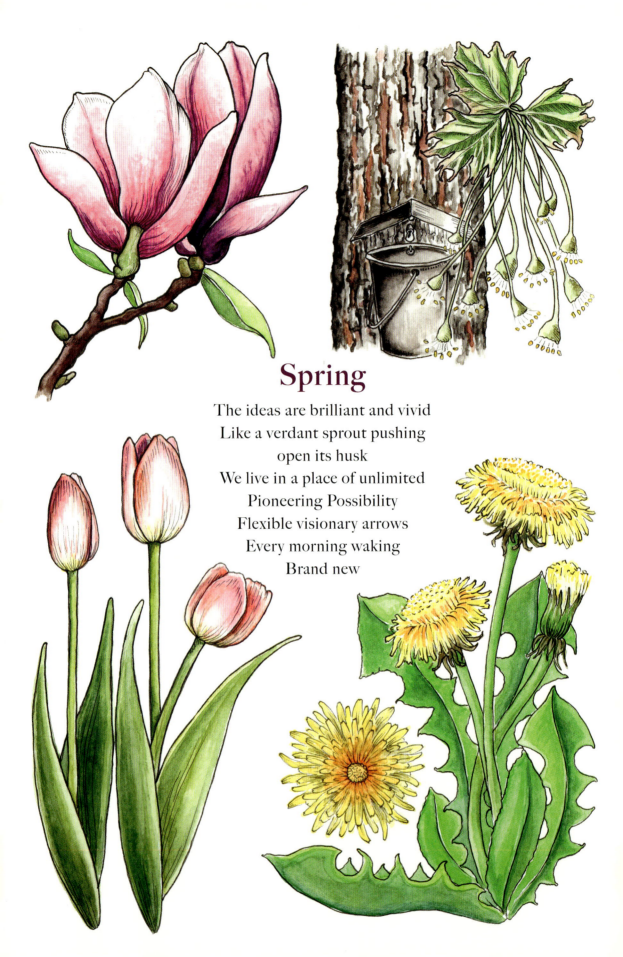

Spring

The ideas are brilliant and vivid
Like a verdant sprout pushing
open its husk
We live in a place of unlimited
Pioneering Possibility
Flexible visionary arrows
Every morning waking
Brand new

Recipes through the Seasons

Embrace the Dragon

alterative • bitter tonic • cardiovascular tonic
• demulcent • liver tonic • nutritive

Bring forth the fires of transformation in the year of the dragon! Kylie Smithline of Ki Ceramics in Biddeford, Maine, makes unique pottery, and I formulated this smoky Paloma-esque nonalcoholic fizzy drink to match her cups (take a look at the beautiful cups on page 28). It includes burdock root and aloe for detoxification.

Makes 1 drink

4 ounces (120 ml) mixed citrus juice
3 ounces (90 ml) celery-beet juice (see the note)
1 ounce (30 ml) aloe juice
1 ounce (30 ml) agave syrup
3 dropperfuls smoke bitters
Pinch of applewood-smoked sea salt
1 dropperful burdock root tincture
1 dropperful Boswellia tincture
2 ounces (60 ml) mineral water

Put the juices, agave syrup, smoke bitters, sea salt, and tinctures into a shaker tin and shake. Pour into a drinking vessel of choice without ice. Top with the mineral water.

NOTES

I make this drink with a blend of seasonal grapefruit, Meyer lemon, and orange in late winter and early spring, but you can use the citrus juice blend of your choice.

You can make your own celery-beet juice or buy bottled celery juice and bottled beet juice and combine them in equal parts.

I use smoke bitters by Vena's Fizz House in Portland, Maine.

Everyday Aperitif

alterative • antimicrobial • aromatic • bitter tonic • carminative • nervine

Many of the elixir recipes in this book might be considered aperitifs, particularly the bitters and soda recipes or any that are oxymel bases. I call this recipe Everyday Aperitif because it works well for making in a large batch that will last a month or so in the refrigerator. I like to bottle it into a fancy vintage decanter and keep it on hand for daily use.

Makes 1 quart (960 ml)

- 4 ounces (120 ml) balsam fir and pine hydrosol (see the note)
- 10 ounces (300 ml) Digestivo Oxymel (recipe follows)
- 16 ounces (480 ml) grapefruit juice
- 2 ounces (60 ml) ginger juice

To make the aperitif, simply combine all ingredients in a glass decanter or a quart-sized Mason jar. Shake to incorporate. Serve over ice with club soda and garnish as desired.

NOTE
I use Winter Woods hydrosol from Wild Sings the Bird.

Digestivo Oxymel

The quantities listed below are for dried herbs. Double the amounts if you use fresh herbs.

Makes 1 pint (480 ml)

- 1 cup (240 ml) raw apple cider vinegar
- 1 tablespoon artichoke leaf
- 1 tablespoon rosemary
- 1 tablespoon chamomile
- 1 tablespoon fennel seeds
- 1 tablespoon cardamom pods
- 1 tablespoon organic grapefruit peel
- 1 cup (240 ml) raw unfiltered honey

Gently heat the apple cider vinegar in a pot then mechanically blend with the artichoke leaf, rosemary, chamomile, fennel, cardamom, and grapefruit peel. Add the honey to dissolve. Macerate this herbal-infused vinegar-and-honey solution for 2 weeks in a glass jar with a noncorrosive lid. Strain. Store in the refrigerator and use within 6 months.

About Aperitifs

With a name that derives from Latin *aperire*, meaning "to open," aperitifs open the digestion and are best to drink before enjoying a meal. The aperitivo hour is a social experience that originated in Italy in the 1700s. It takes place before dinner and prepares the body to digest.

Aperitifs include bitter herbs that are choleretics and cholagogues, increasing the production and secretion of bile, as well as pancreatic enzymes. Aromatic herbs and spices or carminatives are often included for flavor. These relax the smooth muscles of the GI tract and reduce the risk of flatulence.

Bitters & Soda

alterative • bitter tonic • blood sugar regulating • carminative • grounding • hypoglycemic • liver tonic

Sometimes the simplest recipes can be the most potent. There are countless variations on Bitters and Soda drinks, depending on the types of bitters you have on hand, but here is a recipe for my favorite, with three variations on the theme, including a unique topping or garnish for each. This is my go-to for a low-alcohol night on the town and is also considered an aperitif.

Makes 1 serving

VARIATION #1
1 ounce (30 ml) grapefruit juice
3 dropperfuls Cardamom Bitters (recipe follows)
8 ounces (240 ml) club soda

For this variation, use an atomizer to mist St-Germain elderflower liqueur over the top of the finished drink. Garnish with an edible white flower such as elderflower, yarrow, or Queen Anne's lace.

VARIATION #2
½ ounce (15 ml) lime juice
1 ounce (30 ml) ginger beer
8 ounces (240 ml) club soda

For this variation, tear several mint leaves and push them down into the liquid in the glass so they are underneath the ice. Float on a capful of Angostura bitters by pouring it over the back of a bar spoon. Clap a fresh mint leaf in your hands to bruise it and place on top as the garnish.

VARIATION #3, ALCOHOL-FREE
1 teaspoon Wormwood Vinegar Bitters (recipe follows)
1 ounce (30 ml) Fennel Honey Syrup (recipe follows)
8 ounces (240 ml) club soda

For this variation, gather a few fresh fennel flowers (that have begun producing pollen, if possible). Float the flowers atop the finished drink.

To make a Bitters and Soda, fill a collins glass or Mason jar with ice and build in the glass, gently swizzling the ingredients with a bar spoon or straw prior to drinking. Garnish each variation as described above.

Cardamom Bitters

Makes 2 ounces (60 ml)
Dried cardamom pods
Overproof spirit

Fill a 2-ounce tincture dropper bottle halfway with dried cardamom pods. Cover with overproof spirits and allow to infuse for at least 2 weeks prior to using.

Wormwood Vinegar Bitters

I love vinegar bitters because they offer the medicinal benefits of sour flavor and probiotics (if made from raw vinegar).

Makes 1 pint (480 ml)
Fresh wormwood (*Artemisia absinthium*) flowers
Raw apple cider vinegar

Wormwood flowers fresh from the garden are best for bitters. Chop up some flowers and fill a pint-sized glass jar. Pour raw apple cider vinegar over the flowers, making sure the plant matter is covered completely. Cover the jar with a non-corrosive (non-metallic) lid and macerate 2 to 4 weeks before straining.

Fennel Honey Syrup

Makes 1 pint (480 ml)
8 ounces (240 ml) boiling water
1 tablespoon fresh or dry fennel flowers
Raw unfiltered honey

Pour the boiling water over the fresh or dry fennel flowers in a heat-safe glass jar or French press. Cover to steep. Strain after 15 minutes into a measuring glass. Add an equal volume of raw unfiltered honey and mix. Store the syrup in the refrigerator and use within 1 month.

Spring Tonic #1

alterative • bitter tonic • carminative • liver tonic • lymphatic • stimulant

The transition from winter into spring can be difficult for the body, and spring tonics can help make the shift more graceful. In the Northeast, aralia (*Aralia nudicaulis*) is an abundant rhizome covering the forest floor that is made apparent as the earth is waking up. It has a long history of use as a spring tonic.

Makes 2 drinks

2 ounces (60 ml) Spring Tonic Oxymel (recipe follows)
2 ounces (60 ml) Aralia Root and Ginger Tea (recipe follows)
6 ounces (180 ml) sparkling mineral water
Wild violets, for garnishing

Fill two rocks glasses with ice. Put 1 ounce (30 ml) of the Spring Tonic Oxymel, 1 ounce of the Aralia Root and Ginger Tea, and 3 ounces (90 ml) of the mineral water in each of the two glasses. Stir gently and garnish with violets.

Spring Tonic Oxymel

Makes 1 pint (480 ml)

½ cup (20 g) chopped stinging nettle (*Urtica dioica*) shoots
¼ cup (25 g) raw dandelion root
¼ cup (25 g) raw burdock root
½ cup (120 ml) raw unfiltered apple cider vinegar
1½ cups (360 ml) raw, unfiltered honey

Put all the ingredients in a quart jar and cover with a non-metallic cover. Shake the jar well until the honey is dissolved. Top with more vinegar if necessary to cover the herbs in the jar. Let macerate for 2 to 3 weeks, then strain and store in the refrigerator and use within 6 months.

Aralia Root & Ginger Tea

Makes about 2 cups (480 ml)

Fresh aralia rhizomes
Fresh gingerroot

Chop about ½ cup each of fresh aralia rhizomes and gingerroot. Add to a small pot with 1 quart (960 ml) of water and bring to a boil. Boil for 10 minutes, then reduce to a simmer for another 10 minutes. Strain and allow to cool fully before using it in a Spring Tonic #1.

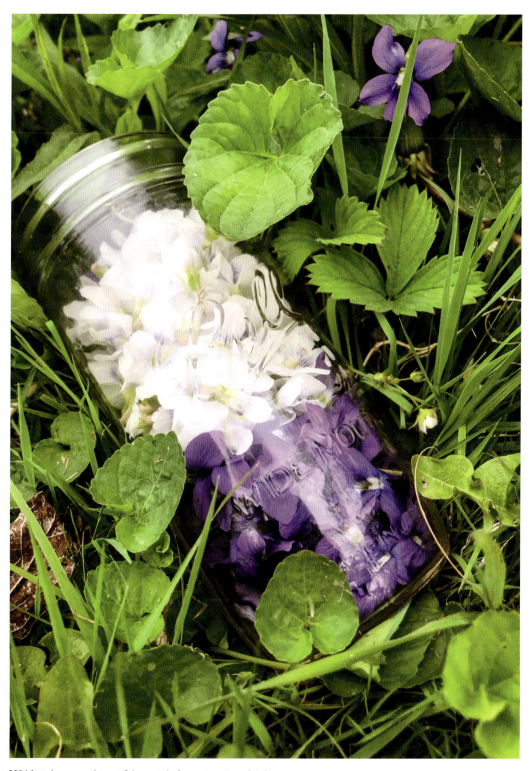

Wild violets are a beautiful garnish for springtime drinks.

Botanical Bar Craft

The Mosscat

alterative • aromatic • carminative • nutritive • stimulant

This is a recipe made for carrying the vitality and nutrition of spring greens. Some suitable foraged greens to add to this juice are chickweed (*Stellaria media*), claytonia, violet leaves, and dandelion greens. Use the ones popping up in your yard! The vegetables chosen are a little juicier and help stretch out the potent flavor and effect of the wild weeds. The mint and parsley improve palatability. Drink the juice as is or top with sparkling lemon ginger kombucha for a stimulating nonalcoholic cocktail.

Makes 4 servings

1 cucumber, ends cut off
½ bunch celery
1 apple, coarsely chopped
1 handful edible spring weeds
Several sprigs fresh mint
Several sprigs fresh parsley
Thumb-sized piece gingerroot
1 organic lemon, halved
4 ounces (120 ml) cold lemon-ginger kombucha

Using a juicer, juice the cucumber, celery, apple, spring weeds, mint, parsley, and gingerroot. Use a citrus juicer to juice the lemon, and add the lemon juice to the other juices. Fill a cocktail glass two-thirds of the way full with this juice mixture. Top with the kombucha.

NOTE
If you don't have a juicer, you can substitute a high-quality store-bought green juice for the spring weeds, mint, and parsley.

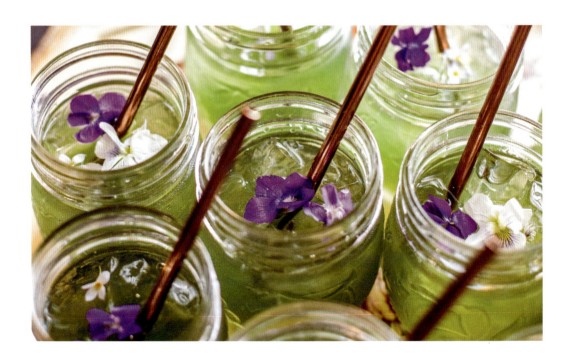

Recipes through the Seasons

Ephemeral Beauty

aromatic • carminative • lymphatic • nutritive

The woodland nymph is perched on the mossy ledge by the river, sipping a wild spring spritzer in an enchanted forest. This recipe was formulated to serve at a natural-beauty-focused event. The taste is reminiscent of water rushing down a mountainside in the spring.

Makes 1 drink

1 dropperful trillium flower essence
3 ounces (90 ml) Forest Green Juice (recipe follows)
3 ounces (90 ml) sparkling mineral water
Wild violets, for garnish

Add the trillium flower essence to the Forest Green Juice and stir. Pour over ice in a rocks glass and top with the mineral water. Garnish with a sprinkle of wild violets.

This recipe is also appropriate for batching. When I made this for the event, I blended a large amount of the Forest Green Juice and placed it in a large glass decanter with a spigot. I added the flower essence and large chunks of clean quartz into the vessel as well. I then poured directly over ice into rocks glasses, topped each one with sparkling mineral water, and sprinkled on a garnish of wild violets.

NOTE
I did not harvest the trillium, as it is on the United Plant Savers Species At-Risk List. To make the flower essence, I gently tipped the stem to soak the living flower's energy into clean stream water for 6 hours.

Forest Green Juice

Makes about 2 quarts (1.9 L)

Generous handful (about 1 cup) fresh stinging nettle (*Urtica dioica*) leaves
Generous handful (about 1 cup) chickweed flowers, leaves, and stems
Generous handful (about 1 cup) balsam fir tips
¼ cup (60 ml) raw unfiltered honey

Blend the young stinging nettle, chickweed, balsam fir tips, and honey with 2 quarts (1.9 liters) of water in a high-performance blender. Strain. This juice can be kept in the refrigerator for up to 3 days. It can also be frozen for later use.

NOTE
The Forest Green Juice can be made with whatever spring greens and edible conifer tips you happen to have on hand.

Heart of Venus

antidepressant • aphrodisiac • cardiovascular tonic
• demulcent • liver tonic • nervine • nutritive

I started with a nonalcoholic chocolate "Martini" and added spring botanicals and floral aroma. Then I collected water from a local spring. This drink softens the heart to promote open, honest connection with nature, self, and others.

Makes 4–6 Martinis

2 cups (480 ml) springwater, divided
1 tablespoon roasted dandelion root
1 tablespoon marshmallow root powder
1 cup (240 ml) raw dairy cream
½ cup (100 g) chopped cacao paste
¼ cup (60 ml) barrel-aged maple syrup
¼ cup (60 ml) wild rose hydrosol or culinary-grade rose water
¼ cup (60 ml) Wild Rose Elixir (page 139)
4–6 dropperfuls Reishi Tincture (page 189) (see the note)
3 dropperfuls magnolia flower essence
Apple blossoms, for garnishing

First make dandelion root tea by boiling 1 cup of the springwater and pouring it over the roasted dandelion root. Leave it to steep for 15 minutes, covered. While it steeps, put the marshmallow root powder in the remaining cup of cold springwater to soak.

After about 15 minutes, strain the dandelion root tea. Gently heat the cream and place it in a blender with the dandelion tea, marshmallow tea, cacao paste, maple syrup, wild rose hydrosol, Wild Rose Elixir, Reishi Tincture, and magnolia flower essence. Garnish with apple blossoms.

NOTE
The Reishi Tincture contains alcohol. You may omit this tincture if you're abstaining from alcohol completely.

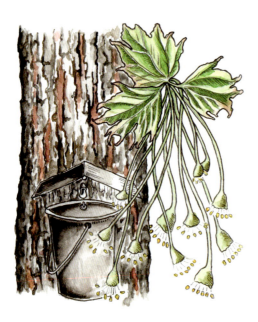

Like Bunny Rabbits

adaptogen • antidepressant • aphrodisiac • cardiovascular tonic
• nervine • nutritive • stimulant

This luscious drink is a chocolate-covered Strawberry Martini with damiana and schisandra. Originally created for a Valentine's Day event, I used strawberry powder made by the same farmer who grew the strawberries I had picked and frozen the previous summer.

Makes 4 drinks

2 tablespoons freeze-dried strawberry powder
2 tablespoons schisandra berry powder
¼ cup (65 g) frozen strawberries
¼ cup (25 g) raw, chopped cacao paste
¼ cup (10 g) damiana leaf
2 vanilla beans, scraped (see the note, page 127)
1 teaspoon cayenne powder
¼ cup (60 ml) raw unfiltered honey

NOTE
You can add a splash or two of cream or spike the drink with vanilla bean vodka if desired. Add either or both these ingredients to the cocktail shaker just before mixing.

Mix the strawberry and schisandra powders together in a shallow bowl; set aside.

Bring 3 cups (720 ml) of water to a boil. Add the frozen strawberries and boil for 10 minutes, then add the cacao and allow it to dissolve. Shut off the heat and add the damiana. Cover and steep for 15 minutes. Strain. Scrape the seeds from the vanilla beans into the strained liquid and add the cayenne powder. Add the honey and allow to dissolve. Shake this preparation.

Rim a coupe glass by wetting one side of the glass with a wet paintbrush or by dipping one side of the glass in water. Then turn the glass upside down and dip the rim into the mixed berry powders (the powder will cling to the wet side of the glass only). Strain the cocktail into the glass.

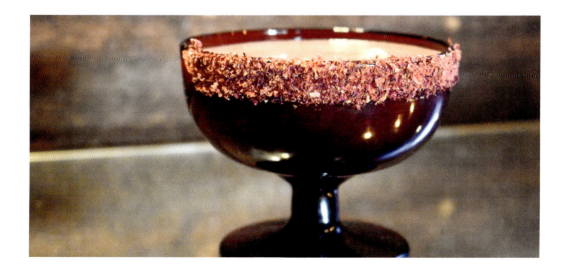

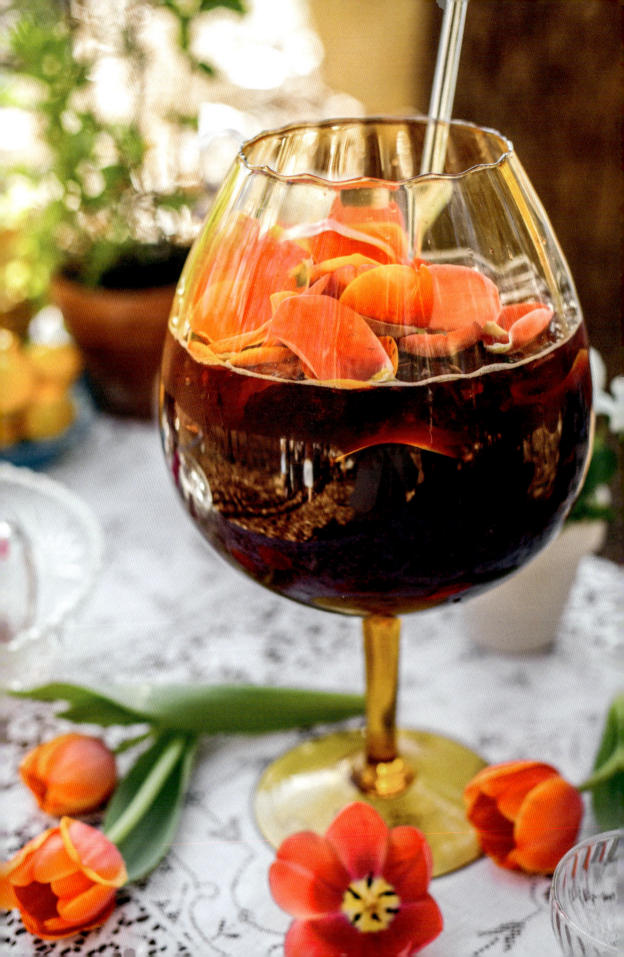

Recipes through the Seasons

Pregnancy Punch

antioxidant • blood builder • carminative • nervine • nutritive

Chock-full of blood-building botanicals that are safe for pregnancy, this is an ideal recipe to bring to the next baby shower you're invited to.

Fills a small punch bowl

FOR THE RED RASPBERRY LEAF & STINGING NETTLE TEA

2 tablespoons dried red raspberry leaves
4 tablespoons chopped fresh nettle leaves or 2 tablespoons dried stinging nettle (*Urtica dioica*)
1 tablespoon apple cider vinegar

FOR THE "RUM-SPICED" MOLASSES

8 ounces (240 ml) molasses
1 tablespoon ground cinnamon
1 tablespoon cardamom
1 tablespoon vanilla extract
1 teaspoon ground cloves
1 teaspoon ground ginger

FOR THE PREGNANCY PUNCH

1 quart (960 ml) Red Raspberry Leaf and Stinging Nettle Tea
1 pint (480 ml) "Rum-Spiced" Molasses
1 quart (960 ml) 100 percent juice blend: pomegranate, blueberry, and purple carrot or similar blend
8 ounces (240 ml) lime juice
4 ounces (120 ml) ginger juice
2 ounces (60 ml) Wild Rose Elixir (page 139)
8 ounces (240 ml) culinary-grade rose water
16 ounces (480 ml) sparkling apple cider
8 ounces (240 ml) club soda
Flowers, for decoration around the bowl

The night before you plan to serve the punch, make the Red Raspberry Leaf and Stinging Nettle Tea: Pour 1 quart (960 ml) of boiling water over the red raspberry leaves and stinging nettle. Add the apple cider vinegar and leave to steep, covered, overnight to fully extract the minerals from the herbs. The following morning, strain into a 1-quart jar.

When it's time to prepare the punch, first make the "Rum-Spiced" Molasses: Combine 8 ounces (240 ml) of hot water with the molasses. Add the cinnamon, cardamom, vanilla extract, cloves, and ginger. Stir until well mixed.

To make the punch, pour the Red Raspberry and Stinging Nettle Tea and the "Rum-Spiced" Molasses into the punch bowl. Then add the juice blend, lime juice, ginger juice, Wild Rose Elixir, rose water, sparkling apple cider, and club soda. Add ice and stir gently. Place tulip petals around the base of the punch bowl and in individual glasses of punch, if desired.

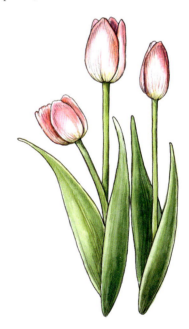

Street Smarts

nervine • nootropic • nutritive

This recipe is a toast to the astounding adaptability and resilience of the plant kingdom, to invasive plant medicine, and to our own adaptability through regular consumption of these wise plants that mirror us, growing on the borders of our lives.

Makes 1 drink

Dried ground sumac powder, for the rim
8 ounces (236 ml) Street Smarts Decoction (recipe follows)
3 dropperfuls Street Smarts Tincture (recipe follows)
Club soda
Lilac, for garnishing

Place the sumac powder in a shallow bowl and some water in a second bowl. Dip the rim of a rocks glass in the water first, then the powder. Combine the Street Smarts Decoction and Street Smarts Tincture in a cocktail shaker. Shake and strain over ice into the rimmed glass. Top with club soda.

Street Smarts Decoction

Makes 1 quart (960 ml)

1 cup (100 g) chopped Japanese knotweed (*Reynoutria multiflora*) shoots
1 cup (35 g) dried hibiscus flowers
½ cup (45 g) wild rose petals
Raw unfiltered honey

Simmer the Japanese knotweed shoots in 2 quarts (1.9 L) of water until they turn mushy. Add the hibiscus and wild rose. Steep, covered for 15 minutes. Strain and sweeten with honey to taste. (I use 4 tablespoons.) Store this decoction in the refrigerator and use within 3 days or freeze for later use.

Street Smarts Tincture

Makes 4 ounces (120 ml)

Fresh or dried ginkgo (*Ginkgo biloba*) leaves
Fresh or dried dandelion root
Fresh or dried mugwort (*Artemisia vulgaris*) leaves
Overproof spirit

To make this tincture yourself, place approximately equal amounts of fresh or dried ginkgo leaves, dandelion root, and mugwort leaves in a 4-ounce glass jar. Cover with overproof spirits and macerate for 4 weeks. Strain into a glass tincture bottle. You can also purchase individual tinctures and combine them in equal parts.

Sugar on Snow

There is a beautiful tradition here in Maine of pouring freshly boiled maple syrup over snow for kids and the child-at-heart to enjoy as fun, sticky taffy. This recipe is inspired by sugar on snow—it is early spring captured in a glass!

Makes 1 cocktail

Apple Cider Caramel (recipe follows), for the rim
Laphroaig or another very peaty scotch, for rinsing
1½ ounces (45 ml) birch-infused rye
¼ ounce (7.5 ml) Glenmorangie A Tale of the Forest Scotch
¼ ounce (7.5 ml) Winter Amaro (page 140)
¾ ounce (22.5 ml) lemon juice
¾ ounce (22.5 ml) maple syrup
2 ounces (60 ml) sparkling mineral water
2 ounces (60 ml) carbonated maple sap (optional)
Birch twigs, for garnishing

Place some room-temperature caramel into a shallow bowl for easy use. Rinse a rocks glass with the Laphroaig. Dip the rim of the glass into the caramel and then fill the glass with ice. Put the rye, scotch, Winter Amaro, lemon juice, and maple syrup into a cocktail shaker with ice and shake. Strain into the glass. Top with the sparkling mineral water and carbonated maple sap, if using. Garnish with birch twigs.

NOTES

I use Old Forester rye and Gerolsteiner Sparkling Mineral Water.

To carbonate sap, place some sap in a soda-making device such as a SodaStream or iSi brand soda maker. Commercial sap soda is also available.

Apple Cider Caramel

All it takes to make apple cider sap is some cider and a lot of patience. Put about a gallon (4 liters) of apple cider into a very large pot and heat to boiling. Boil the cider hard for 30 to 45 minutes, then reduce to a gentle boil and let it cook for about 2 hours more. Check and stir occasionally, watching for the liquid to become a thick syrup with a caramel-like consistency. Be sure to remove it from the heat before it reaches the hard candy stage. You'll end up with about a cup (240 ml) of caramel. A woodstove would be great for this recipe, but it would be a multiday process to cook down the sap. Extra caramel can be stored in the refrigerator and used within 3 months.

Cheshire Cat

"Curiouser and curiouser." This fun and fresh cocktail is a nod to this famous trickster character from *Alice's Adventures in Wonderland*, invented by the wild imagination of Lewis Carroll. "We're all mad here."

Makes 1 cocktail

Several fresh spilanthes blossoms, for the rim
Bee pollen, for the rim
2 ounces (60 ml) cucumber-infused Barr Hill Gin (bonus points if the cucumbers are from your garden)
1 ounce (30 ml) lemon juice
1 ounce (30 ml) Garden Honey Tea Syrup (recipe follows)
¾ ounce (22.5 ml) Sugar Snap Pea Juice (recipe follows)
Sprig of sweet alyssum, for garnishing
Rosemary bitters, for misting

Use a food processor to combine the spilanthes blossoms with the bee pollen until powdered. Transfer this "spilanthes pollen" to a small, shallow bowl for easy use. Wet the rim of a Martini glass by dipping in water or rubbing with a cut lemon wedge. Then upturn the glass and dip the rim in spilanthes pollen. Put the gin, lemon juice, honey tea syrup, and pea juice in a cocktail shaker and shake. Strain into the rimmed glass. Attach the sweet alyssum sprig to the rim with a tiny clothespin. Mist the surface of the drink with the bitters.

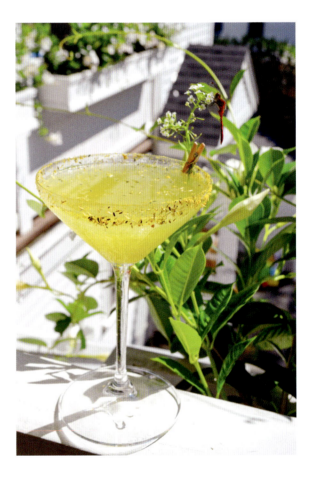

Cucumber Infused Gin

Makes 1 quart (960 ml)

Several small cucumbers

Barr Hill gin

Chop several small garden cucumbers into thin slices, then half or quarter these slices. Add to a quart-sized jar and pour Barr Hill Gin over them, ensuring they are completely covered. Allow to infuse for several days.

Garden Honey Tea Syrup

Use fresh herbs to brew the tea for this syrup.

Makes 1 pint (480 ml)

1 sprig dill

1 sprig lavender

1 sprig rosemary

1 sprig thyme

1 cup (240 ml) raw unfiltered honey

Chop the dill, lavender, rosemary, and thyme. Loosely fill a Mason jar about halfway with the herbs. Cover with 1 cup (240 ml) of hot water. Let steep, covered, for 20 to 30 minutes. Strain into a measuring glass and add an equal amount of the honey. Stir or shake to dissolve. Store the syrup in the refrigerator and use within 1 month.

Sugar Snap Pea Juice

Makes about 2 cups (480 ml)

Sugar snap peas

Place about 1 cup (63 g) sugar snap peas in a high-performance blender with 2 cups (480 ml) water. Blend at the highest setting and then strain out the solids. Store the juice for several days in the refrigerator or freeze for later use.

Transcendental Lilac

The aroma of lilacs is both elusive and transcendent. It evokes the memory of many Mays, the hopes and wishes of springs past.

Makes 2 cocktails

12 ounces (360 ml) coconut cream
½ cup (20 g) fresh lilac flowers, plus extra for garnishing
2 ounces (60 ml) Sweetfern Honey Syrup (recipe follows)
3 ounces (90 ml) Barr Hill Gin

On low heat, gently heat the coconut cream and fresh lilac flowers. Cover the pot and infuse on low heat for several hours.

After infusing, strain out the flower residue and allow the cream to cool. Combine the floral cream, Sweetfern Honey Syrup, and gin with ice in a mixing glass. Stir gently and strain into a coupe. Garnish with fresh lilacs.

Sweetfern Honey Syrup

Sweetfern (*Comptonia peregrina*) is a sweet-swelling aromatic shrub-like plant native to Maine.

Makes 8 ounces (240 ml)

Fresh sweetfern buds and leaves
Raw unfiltered honey
Hot (not boiling) water

To make this syrup, chop up fresh sweetfern buds and leaves and place into a 4-ounce glass jar. Cover with raw unfiltered honey and let infuse for several weeks. Prior to straining, mix with an equal amount of hot but not boiling water. Then strain the syrup. This can be kept in the refrigerator for 1 month.

Victory Garden

During the Victory Garden campaign initiated during World War II in response to food shortages, people planted gardens in their yards and in public parks to help feed one another and as an act of patriotism. I love the idea of gardening being patriotic, and so I created this drink! Here in Maine, strawberries and rhubarb are both ready for harvest right around Independence Day.

Makes 1 cocktail

4 ounces (120 ml) rhubarb wine
2 ounces (60 ml) Cardamaro aperitif
3 ounces (90 ml) sparkling mineral water
3 ounces (90 ml) sparkling rosé
White pansies, for garnishing
Strawberries, sliced in half vertically, for garnishing
3 dropperfuls chamomile bitters, for garnishing
Bluet (*Houstonia caerulea*) blossoms, for garnishing

Build the drink in a large glass goblet or burgundy glass filled with ice, starting with the wine and then adding the Cardamaro, mineral water, and sparkling rosé. Use a paper straw (navy blue in color if possible) to push some of the pansies and strawberry halves into the drink for ornament. Put the 3 dropperfuls of the bitters on top for the nose and garnish with a little bunch of bluets.

NOTE
I use Victoria rhubarb wine by eighteen twenty wines in Maine and a biodynamically grown Brut Rosé from Roederer Estate.

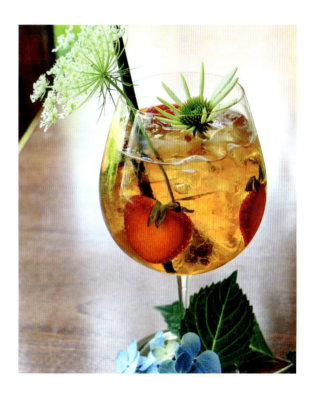

Poets & Outlaws

This riff on the classic Hemingway Daiquiri is dedicated to the creative and spiritual rebels of society. What makes this cocktail edgy? Is it the deep thorns of the hawthorn branches, the flowers with an aroma of death…or the cyanide in the cherry bark?

Makes 1 cup (240 ml)

1½ ounces (45 ml) light rum
¾ ounce (22.5 ml) Very Cherry, Thorns, and Flowers Syrup (recipe follows)
¾ ounce (22.5 ml) freshly squeezed grapefruit juice
¼ ounce (7.5 ml) lime juice
¼ teaspoon almond extract
Cocktail cherry, for garnishing

Put the rum, syrup, grapefruit juice, lime juice, and almond extract in a cocktail shaker and shake it up, baby! Serve up in your choice of a Martini glass. Garnish with a good cherry.

NOTE
I use Filthy brand wild Italian black cherries.

Very Cherry, Thorns & Flowers Syrup

Makes 1 quart (960 ml)

¼ cup (50 g) tart cherries, fresh or frozen
¼ cup (25 g) hawthorn (*Crataegus* spp.) flowers
1 tablespoon chopped wild cherry bark (*Prunus serotina*)
Several wild cherry blossoms
2 cups (400 g) organic sugar

Simmer the cherries in 1 quart (960 ml) of water for 20 minutes. Shut off the heat. Add the hawthorn flowers, wild cherry bark, and cherry blossoms; cover to steep for another 15 minutes. Strain and dissolve the sugar into the fruity liquid. Store in the refrigerator and use within 1 month.

Preserved Cocktail Cherries

If you live in a locale that grows cherries, I highly suggest picking some at their height of freshness and preserving them. It is tedious to pit cherries and a bit finicky to do it without ruining the fruit. I recommend squeezing each ripe cherry and using the pointy edge of a chopstick to enlarge the hole at the stem end and fish out the pit.

Fill a jar with pitted sweet or tart cherries. Make a rich simple syrup by combining 2 parts sugar to 1 part water. Add enough of this syrup to the jar to cover the cherries. I store them in the refrigerator, but they can also be preserved by water-bath canning. Add 1 tablespoon lemon juice per pint (400 g) of cherries if you plan to can them.

I also like to add spices, such as chai spices, to a syrup for preserved cherries for stellar results. To make a chai-spiced syrup, combine 1 tablespoon each ground cinnamon, diced fresh gingerroot, and cardamom pods along with 1 teaspoon whole cloves in 1 quart (960 ml) water. Simmer for 15 minutes on medium-high heat. Pour the hot decoction into a measuring cup. Multiply that volume by 2—that's the amount of sugar to add to the decoction. Leave the spices in the decoction and pour over fresh, pitted cherries in a glass jar.

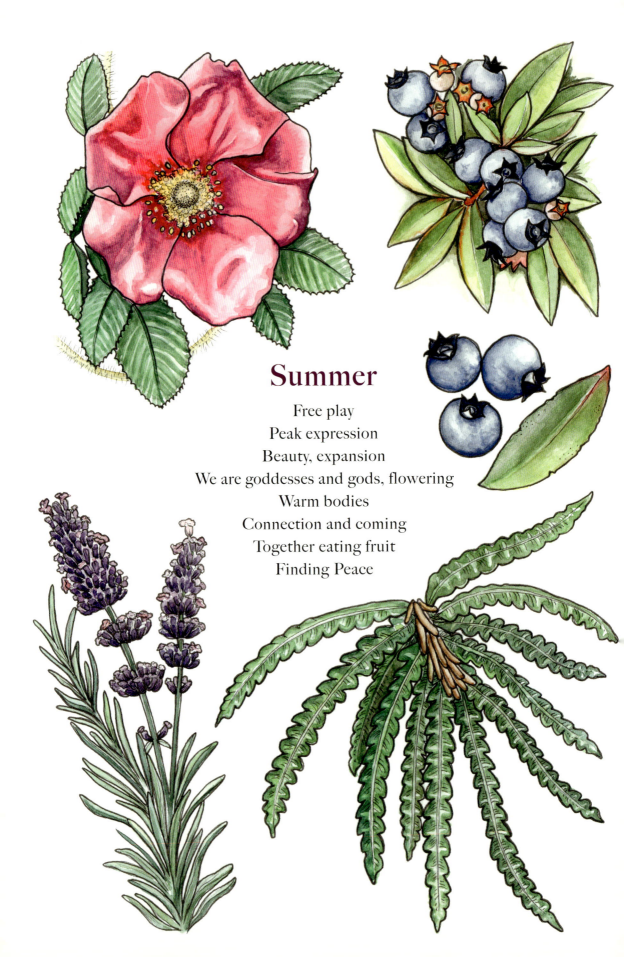

Summer

Free play
Peak expression
Beauty, expansion
We are goddesses and gods, flowering
Warm bodies
Connection and coming
Together eating fruit
Finding Peace

Recipes through the Seasons

Ruby Throat Sunset

antiviral • astringent • carminative • cooling • nervine • nutritive

This drink was inspired by the beloved hummingbirds who love to drink the nectar from bee balm flowers. Summer is watermelon season, and fresh watermelon juice makes this drink unforgettable.

Makes 1 drink

Fresh bee balm petals, for the rim
Sea salt, for the rim
4–5 fall raspberries
3 ounces (90 ml) watermelon juice
1 dropperful St. John's wort tincture
½ ounce (15 ml) culinary-grade rose water
¼ ounce (7.5 ml) lime juice
¾ ounce (22.5 ml) honey simple syrup

To make the infused salt for the rim: Pulse equal parts of the bee balm petals and sea salt in a food processor or spice grinder, then place the mixture in a shallow bowl. Put some water in another shallow bowl. Upturn a glass and dip the rim first in the water and then in the salt.

Put the raspberries in a shaker tin and muddle (smash) them. Then add the watermelon juice, tincture, rose water, lime juice, and simple syrup. Shake with ice. Double-strain into the rimmed glass.

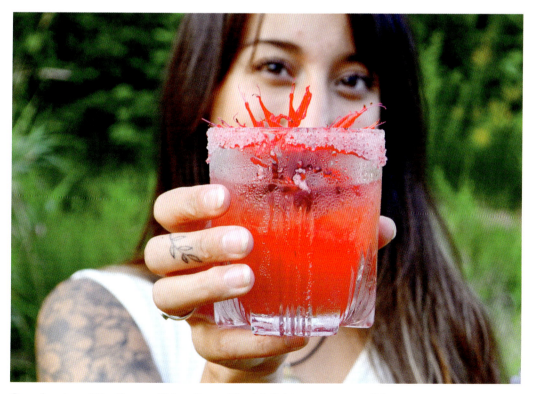

One of my beautiful colleagues, Briana Betts of Seed & Spirits, toasting to collaboration over competition.

Babe in the Woods

anti-cancer • anti-inflammatory • antioxidant • cardiovascular tonic
• immune tonic • nutritive

This cocktail's name is an idiom or expression referring to a naive or innocent person—a baby lost in the woods. Celebrate the beautiful fool in love with this sweet summer sip.

Makes 1 drink

1 ounce (30 ml) sweet Annie hydrosol
6 ounces (180 ml) Blueberry-Chaga Elixir (recipe follows)
½ ounce (15 ml) lemon juice

Combine all ingredients in a shaker tin. Shake and strain up into a small decorative cocktail glass of your choice.

Blueberry-Chaga Elixir

Chaga mushrooms are rich in antioxidants, and so are blueberries, giving this elixir some impressive healing potential. Packaged chaga chunks are available at specialty stores or online.

Makes 1 quart (960 ml)

6–8 small chunks chaga mushroom
2 cups (240 g) wild blueberries
Maple syrup

Decoct the chaga chunks in 4 quarts (3.8 liters) of water on medium-high heat for 20 minutes, and then simmer on low heat for 40 minutes. Cover the pot after the initial boiling. The result should be an opaque black liquid. Use a small strainer to pull out the chaga chunks (they can be reused). Add another 2 cups (480 ml) of fresh water and the wild blueberries to the liquid in the pot and bring back to a boil for 5 to 10 minutes. Blend with an immersion blender. Strain into a large glass measuring cup, note the volume, and then pour into a glass jar. Sweeten with the maple syrup in a 1:4 syrup-to-liquid ratio, or to taste. (This elixir should be sweet.) This will keep in the refrigerator for a couple of weeks.

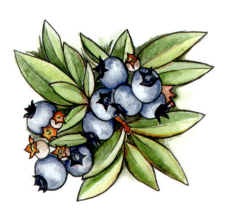

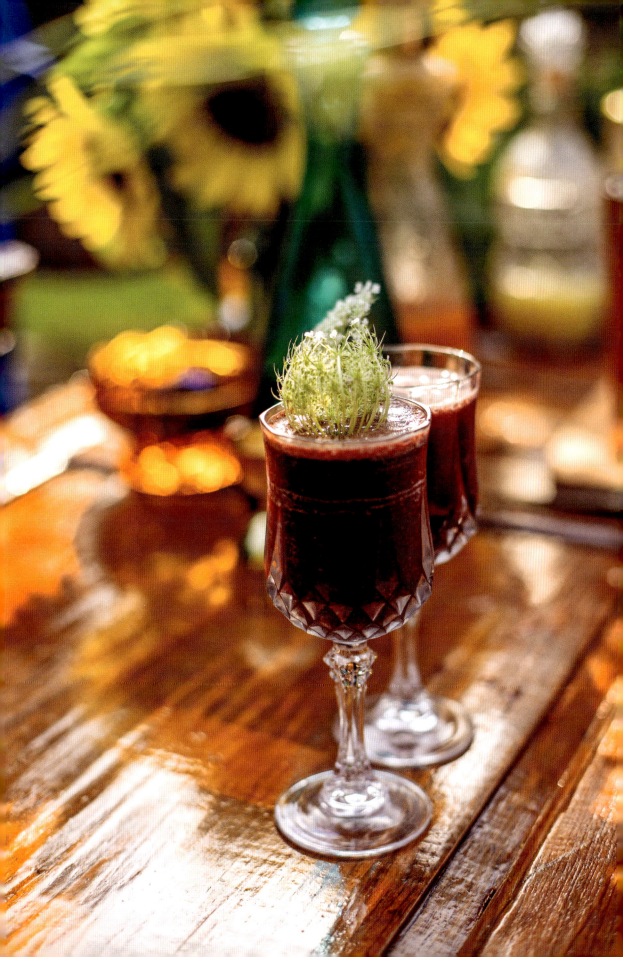

Juice of Life

astringent • athletic performance • cooling • nervine • nutritive

This vivid pink cocktail is Margarita-ish and easy to drink. It's deeply thirst quenching after a long walk in the desert, with electrolytes from the salted rim.

Makes 1 drink

Cardamom-Rose Sea Salt (recipe follows), for the rim
3 ounces (90 ml) cactus water
½ ounce (15 ml) culinary-grade rose water
2 ounces (60 ml) prickly pear purée or strawberry purée
1 ounce (30 ml) agave syrup
½ ounce (15 ml) lime juice
1–3 dropperfuls Oak Extract (recipe follows) (optional)
Club soda
Prickly pear (*Opuntia* spp.) flower or wild rose, for garnishing

First, rim a rocks glass with the Cardamom-Rose Sea Salt: Use a cut lime wedge to wet the rim of the glass, then overturn the glass and dip the rim into a shallow bowl filled with the infused salt. Set aside. Combine the cactus water, rose water, prickly pear purée, agave syrup, lime juice, and Oak Extract in a cocktail shaker with ice and shake, shake, shake. Pour the contents of the shaker, including the ice, into the rimmed glass. Add a little splash of club soda. Garnish with a wild rose or cactus flower.

Cardamom-Rose Sea Salt

Makes about 1¼ cups (325 g)

1 cup (236 g) sea salt
1 cup (90 g) fresh rose petals
2 teaspoons cardamom powder

Put all the ingredients into a small food processor and pulse until the salt is very pink and no pieces of rose petal are evident. Store in an airtight container in a dry place. The salt will retain the pink coloration for about 6 months.

Oak Extract

Oak extract, a source of tannins, is ubiquitous in zero-proof spirits and alcohol alternatives because oak is a natural flavor in many barrel-aged spirits from tequila to whiskey, as well as wine. Tannins lend added complexity and interesting mouthfeel to nonalcoholic drinks. You can make an oak extract using chopped leaves and bark of any type of oak (*Quercus* spp.).

Makes 4 ounces (120 ml)

Fresh oak leaves and bark
1 tablespoon food-grade vegetable glycerin
100-proof clear spirit

Fill a 4-ounce jar halfway with fresh plant material and cover it with 1 tablespoon food-grade vegetable glycerin and 100-proof clear spirit. Let sit for 2 to 4 weeks, shaking the jar when you remember to. Then strain the extract and transfer it into a tincture dropper bottle.

Nootropical Paradise

nervine • nootropic • nutritive

This is a purple Piña Colada with brain power! Enjoy this delightful riff on a classic while relaxing on your next tropical vacation.

Makes 2 drinks

8 ounces (240 ml) fresh pineapple juice
4 ounces (120 ml) coconut cream
¼ cup (50 g) frozen pineapple
2 teaspoons butterfly pea flower powder
2 dropperfuls Cerebrum Tonic by Anima Mundi Herbals

Add all the ingredients to a mechanical blender with a few ice cubes and blend to the consistency of a slushy. Pour into glasses of your choice and garnish as desired.

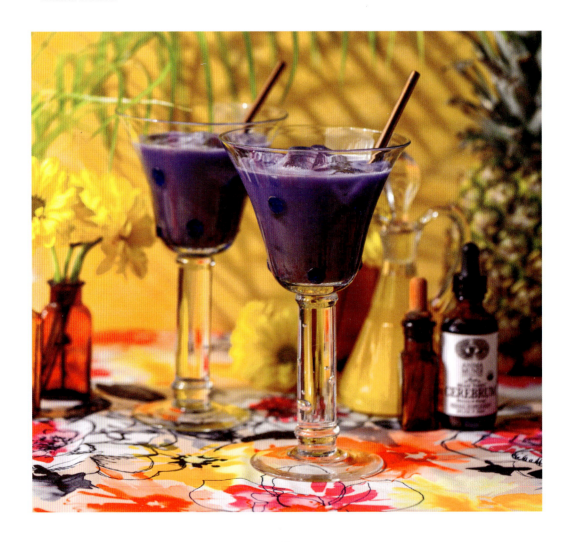

Recipes through the Seasons

Altar & Intent

anti-inflammatory • antioxidant • carminative • nervine

This very aromatic spiritual potion was formulated for the women's herb retreat at Earth Spiral Apothecary in Maine. This cordial is full of the flavors of berries, cherries, and flowers that are ripe in Maine in late July.

Makes 1 quart (960 ml)

½ cup (95 g) tart cherries, fresh or thawed
½ cup (95 g) wild blueberries
20 fresh organic aromatic rose petals or 2 tablespoons dried petals
2 tablespoons lavender flowers
Several types of fresh herb sprigs (see the note)
Raw unfiltered honey
Calendula blossoms, for garnishing
Sweet Annie hydrosol, for misting

Place the cherries and blueberries in a small pot with 2 quarts (1.9 liters) of water and bring to a boil. Simmer on medium heat until the fruit breaks down, then use an immersion blender to complete the process. Shut off the heat. Add the rose petals, lavender flowers, and herb sprigs to the pot; cover and allow to steep for 20 to 30 minutes. Strain and add honey to taste. (I recommend 1 tablespoon per 4 ounces / 120 ml of liquid.) Pour into small cocktail or cordial glasses. Garnish with the calendula blossoms and use an atomizer to mist the sweet Annie aromatics on top. This is best drunk gently chilled: Cool in the refrigerator prior to serving, or stir with ice.

NOTE
I use sprigs of St. John's wort, lemon balm, yarrow, peppermint, and mugwort, but feel free to use the aromatic herbs you have available in your garden.

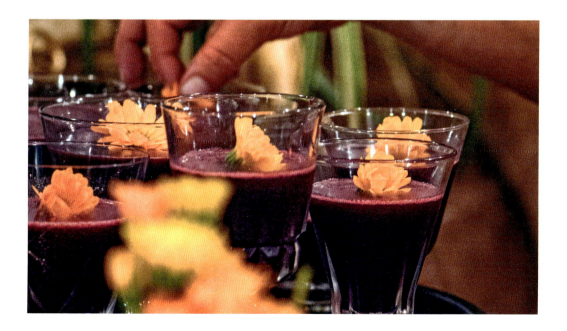

Wildfire Hearts

This drink from the summer 2023 menu I created for the White Barn Inn is an elevated Paloma variation. It is an ode to the wild beach rose growing abundantly on the rocky coast of Maine.

Makes 1 cocktail

1 teaspoon beet powder, for the rim
1 teaspoon hibiscus powder, for the rim
2 ounces (60 ml) Wild Rose Tequila (recipe follows)
1 ounce (30 ml) fresh grapefruit juice
½ ounce (15 ml) Hibiscus Agave (recipe follows)
¼ ounce (7.5 ml) lime juice
1 teaspoon beet juice
Pinch applewood-smoked sea salt
Club soda

FOR GARNISHING

Grapefruit wedge
Confectioners' sugar
Wild rose (*Rosa rugosa*) blossom

Mix together the beet powder and hibiscus powder. Place the powder into a shallow bowl. Put some water in a second shallow bowl. Dip the rim of a collins glass into the water first, then the powder, and then fill the glass with ice. Put the infused tequila, grapefruit juice, Hibiscus Agave, lime juice, beet juice, and sea salt in a shaker tin. Shake and strain over ice into the rimmed glass. Top with club soda.

Prepare the grapefruit wedge by dipping it in confectioners' sugar and heating until charred with a butane torch. Place it on top of the cocktail with a rose for an over-the-top garnish game!

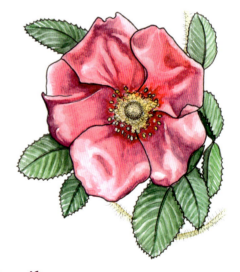

Wild Rose Tequila

Makes 1 bottle

Wild rose petals
Tequila
Mezcal (optional)

Collect wild rose petals and place them in a glass jar. Cover with tequila, or with a 50:50 blend of tequila and Mezcal if you like smoky flavor. Let infuse for at least a week prior to straining and using. This infusion is shelf-stable and does not need to be refrigerated.

Hibiscus Agave

Makes 1 pint (480 ml)

8 ounces (240 ml) hot water
1 tablespoon dried hibiscus
Agave nectar

Make hibiscus tea by pouring the hot water over the dried hibiscus. Let steep for 10 to 15 minutes and then strain. While the tea is still warm, add an equal volume of agave nectar to dissolve. Store this mixture in the refrigerator and use within 1 month.

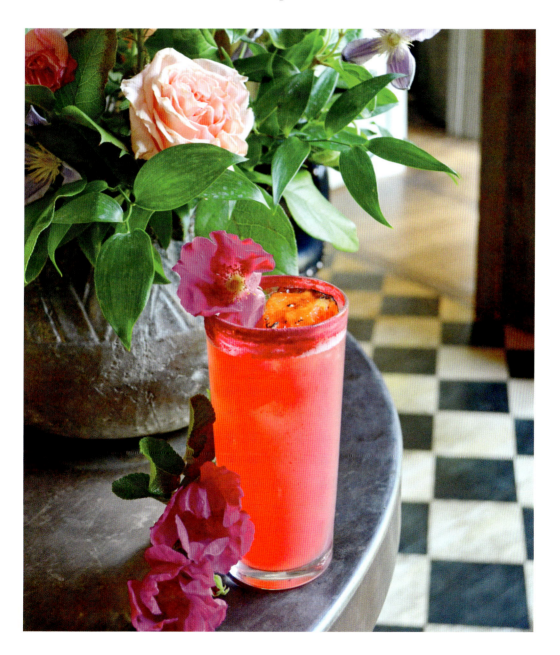

The Visionkeeper

The Visionkeeper features local peaches with honey, vanilla, and spice. The dreamy aromatics of fresh tulsi mingle with mugwort for a vivid, perception-enhancing experience.

Makes 1 cocktail

FOR THE VANILLA GINGER HONEY SYRUP

2 ounces (60 ml) raw, unfiltered honey
1 teaspoon vanilla extract
1 teaspoon ground ginger

FOR THE VISIONKEEPER

1 teaspoon Spicy Pink Salt, for the rim (recipe follows)
1 freestone peach, cut in quarters
1½ ounces (45 ml) Mugwort Infused Gin (recipe follows)
1 ounce (30 ml) lemon juice
1 ounce (30 ml) Vanilla Ginger Honey Syrup
Fresh tulsi sprig, for garnishing

First, make the Vanilla Ginger Honey Syrup. Combine the honey with 2 ounces (60 ml) of warm water in a small jar or glass measuring cup. Allow the honey to dissolve. Add the vanilla extract and ginger powder and stir to incorporate the syrup. Set aside (this is enough syrup to make 4 Visionkeeper drinks).

Put the Spicy Pink Salt into a shallow bowl, and some water in a second shallow bowl. Dip the rim of a cocktail glass first into the water and then into the salt. Muddle (smash) three of the peach quarters at the bottom of a shaker tin. (Set aside the remaining quarter for garnishing.) Add the infused gin, lemon juice, and 1 ounce (30 ml) of the Vanilla Ginger Honey Syrup to the shaker tin. Shake and double-strain into the rimmed glass. Garnish with the fresh tulsi and the last quarter of the peach. If you like, sprinkle some spicy salt on the peach garnish, too!

Spicy Pink Salt

Makes 6 ounces (170 g)

Pink salt
2 teaspoons ground cardamom
2 teaspoons rose petal powder
Cayenne powder

Fill a 6-ounce bowl with pink salt and add 2 teaspoons each ground cardamom and rose petal powder. Also add ½ teaspoon cayenne (or more if you would like it spicier). Mix the spices gently with the salt. Store leftover salt in a cool, dry place.

Mugwort Infused Gin

Makes 1 bottle

Fresh mugwort (*Artemisia vulgaris*) leaves and flowers or dried mugwort
Gin

Pick fresh mugwort preferably when it's flowering in late summer or early fall. Chop up the fresh flowering herb and fill a quart Mason jar three-quarters of the way full. If fresh mugwort is not available, you can use dried, but fill the jar only halfway. Cover the plant material with gin. Let infuse for at least a week prior to straining and using. This infusion is shelf-stable and does not need to be refrigerated.

NOTE
I use Barr Hill Gin, as it is made with raw unfiltered honey.

Gates of Immortality

Reishi mushroom has been used as an elixir of immortality for more than a thousand years in Traditional Chinese Medicine. In this apothecary variation on the traditional Whiskey Smash, the antioxidant and anti-inflammatory power of dark berries and mint, as well as the graceful wild beauty of elder and hawthorn, are the perfect complement to the reishi.

Makes 1 cocktail

Handful mixed fruit: wild blueberries, raspberries, and sweet cherries
1½ ounces (45 ml) bourbon
1 ounce (30 ml) fresh lemon juice
½ ounce (15 ml) honey syrup
¼ ounce (7.5 ml) elderflower liqueur
1 dropperful Reishi Tincture (recipe follows)
Several drops Hawthorn Flower Essence (recipe follows)
Club soda
2 sprigs fresh peppermint, for garnishing

Muddle (smash) the berries and cherries in a shaker tin and then add the bourbon, lemon juice, honey syrup, liqueur, Reishi Tincture, and flower essence. Shake it all up and double-strain into a collins glass or Mason jar over ice. Top with the club soda. Give the mint sprigs a little fondle or clap before placing them as a garnish.

NOTE
You can substitute hawthorn tincture if you did not make any hawthorn flower essence in the springtime.

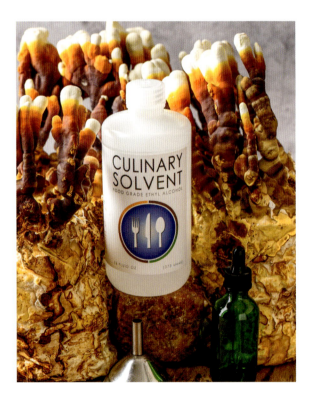

This was a fun project, growing mushrooms on my kitchen countertop and then making double-extracted Reishi Tincture using reishi fruiting blocks from North Spore.

Reishi Tincture

Mushrooms contain both polysaccharides, which are water-soluble, and beta-glucans, which are alcohol-soluble. Because of this, I make a double extraction tincture to capture both components. Basically, you make two extracts to combine together.

Makes 1 pint (480 ml)
Fresh reishi mushroom, chopped
95 percent ethanol

Chop fresh reishi mushroom to fill a ½-pint jar and cover with 95 percent ethanol. Also begin drying some reishi mushrooms for the water-based decoction. Let the mushrooms in ethanol sit to extract for 4 weeks, shaking occasionally. By the time the alcohol tincture is ready to be strained and pressed, the mushrooms will be dry and ready to extract in water. Add the dried mushrooms to a slow cooker with enough water to cover. Heat on high for 1 to 2 hours, then lower the temperature and let simmer for about 8 hours. Strain the hot extract. Combine the alcohol tincture and water extract at a 50:50 ratio.

Hawthorn Flower Essence

Makes 1 pint (480 ml)
Hawthorn blossoms
Well water or spring water
Brandy

The process of making a flower essence is an integral part of its medicine. The process involves meditating and resonating with the flower in its environment. For the essence, you will gather hawthorn (*Crataegus* spp.) blossoms, which open in springtime in Maine around the same time as apple blossoms.

On a sunny day, prepare a small glass bowl of well or spring water and check to be sure that your garden clippers are clean. Sit with the hawthorn tree and observe its blooms bustling with bees. Breathe and meditate with the tree for 10 to 20 minutes. Then, without touching the flowers, use the clippers to cut a small bunch of them into the glass bowl. Place the bowl under the tree and leave it sitting there for several hours. When you return to gather the flowers' essence, bring along a little brandy, a funnel, and a dark-amber bottle. Using the funnel, fill the amber bottle halfway with the magic water from the glass bowl. Then fill to the top with brandy.

Fields of Gold Mead

This recipe tastes like an August stroll through a meadow of blooming goldenrod in Maine. Mead is my favorite way to put up the abundant flavors of summertime. There is nothing quite like opening a bottle of this mead in the wintertime, with aromas representing the wild places you frolicked through in the season past.

Makes 1 gallon (3.8 liters)

2 quarts (140 g) mixed huckleberries, blackberries, and wild blueberries
1 bunch sweetfern (*Comptonia peregrina*)
1 bunch flowering goldenrod (*Solidago canadensis*)
3 pounds (1.4 kg) raw unfiltered honey
Champagne yeast

Use a food-safe sanitizer to sanitize a 1-gallon glass carboy with an air lock, and set the carboy aside. Bring 1 gallon (3.8 liters) of water to a boil in a large pot. Add the berries to the water. (Set a handful of berries aside if you plan to capture yeast, as described in the sidebar.)

Simmer the berries for about 10 minutes, using an immersion blender to emulsify. Pull leaves and flowers off the stems of the sweetfern and goldenrod and add them to the pot. Shut off the heat and cover. Steep for 10 minutes.

Strain the hot fruit-herb tea into another large clean pot. Add the honey to dissolve. Use a large glass measuring cup to transfer the fruity honey syrup into the carboy. Let cool to room temperature, put in the yeast, and cover with the air lock (filled to the marked line with water).

The speed of fermentation depends on temperature, but you should begin to see some bubbling action in the bottle that will create larger bubbles in the air lock within a day or two. The bubbling will increase, peak, and then die off as the yeast consumes the available sugars in the fruity syrup. When you no longer see the air lock bubble, the transformation into mead is complete. Either screw on the cap of the carboy or transfer the mead into swing-top glass bottles. Burp the bottles occasionally after bottling to check pressure.

CAUTION
Do not bottle the mead prematurely, or the pressure as fermentation proceeds can cause the liquid to spurt up out of the bottles, which can stain the ceiling!

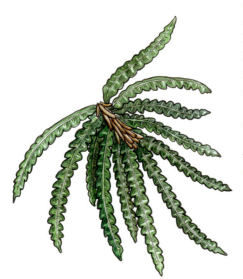

How to Capture Wild Yeast

You can use wild yeast in your mead making rather than buying champagne yeast. I have been brewing for years, so wild yeast strains are alive and well in the air of my apartment. You will need to plan ahead, as it takes about a week to capture the yeast.

Place a handful of unwashed fresh wild berries in a glass jar. Squish the berries, and then cover them with water and add a couple of tablespoons of any kind of sugar. Cover the jar with a cloth and let it sit on the countertop at room temperature for about a week. Stir and check up on it every couple of days to see if it is activating.

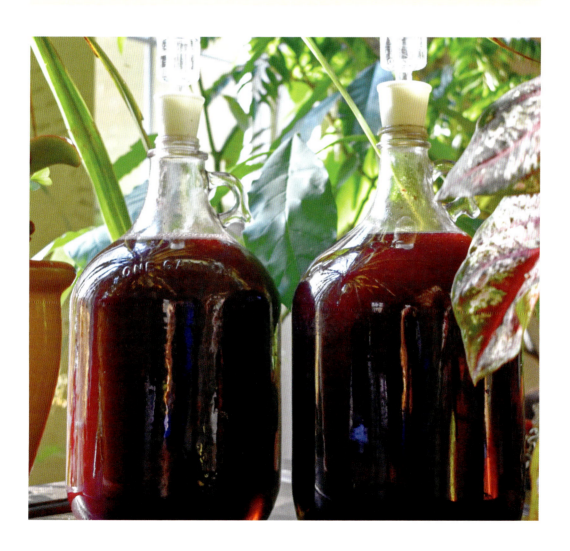

"Fields of Gold" Mead Spritzer

Here's a basic spritzer recipe that features homemade Fields of Gold Mead. You can substitute any mead or wine of your choice. I usually try a little bit of mead upon bottling and drink it in the garden in the late summer to celebrate harvest season.

Makes 1 drink

3 ounces (90 ml) mead
5 ounces (150 ml) club soda
½ ounce (15 ml) lemon juice (optional)
Fresh blackberries, for garnishing
1 sprig goldenrod, for garnishing

Build this drink by combining the mead, club soda, and lemon juice in a wineglass with ice. Garnish with a few blackberries and the goldenrod sprig, and serve with a straw.

Effervescence: Rising to the Occasion

What makes bubbles? Why are some fermented beverages naturally fizzy and not others? The bubbles are carbon dioxide gas resulting from the breakdown of carbohydrates or sugars, usually by yeast. When a bottle is corked or sealed, often some fermentation and breakdown continue, and the gas is trapped. A little is good, but too much can cause unwanted explosive escape!

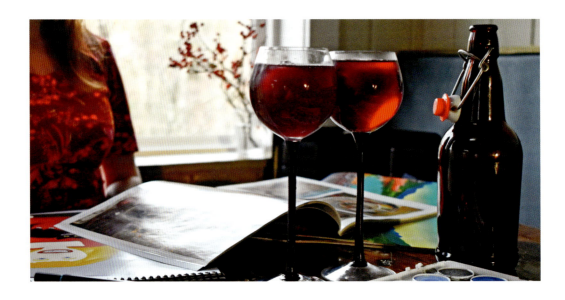

Recipes through the Seasons

Kava Hula Girl

antispasmodic • hypnotic • nervine • nootropic • nutritive • relaxant

This one is a showstopper! I served this delicious creamy nervine tonic in the hull of a local Maine melon.

Makes 2-plus servings

1 quart (960 ml) coconut milk
3 tablespoons (15 g) kava root
1 tablespoon cinnamon chips
1 tablespoon sunflower lecithin powder
4 ounces (120 ml) maple syrup
1 ounce (30 ml) culinary-grade rose water, plus more for misting
Whole, ripe muskmelon
Freshly grated nutmeg, for garnishing
Vanilla extract, for misting
1 blooming sunflower head, for garnishing

Combine the coconut milk and 1 cup (240 ml) of water in a small pot and heat until just under boiling. Add the kava root and cinnamon chips. Simmer at medium-high for 20 minutes. Strain into a blender pitcher and add the sunflower lecithin, maple syrup, and rose water. Cut the melon in half. Remove the seeds and then scrape the melon pulp into the blender as well, but set aside the hulls—they will be your serving vessels. After fully blending, pour the resulting thick liquid into the hollow melon rinds. Garnish with the grated nutmeg. Combine the vanilla extract and more rose water in equal parts in an atomizer and mist the surface of the drink. Cut the sunflower head in half and prop it on edge as decoration.

NOTE
Lecithin is a foaming agent that has both hydrophilic and lipophilic aspects, so it also acts as an emulsifier. Sunflower lecithin is typically non-GMO and is a source of phosphatidylcholine, which has possible positive effects for digestion, cognition, cholesterol balance, and liver health.

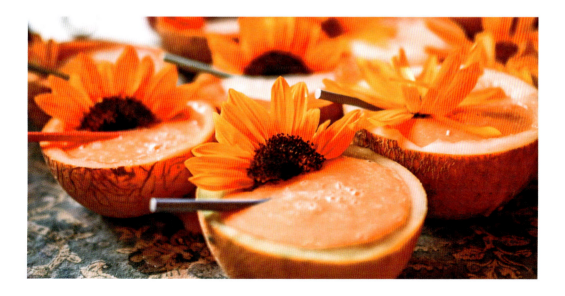

Elderflower Collins

This elderflower series is inspired by my dear friend Carol, who is a wise and feisty woman in her eighties with a very green thumb. The girls and I often go to Carol's house to harvest medicinal herbs and sit among the plants, chatting over a glass of wine and basking in the glory of her garden!

Makes 2 cocktails

Fresh mint leaves
2 ounces (60 ml) vodka
1½ ounces (45 ml) lemon juice
1 ounce (30 ml) elderflower liqueur
3 ounces (90 ml) club soda
4 ounces (120 ml) Carol's Elderflower Champagne (recipe follows)
Fresh elderflowers, for garnishing

Fill a burgundy or goblet-style glass with ice. Tear the mint leaves and place in the bottom of the glass. Add the vodka, lemon juice, elderflower liqueur, club soda, and champagne, stirring gently to incorporate. Garnish with fresh elderflowers.

Carol's Elderflower Champagne

Makes 1 bottle

¾ cup (180 ml) honey
6 large elderflowers
2 organic lemons

Bring 1 cup (240 ml) of water to a boil, add to the honey, and allow to dissolve. Set aside. Strip the lacy white elderflowers into 7 cups (1.7 liters) of water in a ½-gallon Mason jar. Peel the lemons and chop the zest. Juice the pulp and add the juice and zest to the jar. Add the liquefied honey, cover the jar with a piece of fabric, and secure it with a rubber band. The flowers and zest should be fully covered by the liquid in the jar to prevent molding. Let sit at room temperature. The mixture will become fizzy within a few days from the natural yeast present on the flowers. After 1 week, transfer to a swing-top bottle and refrigerate. Drink within 1 month.

Mojito Popsicles

A cocktail-flavored popsicle that is refreshing and relaxing on a hot day. Plus, each one boasts a bonus of electrolytes. A great way to recharge when you overheat.

Makes 6 Popsicles

2 tablespoons fresh spearmint leaf or 1 tablespoon dried leaf
Fresh mint sprigs
1 cup (240 ml) coconut water
¼ cup (60 ml) lime juice
2 tablespoons elderflower liqueur
Pinch sea salt

Brew spearmint tea by pouring 1 cup (240 ml) of boiling water over the spearmint leaf. Steep, covered, for 15 minutes. Strain and let the tea cool to room temperature. Place a mint sprig in each of the cavities of a Popsicle mold. Mix ¾ cup (180 ml) of the spearmint tea with the coconut water, lime juice, liqueur, and salt in a pitcher, then pour the mix into the molds. Put Popsicle sticks in place and freeze until solid.

Crimes of Passion

Passionflower, green coffee, and vanilla dance with sea buckthorn and tulsi on long summer nights. Fruity, floral, and fun!

Makes 1 cocktail

FOR THE MIXED FRUIT PURÉE
⅓ cup (80 ml) sea buckthorn purée
⅓ cup (80 ml) mango purée
⅓ cup (80 ml) passionfruit purée
½ teaspoon turmeric powder

FOR THE CRIMES OF PASSION
Popping candy, for the rim
Passionflower, edible orchid, or whatever edible flower you have available, for garnishing
Passionflower (*Passiflora* spp.) vine clipping, for garnishing (optional)
2 ounces (60 ml) vanilla bean vodka
2 ounces (60 ml) Mixed Fruit Purée
1 ounce (30 ml) very simple syrup (1:1 sugar and water)
2 dropperfuls Tulsi Glycerite (recipe follows)
1 dropperful Green Coffee Tincture (recipe follows)
1 teaspoon orange blossom water

To make the Mixed Fruit Purée: Put the purées and the turmeric powder in a blender and blend until the powder is incorporated. (This is enough to make four Crimes of Passion cocktails.) Set aside.

Put a small amount of popping candy in a shallow bowl and some water in a separate shallow bowl. Rim your chosen Martini glass with the popping candy by first dipping the rim of the glass in water, then the candy. Clip the passionflower and vine onto the glass with a tiny clothespin. Set the glass aside.

Shake the vanilla bean vodka, Mixed Fruit Purée, simple syrup, Tulsi Glycerite, Green Coffee Tincture, and orange blossom water in a shaker with ice and strain into the rimmed glass. Serve up!

NOTES
For the popping candy, I use Culinary Crystals Unflavored Popping Candy. Or you can try making your own.

I use Cold River Vodka, which is distilled from Maine potatoes.

The tulsi glycerite may be purchased rather than made from scratch.

Tulsi Glycerite

Makes 8 ounces (240 ml)
8 ounces (240 ml) food-grade glycerin
Fresh flowering tulsi (*Ocimum sanctum*)

Put the food-grade glycerin in a blender with a large handful of fresh flowering tulsi. Blend on low until fully incorporated. Transfer to an 8-ounce glass jar. Let infuse for 2 to 4 weeks, then strain and bottle into a tincture bottle.

Green Coffee Tincture

Makes 4 ounces (120 ml)

Green (unroasted) coffee beans
Overproof rum

Fill a 4-ounce glass jar with green coffee beans. Cover with overproof rum. Let infuse for 2 to 4 weeks and strain into a tincture bottle.

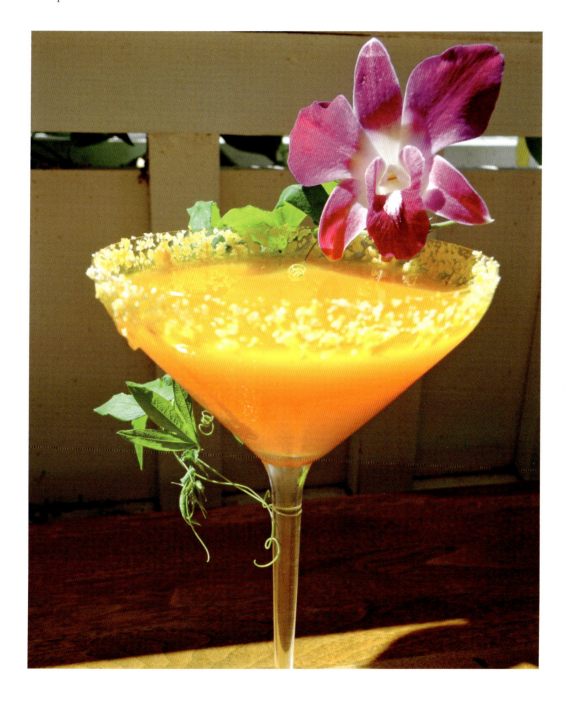

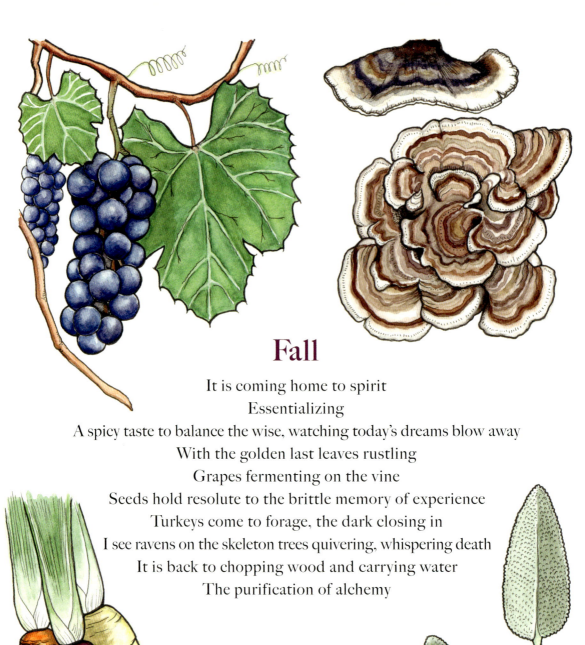

Fall

It is coming home to spirit
Essentializing
A spicy taste to balance the wise, watching today's dreams blow away
With the golden last leaves rustling
Grapes fermenting on the vine
Seeds hold resolute to the brittle memory of experience
Turkeys come to forage, the dark closing in
I see ravens on the skeleton trees quivering, whispering death
It is back to chopping wood and carrying water
The purification of alchemy

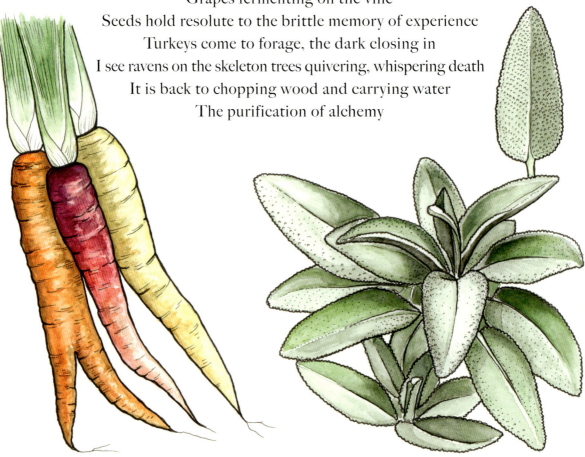

Recipes through the Seasons

"Elderberry Sour"

antioxidant • antiviral • immune tonic

A tasty tea-tini to sip on as the threat of cold and flu season approaches. This tonic tastes like a medicinal lemonade.

Makes 1 drink

1 tablespoon tulsi (*Ocimum sanctum*)
1 teaspoon hyssop (*Hyssopus officinalis*)
1½ ounces (45 ml) lemon juice
1½ ounces (45 ml) Chai-Spiced Elderberry Syrup (page 146)
1 dropperful elecampane tincture (optional)
Absinthe, for rinsing (optional)
1 sage sprig, for garnishing

Pour 8 ounces (240 ml) of hot water over the tulsi and hyssop in a tea press or jar. Steep, covered, for 10 to 15 minutes. Strain and allow to cool to room temperature.

Shake 6 ounces (180 ml) of the cooled tulsi-hyssop tea with the lemon juice, elderberry syrup, and elecampane tincture (if using) vigorously with ice. Strain into a coupe glass rinsed with absinthe. Garnish with the sage sprig.

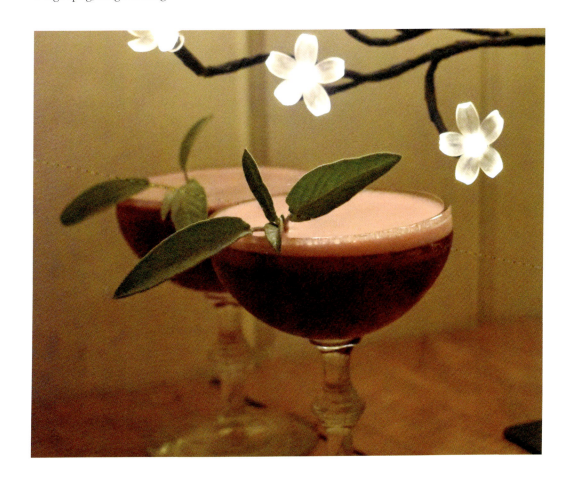

Dreaming with Morpheus

nervine • oneirogen • relaxant

Did you know that your body makes its own morphine, which plays a role in relaxation and pain perception? Named after Morpheus, the Greek god of dreams, this tonic is a trifecta, offering relaxant effects across three systems, binding to the body's natural opiate receptors and to GABA receptors and interacting with the endocannabinoid system.

Caution: Do not combine this drink with alcohol or opiates.

Makes 1 drink

FOR THE DREAMER'S TEA
Pinch dried California poppy
Pinch dried butterfly pea
Pinch dried mugwort
Pinch dried lavender

FOR THE DREAMING WITH MORPHEUS
2 ounces (60 ml) club soda
6 ounces (180 ml) Dreamer's Tea
1 dropperful Wild Lettuce Tincture (recipe follows)
5 mg hemp-derived CBD
½ ounce (15 ml) lemon juice
½ ounce (15 ml) Cinnamon-Vanilla Honey Syrup (recipe follows)
¼ teaspoon almond extract
¼ teaspoon orange flower water
½ ounce (15 ml) heavy cream
1 egg white
Poppy seeds, for garnishing

Brew the Dreamer's Tea: Put the dried herbs into a tea press and cover with 16 ounces (480 ml) of hot water. Stir and place a lid on the press. Let steep for 10 minutes. Strain the tea and set aside.

Fill a collins glass with ice, add the club soda, and set aside. In a shaker tin, combine 6 ounces of the Dreamer's Tea along with the Wild Lettuce Tincture, CBD, lemon juice, honey syrup, almond extract, orange flower water, heavy cream, and egg white. Because this tonic is a fizz, it requires a lot of shaking (total of 3 to 4 minutes). Shake it first without ice and then with. Strain the very foamy mix into the collins glass. Top with a sprinkle of poppy seeds.

NOTES
For a 100 percent alcohol-free version of this recipe, make a vinegar tincture of the wild lettuce, or leave out the tincture altogether.

I recommend using a farm-to-bottle CBD product rather than one made from an isolate. I use CBD oils from Rooted Heart Remedies and Sunsoil. The important thing is to seek out a product made from whole plants, not from an isolate.

Wild Lettuce Tincture

Makes 4 ounces (120 ml)

85 percent ethanol
15 percent vinegar
Fresh wild lettuce (*Lactuca virosa*) flowering tops, finely chopped

Use 85 percent ethanol, 15 percent vinegar for extracting the alkaloids from fresh flowering tops of *Lactuca virosa*. For 4 ounces (120 ml), this is roughly 3½ ounces (105 ml) of alcohol for the solvent and ½ ounce (15 ml) of vinegar. Fill a 4-ounce jar halfway full with finely chopped plant material and cover with the alcohol-vinegar mix and then a non-corrosive lid. Macerate for 4 weeks. Strain, then transfer to a tincture bottle.

Cinnamon-Vanilla Honey Syrup

Makes 1 pint (480 ml)

3 cinnamon sticks
1 cup (240 ml) raw unfiltered honey
Pinch sea salt
2 vanilla beans, scraped (see the note, page 127)

Heat 2 cups (480 ml) of water, add the cinnamon, and simmer for 30 minutes, adding more water if necessary. After simmering, there should be about 1 cup (240 ml) of cinnamon tea. Strain into a measuring glass. Add the honey and dissolve. Add the sea salt and vanilla seeds. This syrup will keep up to a month in the refrigerator.

The Queen's Fortress

aromatic • hypnotic • nervine • relaxant

This is the ultimate nervine trophorestorative to assist with burnout and nervous system exhaustion. Because this tonic has sedative effects, it's best to drink it shortly before bed. Good hot or cold, it feels like a hug and a blanket in a glass!

Makes 1 drink

FOR THE ASHWAGANDHA DECOCTION
1 tablespoon ashwagandha root powder
Pinch ground cinnamon
Pinch ground cloves

FOR THE QUEEN'S FORTRESS
8 ounces (240 ml) Ashwagandha Decoction
4 ounces (120 ml) oat milk
¾ ounce (22.5 ml) maple syrup
½ teaspoon licorice root
½ ounce (15 ml) tulsi hydrosol
1 dropperful Skullcap Glycerite (recipe follows)
1 dropperful Milky Oat Tincture (recipe follows)
1 dropperful passionflower tincture
1 dropperful Wild Rose Elixir (page 139)
1 dropperful or 5 mg CBD
Whole nutmeg, for garnishing
Fresh tulsi, for garnishing (optional)

Begin by making the Ashwagandha Decoction. Add the ashwagandha powder to 8 ounces (240 ml) of water and simmer for 5 minutes on medium-high heat. Add the cinnamon and cloves. If you plan to serve the Queen's Fortress warm, also add the oat milk and maple syrup to the hot decoction and allow it all to warm. Then remove from the heat and add the licorice root, tulsi hydrosol, Skullcap Glycerite, Milky Oat Tincture, passionflower tincture, Wild Rose Elixir, and CBD. Use a hand blender to froth. Pour into a mug and garnish with freshly grated nutmeg.

If you'll be drinking this cool, let the Ashwagandha Decoction cool, and then transfer it into a mixing glass with ice. Add the rest of the ingredients, stir, and strain into a cocktail glass. Garnish with grated nutmeg and a sprig of tulsi.

NOTE
You can substitute dried cut and sifted ashwagandha root for the ashwagandha powder, but allow it to steep for 15 minutes.

Skullcap Glycerite

Makes 4 ounces (120 ml)

Fresh skullcap (*Scutellaria lateriflora*) flowering tops

Food-grade vegetable glycerin

Chop fresh flowering tops of skullcap and place in a 4-ounce glass jar. Fill the jar three-quarters of the way full with chopped plant material and cover with food-grade vegetable glycerin. Cover the jar and let macerate for 4 weeks before straining and bottling in a tincture bottle. Glycerites should be stored in a cool, dry place and used within 1 year.

Milky Oat Tincture

Milky oats are the supreme nervous system tonic. They come from the same plant—*Avena sativa*—as the oatmeal we eat for breakfast, but for milky oats, *A. sativa* is harvested when the seed is milky when squished (not hard). It is very important to use fresh milky oat tops for this tincture.

Makes 4 ounces (120 ml)

Milky oats

Overproof spirit

Fill a 4-ounce jar halfway with milky oats and cover with overproof spirit. Transfer to a blender to whiz it up until all the seeds are broken, then put the mixture back in the jar. Add more alcohol if needed to make sure all the plant matter is covered. Place a lid on the jar. Let this extract for 4 weeks, shaking occasionally. Strain into a tincture bottle for easy use.

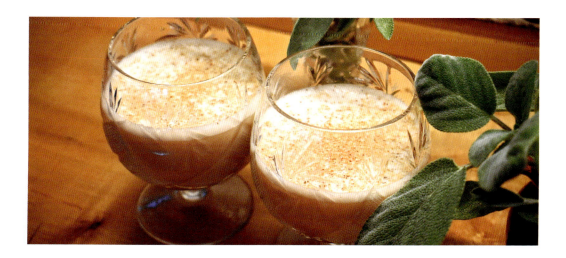

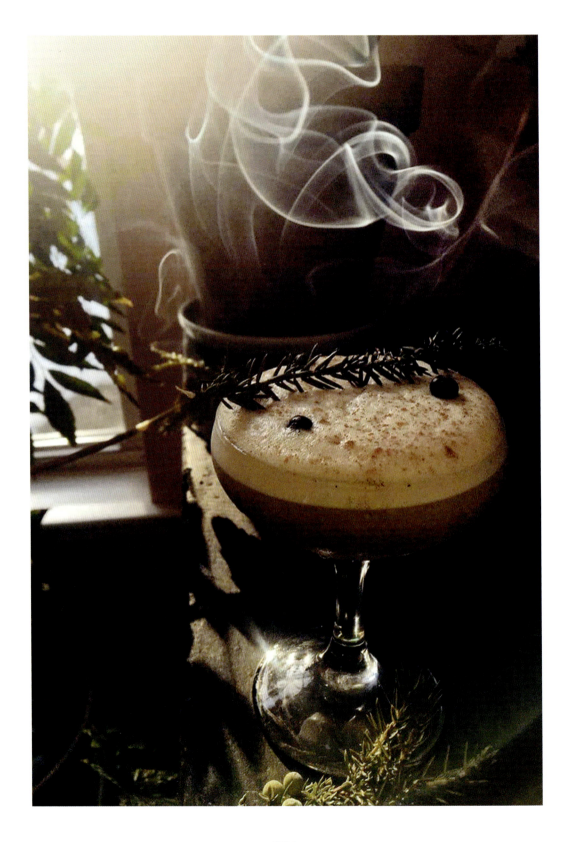

Recipes through the Seasons

The Common Sage

antioxidant • aromatic • carminative • nervine • nootropic

Drink sage to be sage. This wise mint family plant will help you focus. Garden sage is a nootropic, enhancing cognitive function through its antioxidant properties.

Makes 1 drink

6 ounces (180 ml) brewed Earl Grey tea
4 ounces (120 ml) Lavender Sage Honey Tea Syrup (recipe follows)
2 ounces (60 ml) oat milk
½ ounce (15 ml) lemon juice
1 egg white
¼ ounce (7.5 ml) juniper hydrosol, or ½ ounce (15 ml) juniper berry tea, or several drops juniper extract
1–2 dropperfuls rhodiola tincture
Pinch ground cinnamon
Whole nutmeg, for garnishing
Small sprig dried juniper, for garnishing

Brew some Earl Grey tea and allow it to cool. Put 6 ounces of the tea in a shaker tin with the Lavender Sage Honey Tea Syrup, oat milk, lemon juice, egg white, juniper hydrosol, rhodiola tincture, and cinnamon. Shake first without ice, then with ice. Strain into a coupe. Grate some nutmeg over the surface of the drink. Light the juniper sprig on fire, and when the flame dies but the sprig is still smoldering, place it across the top of the glass and serve.

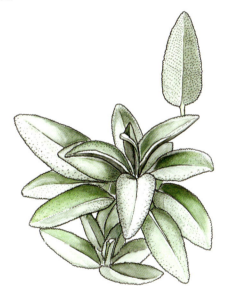

Lavender Sage Honey Tea Syrup

Makes 1 cup (240 ml)

1 tablespoon dried sage or 2 tablespoons fresh
1 tablespoon lavender flowers
Raw unfiltered honey

Pour 8 ounces (240 ml) of hot water over the sage and lavender in a teapot or jar. Cover and steep for 15 minutes. Strain and add honey to taste (make it slightly sweeter than you would want to drink plain).

Juicy

antioxidant • beauty • nervine • nutritive • tissue tonic

As the name suggests, this tonic is meant to promote juiciness—healthy, supple tissues and a youthful glow. Pretty in pink plus vitamins, minerals, and antioxidants. Gentle astringents tone tissues while the rose is the full embodiment of beauty with boundaries.

Makes 1 drink

- 6 ounces (180 ml) Raspberry Leaf and Gotu Kola Tea (recipe follows)
- 2 ounces (60 ml) unsweetened cranberry juice
- 1½ ounces (45 ml) Hawthorn Rose Hip Honey (recipe follows)
- ¼ ounce (7.5 ml) culinary-grade rose water
- 9 drops yarrow tincture or flower essence
- 15 drops Schisandra Tincture (recipe follows) or 1 teaspoon schisandra berry powder dissolved in water

Combine all ingredients in a cocktail shaker with ice and shake it up. Strain into a coupe glass.

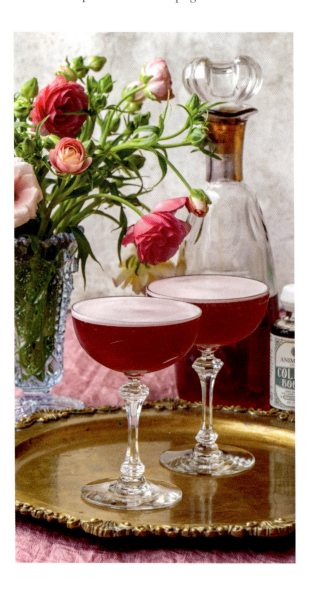

Raspberry Leaf & Gotu Kola Tea

This tea requires a long infusion time to extract the minerals from the raspberry leaves.

Makes 1 cup (240 ml)

1 tablespoon dried raspberry leaves
1 tablespoon gotu kola

Pour 1 cup (240 ml) of boiling water over the raspberry leaves and gotu kola in a ceramic or glass vessel. Cover and allow to infuse for at least 1 hour, and then strain.

Hawthorn Rose Hip Honey

Makes 2 cups (480 ml)

½ cup (50 g) fresh hawthorn (*Crataegus* spp.) berries
½ cup (65 g) rose hips
2 cups (480 ml) raw unfiltered honey

Pulverize the hawthorn berries and rose hips in a mortar and pestle. Transfer into a jar and cover with the honey. Let infuse for 2 to 6 weeks. Store in a covered jar in a cool dark place. When you're ready to use, dissolve the mixture into 2 cups hot water (480 ml) and strain.

Schisandra Tincture

It's ideal to make this tincture from fresh schisandra berries, but they can be hard to find—the vines take as long as seven years from planting to begin bearing fruit.

Makes 4 ounces (120 ml)

Fresh or dried schisandra berries
Overproof spirit

Fill a 4-ounce glass jar with fresh or dried schisandra berries. Cover completely with overproof spirits. Transfer to a blender and pulse, then transfer back to the jar and let extract for 4 to 6 weeks. Shake the jar daily or whenever you think of it. Strain and bottle into a tincture bottle.

Upside-Down Storm

anti-inflammatory • carminative • nutritive • stimulant

Have you ever had a Dark and Stormy? This is the best nonalcoholic version I've come up with!

Makes 1 drink

1 ounce (30 ml) "Rum-Spiced" Molasses (page 167)
6 ounces (180 ml) Ginger Beer (recipe follows)
¾ ounce (22.5 ml) lime juice
1–2 ounces (30–60 ml) club soda
Crystallized ginger, for garnishing
Pineapple sage sprig, for garnishing (optional)

Build in a rocks glass with ice, beginning with the "Rum-Spiced" Molasses and then adding the Ginger Beer, lime juice, and club soda. Swizzle gently and garnish with the crystallized ginger on a cocktail pick, balanced on the rim of the glass. Add a sprig of aromatic pineapple sage if desired.

Ginger Beer

All you need for naturally fermented ginger beer is water, sugar, organic ginger, and time.

Makes 1 pint (480 ml)

½ cup plus 2 tablespoons (125 g) organic sugar
2 tablespoons finely chopped unpeeled gingerroot
4 tablespoons diced gingerroot
1 ounce (30 ml) lime juice
Pinch salt

First make a ginger "bug" by adding 2 tablespoons of the organic sugar and the finely chopped ginger to 2 cups (480 ml) of water in a glass jar. Cover with a piece of fabric, securing with a rubber band or metal canning jar ring.

Let this mixture activate (ferment) for a few days, and then prepare the beer. Simmer the diced ginger in 1 quart (960 ml) of water on medium-high heat for 20 minutes, adding more water if necessary. Strain out the ginger and add the remaining ½ cup (100 g) of the sugar to dissolve. Also strain the ginger bug.

Allow the sweetened ginger tea to cool to room temperature, then add the strained ginger bug. Add the lime juice and salt. Bottle into swing-top bottles and refrigerate.

Recipes through the Seasons

Harvest Gold

adaptogen • carminative • immune tonic • nutritive

I make this sensational hot drink with organic heirloom apple cider, which is basically pure gold. It is mulled with adaptogens, immune tonics, and chai spices. Quintessentially autumnal.

Makes 3 quarts (2.8 liters)

- 1½ quarts (1.4 liters) organic apple cider made from heirloom apple varieties
- 7 astragalus root slices
- 5 turkey tail mushrooms
- 4 tablespoons hawthorn (*Crataegus* spp.) berries
- 3 cinnamon sticks (preferably Ceylon cinnamon)
- 1 tablespoon cardamom pods
- 4 tablespoons dried elderberries
- 5 fresh gingerroot slices
- 1 tablespoon star anise

In a medium-sized pot, combine the cider with all of the remaining ingredients. Bring to a boil, then simmer on medium-high for 40 to 60 minutes, adding up to a quart (liter) of water as it boils off. Pour over a small strainer as you are serving.

NOTE

I prefer to make this recipe in a Crock-Pot when time allows, because the longer infusion time produces a richer-tasting cider. Put all ingredients in the slow cooker and set on high for about 1 hour. Then switch to low and continue heating for 6 to 8 hours. This technique also allows you to keep the mix warm for the duration of a special occasion.

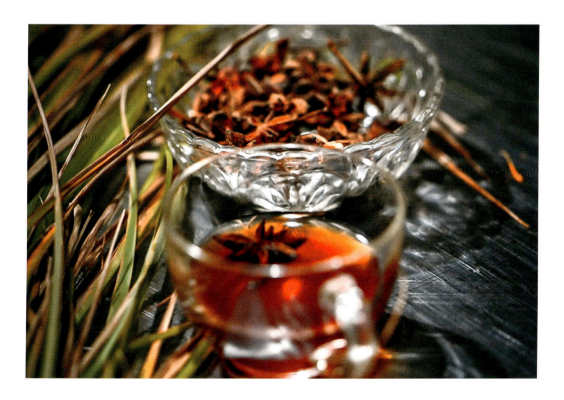

Botanical Bar Craft

Sultry Look

carminative • nutritive • stimulant

Meet me at the orchard at dusk and we can share a sultry look while placing apples in our baskets. Sweet with just the right amount of smoke and spice that might inspire us to build a bonfire.

Makes 1 pint (480 ml)

FOR THE GINGER-CINNAMON CIDER

16 ounces (480 ml) raw unfiltered local apple cider
Several cinnamon sticks
Several slices fresh ginger

FOR THE SULTRY LOOK

Applewood-smoked sea salt
8 ounces (240 ml) Ginger-Cinnamon Cider
½ ounce (15 ml) lemon juice
¼ ounce (7.5 ml) maple syrup
¼ teaspoon vanilla extract
5 ml or 5 dashes smoke bitters
Nasturtium flower, for garnishing

First make the Ginger-Cinnamon Cider: Combine the cider, cinnamon sticks, and fresh ginger with 1 cup (240 ml) of water in a pot on medium-high heat and mull for 15 to 20 minutes. Allow to cool.

To make a Sultry Look, first rim a rocks glass with salt. Put some of the smoked salt in a shallow dish and some water in a second shallow dish. Dip the rim of the glass in the water, then in the salt. Fill the rimmed glass with ice. Put 8 ounces (240 ml) of the Ginger-Cinnamon Cider along with the lemon juice, maple syrup, vanilla extract, and smoke bitters into a shaker tin with more ice and a little pinch of the smoked salt. Shake and strain into the glass. Garnish with the nasturtium flower.

NOTES

To make this drink completely alcohol-free, substitute 1 ounce (30 ml) strongly brewed Lapsang Souchong tea for the bitters.

I use Upta Camp Sea Salt from the Slack Tide Maine company in York and Vena's Fizz House Smoke Bitters.

Euphoria

This is an Espresso Martini made with smoky tequila and the heart-opening aphrodisiacs cacao and damiana. You can make the salted caramel ahead of time to have on hand for garnishing this yummy drink.

Makes 1 drink

1½ ounces (45 ml) Lovers' Tequila (recipe follows)
1 ounce (30 ml) espresso
½ ounce (15 ml) agave syrup
½ ounce (15 ml) heavy cream
2 ml Cardamom Bitters (page 159)
3 fresh raspberries, preferably organic
2 teaspoons Sea-Salted Agave Caramel (recipe follows), for garnishing

Shake the tequila, espresso, agave syrup, heavy cream, and Cardamom Bitters with ice and then strain into a small cocktail glass. Place the raspberries onto a cocktail pick and set it across the top of glass (as shown in the photo of this cocktail on page 48). Drizzle the berries with your caramel. Yum!

Lovers' Tequila

Makes 9-plus ounces (270-plus ml) (enough for 3 drinks)

¼ cup (40 g) chopped raw cacao paste
2 tablespoons damiana leaf
5 ounces (150 ml) reposado tequila
5 ounces (150 ml) Mezcal

Place the cacao paste and damiana in a pint jar and add the tequila and Mezcal to cover. Let infuse for at least 1 week prior to straining.

Sea-Salted Agave Caramel

Makes 2 cups (480 ml)

1 cup (240 ml) agave nectar
½ cup (120 ml) heavy whipping cream
10 tablespoons (142 g) unsalted butter
5 teaspoons sea salt

Place the agave and whipping cream in a medium saucepan and bring to a boil. Boil for about 5 minutes, then remove from the heat and stir in the butter and salt. Transfer to a heatproof container and allow to cool prior to storing in the refrigerator.

Botanical Bar Craft

Siren Call

antioxidant • aperitif • carminative • nervine • nutritive

The rocky coast of Maine with all of its secret inlets is the inspiration for the Siren Call: a mysterious and salty elixir. "Their song is no passing fancy, but a penetrating power, potent enough to break the will of the strongest man."—Homer, *The Odyssey*

Makes 1 drink

FOR THE ANISE HYSSOP & BLUEBERRY LEAF TEA

1 tablespoon anise hyssop (*Agastache foeniculum*)
1 tablespoon blueberry leaves

FOR THE SIREN CALL

2 ounces (60 ml) Anise Hyssop and Blueberry Leaf Tea
2 ounces (60 ml) Seafarer's Oxymel (recipe follows)
1 ounce (30 ml) Beet Kvass (recipe follows)
Large ice cube
2 ounces (60 ml) club soda
1 star anise, for garnishing

First brew the Anise Hyssop and Blueberry Leaf Tea: Pour 8 ounces (240 ml) of hot water over the anise hyssop and blueberry leaves and stir briefly. Cover to keep in the aromatics. Infuse for 20 minutes, then strain the tea (makes enough for about 4 Siren Call drinks). Allow to cool.

In a mixing glass, combine 2 ounces of the tea with the Seafarer's Oxymel, the Beet Kvass, and ice and stir. Put a large ice cube into a rocks glass and strain the mixture into the glass. Top with the club soda and place the star anise on the top of the ice cube. (See the photo of this drink on page 30.)

NOTE

Blueberry leaves don't grow on trees, but you can find them at a local blueberry farm! At the time I formulated this cocktail, blueberry bushes here in Maine had already dropped their leaves. So I bought the leaves from Fields Fields Blueberries, a blueberry grower in Dresden, Maine.

Seafarer's Oxymel

I use beach bay (*Myrica pensylvanica*), also called northern bayberry, to make this oxymel, but you can substitute a different pungent, aromatic edible herb native to the coastal area nearest to where you live. Or regular bay leaves will serve, too. Irish moss is a type of red algae. I use apple cider vinegar from Eden Acres in East Waterboro, Maine, because it is very hard to find organic apples, cider, or cider vinegar in the Northeast, making it as valuable as gold!

Makes 1½ quarts (1.4 liters)

- 1 quart (960 ml) heirloom organic unfiltered raw apple cider vinegar
- 2 cups (480 ml) raw unfiltered honey
- 2 cups (380 g) fresh or thawed wild Maine blueberries or other type of blueberries
- 1 cup (30 g) chopped beach bay leaves or chopped common culinary bay leaves
- ½ cup (5 g) Irish moss (*Chondrus crispus*)

Put all the ingredients in a high-performance blender. Pulse it a few times, then transfer the mixture to a ½-gallon glass jar. Cover the jar with a piece of fabric and secure with a rubber band. Let infuse for 2 to 6 weeks, then strain. This oxymel will keep for 6 months stored in a cool, dark place.

Beet Kvass

This lacto-fermented, probiotic drink made from beets originated in Eastern Europe.

Makes 1 quart (960 ml)

- 2 tablespoons whole caraway seeds
- 1 tablespoon sea salt
- 2 medium unpeeled organic beets

Add the caraway seeds, salt, and 1 cup (240 ml) of boiling water to a glass jar. Stir to dissolve the salt and cover while you wash and chop the beets. Fill a quart-sized Mason jar three-quarters of the way full with the chopped beets and pour in the hot caraway water. Add additional water as needed to ensure that all the beets are covered. Cover the jar with a piece of fabric and secure it with a rubber band. Leave the jar on your kitchen counter for 4 to 8 days. The beets will ferment; bubbles will form, and the liquid will taste slightly sour. Strain and bottle this beautifully pigmented beverage and transfer it into the refrigerator. Best if used within 2 months.

Underground Matrix

The black trumpet is a wild mushroom that is often abundant in late summer here in Maine. It is very flavorful—smoky with rich, earthy overtones. Sautéed in butter is arguably the best way to enjoy mushrooms. I was inspired to carry forward the essence of this mushroom through a savory and sweet, Manhattan-like cocktail. Trust me, you have never tasted anything quite like this…and the experience is well worth the effort.

Makes 1 cocktail

1½ ounces (45 ml) Black Trumpet and Butter-Washed Bourbon (recipe follows)
1½ ounces (45 ml) tawny port
1 teaberry (*Gaultheria procumbens*), for garnishing (optional)

In a mixing glass, combine the infused bourbon and port with ice. Stir about 40 rotations. Garnish with a teaberry, if you like.

Black Trumpet & Butter-Washed Bourbon

To make this infused spirit, I use a technique known to the cocktail community as fat washing.

Makes 1 bottle

1 stick butter
10 black trumpet mushrooms (chopped)
Bourbon

Melt 1 stick of butter in a sauté pan and add about 10 black trumpet mushrooms (chopped); sauté until the mushrooms soften. Transfer the cooked mushrooms and melted butter to a glass jar and cover with a bourbon of your choice. Shake it up and let it set on your kitchen counter to infuse for a few days or up to a week. When you are ready to strain the bourbon, you'll be more successful if the ambient temperature is fairly warm so the butter is not congealed. If necessary, place the jar in a pot of warm water and allow it to heat awhile until the butter in the spirit is melted. Strain and press out the mushrooms. Then place the liquid in the freezer for several hours to allow the separation of fat and alcohol. Strain the infused and washed spirit again through a fine-mesh strainer. Use immediately or store in the refrigerator for up to a month.

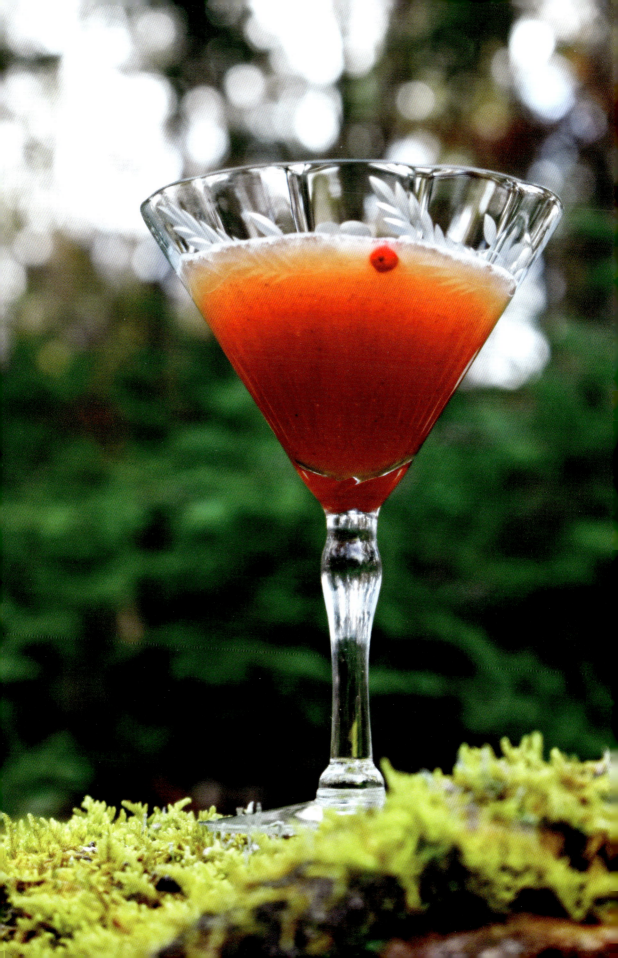

Saving the Sun

This drink was inspired by an abundant year of plums at my favorite local orchard. There were five varieties in shades of purple, yellow, and red.

Makes 1 cocktail

Pink sea salt, for the rim (optional)
1 ounce (30 ml) ginger-infused gin
1 ounce (30 ml) Thai-basil-infused sake
1 ounce (30 ml) Five-Plum Syrup (recipe follows)
¾ ounce (22.5 ml) lime juice
3 dropperfuls lemon balm tincture
Thai basil sprig, for garnishing

If you'll be salting the cocktail glass, rim it with pink salt: First use a lime wedge to wet the rim, then dip the rim in a shallow bowl of the sea salt. Set aside.

Put the gin, sake, Five-Plum Syrup, lime juice, and lemon balm tincture into a cocktail shaker with ice and shake. Strain and garnish with the Thai basil.

NOTE

To infuse gin and sake, place ginger slices directly in a bottle of gin (I use Bimini Gin for this drink) and whole sprigs of Thai basil directly into a bottle of sake 3 to 7 days before you want to use the spirits. Be sure the alcohol fully covers the plant material. Strain the gin and sake before using.

Five-Plum Syrup

Although this is called Five-Plum Syrup, you don't need to have five different kinds of plums! Use what you can find at your local orchards or farmers market.

Makes 1 quart (960 ml)

Fresh plums
2 handfuls chopped fresh lemongrass (optional)
2 handfuls fresh lemon verbena (optional)
Raw unfiltered honey

Chop the plums, removing the pits, and place 2 cups (300 g) in a pot. Cover with 2 quarts (1.9 liters) of water and bring to a boil. Simmer on medium-high until the fruit breaks down. Use a hand blender to speed along the process. Add an extra couple of cups (480 ml) of water and bring the mixture back to high temperature, then remove from the heat. Add the lemongrass and lemon verbena if available, and cover and let steep for 20 minutes. Strain into a large glass measuring cup. Pour into a bowl and add an equal amount of raw unfiltered honey. Dissolve and funnel into a glass bottle. Store in the refrigerator and use within 1 month.

Recipes through the Seasons

Primitivo

The very first cocktail, reimagined. This sangria-esque recipe is inspired by the research and work of Patrick McGovern. In his book *Uncorking the Past*, McGovern describes how he and a team of researchers discovered evidence of the oldest cocktail known: traces of hawthorn, wild grape, rice, and honey on shards of primitive pottery in Jiahu, China.

Makes 1 cocktail

4 ounces (120 ml) Lambrusco
2 ounces (60 ml) unfiltered sake
1 ounce (30 ml) Hawthorn and Bitters Honey Syrup (recipe follows)
Tiny splash sparkling mineral water

Build the drink by placing ingredients in order in a mixing glass. Add ice and stir. To match the theme of the drink, strain into a handmade clay cup.

Hawthorn & Bitters Honey Syrup

Mugwort (*Artemisia vulgaris*) and yarrow (*Achillea millefolium*) are both ancient bittering agents for beer.

Makes 1 pint (480 ml)

¼ cup (20 g) hawthorn (*Crataegus* spp.) berries
1 tablespoon dried mugwort
1 tablespoon dried yarrow
2 cups (480 ml) raw unfiltered honey

Simmer the hawthorn berries in 3 cups (720 ml) of water on medium-high heat for about 20 minutes. Blend with a hand blender and continue simmering for 20 minutes more. Turn off the heat and add the mugwort and yarrow. Cover and infuse for 15 minutes prior to straining into a measuring glass. Add an equal amount of honey and stir to dissolve. Store in the refrigerator and use within 1 month.

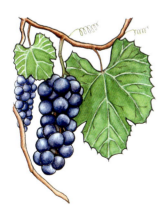

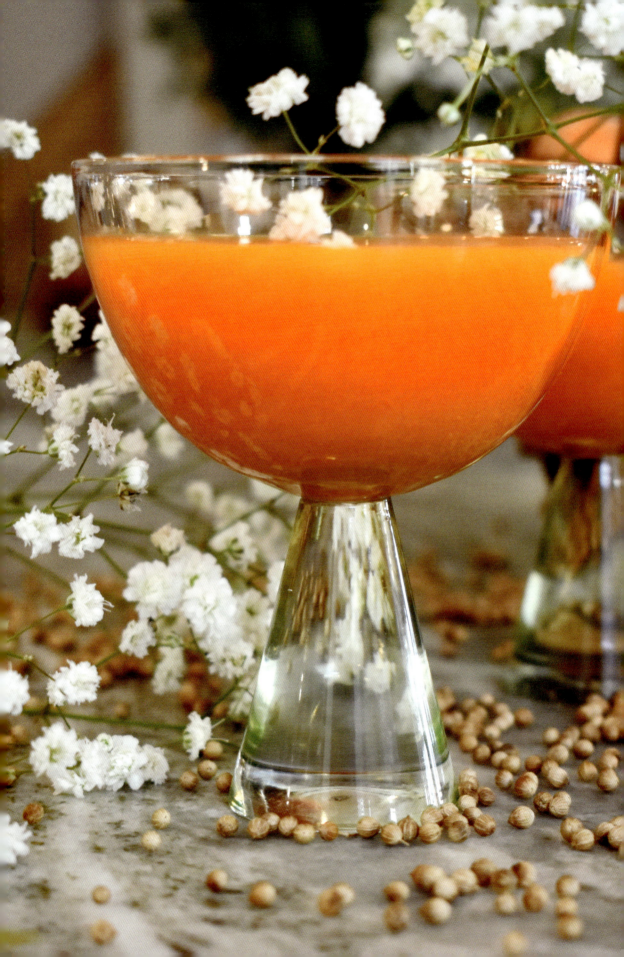

Sweetened by Frost

Roots get sweetened by cooler temperatures in the fall. The brilliant orange of this cocktail pairs perfectly with a vivid foliage display.

Makes 1 drink

1½ ounces (45 ml) rum
6 ounces (180 ml) fresh organic carrot juice
1 ounce (30 ml) Maple Coriander Syrup (recipe follows)
¼ ounce (7.5 ml) lemon juice
3 dropperfuls Chamomile Glycerite (recipe follows)
Sweet Annie flower clusters (*Artemisia annua*), for garnishing

Shake the rum, carrot juice, Maple Coriander Syrup, lemon juice, and Chamomile Glycerite in a shaker tin with ice. Strain over a collins glass filled with ice. Garnish with the sweet Annie.

NOTES

I use Bully Boy Rum Cooperative Volume 2.

It's best to make Chamomile Glycerite using fresh chamomile flowers, not dried. If dried chamomile is the only form available to you, brew some chamomile tea and use it in place of the warm water in the Maple Coriander Syrup recipe below, and omit the Chamomile Glycerite when mixing up a Sweetened by Frost cocktail.

Maple Coriander Syrup

Makes 8 ounces (240 ml)

½ cup (120 ml) warm water
½ cup (120 ml) maple syrup
2 tablespoons coriander seeds

Combine the warm water with the maple syrup. Toast the coriander seeds lightly in a dry pan (cast iron works well) over low heat for about 5 minutes. Blend the liquid with the toasted seeds and then strain. Store the syrup in the refrigerator for up to 1 month.

Chamomile Glycerite

Makes 4 ounces (120 ml)

Fresh chamomile flowers
Food-grade vegetable glycerin

Fill a 4-ounce glass jar halfway with fresh chamomile flowers. Cover with food-grade vegetable glycerin. Transfer to a blender. Blend gently then pour back into the glass jar. Let extract for 2 to 4 weeks before straining into a tincture bottle. Stores at room temperature in a cool, dark place for up to 6 months.

Xocolatl

Xocolatl is a Nahuatl word said to be the root of the word *chocolate*. Nahuatl is the language of the Nahua people and the pre-Hispanic civilizations of ancient Aztecs. *Xocolatl* means "bitter water," and it was the custom to drink this cacao paste simply mixed with water. This traditional beverage was also served with native cornmeal and flowers.

Makes 1 drink

Raw unfiltered honey
Flower confetti, for garnishing (instructions are in the sidebar)
2 ounces (60 ml) cacao-nib-infused tequila/Mezcal
1½ ounces (45 ml) Spiced Chocolate Syrup (recipe follows)
½ ounce (15 ml) Ancho Reyes Ancho Chili Liqueur
½ teaspoon cornmeal

Drizzle a little honey over the back of a bar spoon and onto the outside of a cocktail glass in a diagonal line. Next, sprinkle on flower confetti to stick to the honey. Shake the infused tequila or Mezcal, Spiced Chocolate Syrup, and Ancho Reyes liqueur with ice and strain into the decorated glass. Sprinkle the cornmeal on top.

Spiced Chocolate Syrup

Makes 1 cup

1 cup (240 ml) agave syrup
¼ cup (40 g) dark chocolate callets
1 teaspoon vanilla extract
1 teaspoon ground cinnamon

Gently heat the agave syrup in a small pot. Add the chocolate and stir until just dissolved. Remove the pot from the heat and add the vanilla and cinnamon. Transfer to a heat-safe storage container. Will keep in the refrigerator for 1 month.

Flower Confetti

There are no hard-and-fast rules for making flower confetti. I use orange calendula blossoms, blue bachelor buttons, and pink rose petals, combined in equal amounts. You can feel free to work with any edible flowers you fancy, but for best effect, choose at least two different colors of flowers. Follow the general instructions for drying herbs on page 118. Take special care to avoid exposing the flowers to sunlight while drying, because light will cause bright colors to fade.

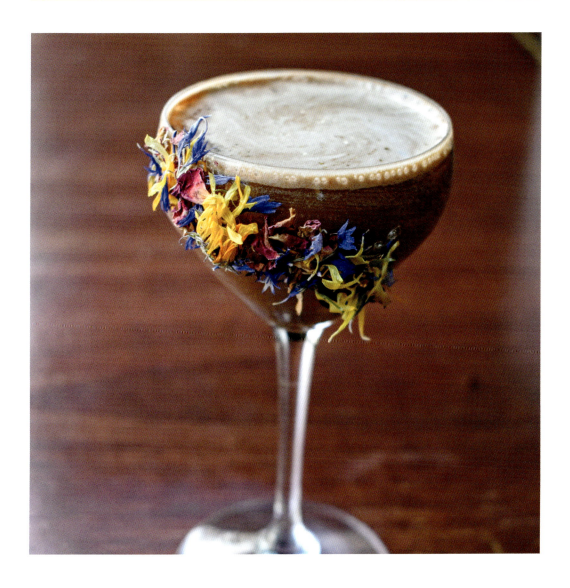

Ambrosia

This cocktail recipe is quintessentially fall with orchard fruit and cozy warming spices. It is a sophisticated after-dinner drink with wonderfully evocative aromatics that ring true to its name: nectar of the gods. *Ambrosios* is an ancient Greek word that means "immortal," of divine origin.

Makes 1 cocktail

- 16 ounces (480 ml) apple cider, for making a reduction
- 1 tablespoon maple sugar, for the rim
- 1 tablespoon cinnamon, for the rim
- 1½ ounces (45 ml) Pear and Cinnamon Stick Infused Calvados (recipe follows)
- ½ ounce (15 ml) allspice dram liqueur
- 2 dropperfuls Cardamom-Orange Bitters (recipe follows)
- 2 dropperfuls Black Walnut Bitters (recipe follows)
- Whole nutmeg, for garnishing

First, make an apple cider reduction by boiling the apple cider until it is reduced to one-quarter its original volume.

Next, mix together the maple sugar and cinnamon in a shallow bowl. Use a lemon wedge to wet the rim of a glass and then dip the rim into the sugar-cinnamon mix. Set the glass aside. Shake 1 ounce (30 ml) of the apple cider reduction with the infused Calvados, allspice dram liqueur, both of the bitters, and ice. Strain up into the rimmed glass. Grate fresh nutmeg over the top.

NOTES

Reducing apple cider concentrates the sweetness as well as the apple flavor.

For the allspice dram liqueur, I use St. Elizabeth brand.

You can substitute store-bought cardamom and/or black walnut bitters for this recipe.

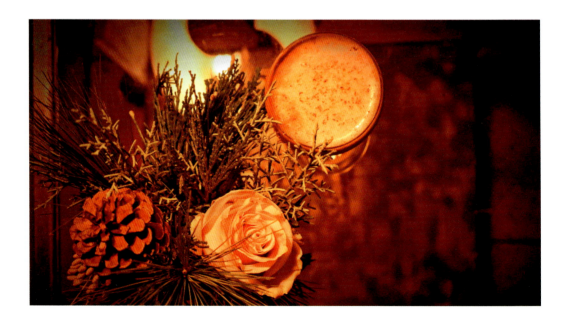

Pear & Cinnamon Stick Infused Calvados

Makes 1 bottle

Ripe pears
4 cinnamon sticks
Calvados

Chop up several ripe pears and place in a quart jar with 4 cinnamon sticks. Cover completely with Calvados. Let infuse for 3 to 7 days prior to straining back into the bottle.

Black Walnut Bitters

Black Walnut Bitters is reminiscent of Nocino, but without the sweetness. Basically, the bitters extracts all the aromatics from the black walnut (*Juglans nigra*) nuts while they are still immature, super sticky, and green! I absolutely adore this smell—it's one of my favorite perfumes.

In Maine, walnuts reach this phase right at the beginning of orchard season in summertime. But walnut ripening varies with regional conditions. I advise finding a black walnut tree in your neighborhood and keeping your eyes on 'em.

Makes 4 ounces (120 ml)

Green walnuts, chopped
Overproof spirit

Fill a 4-ounce jar halfway with chopped green walnuts and cover completely with overproof alcohol. Cover and infuse for 2 to 4 weeks prior to straining.

Cardamom-Orange Bitters

Makes 4 ounces (120 ml)

Cardamom pods
Fresh or dried organic orange peel
Overproof spirit

Fill a 4-ounce jar halfway with equal amounts of cardamom pods and fresh or dried organic orange peel. Cover with overproof spirits of your choice. Let macerate for 2 to 4 weeks prior to straining and transferring into a tincture bottle.

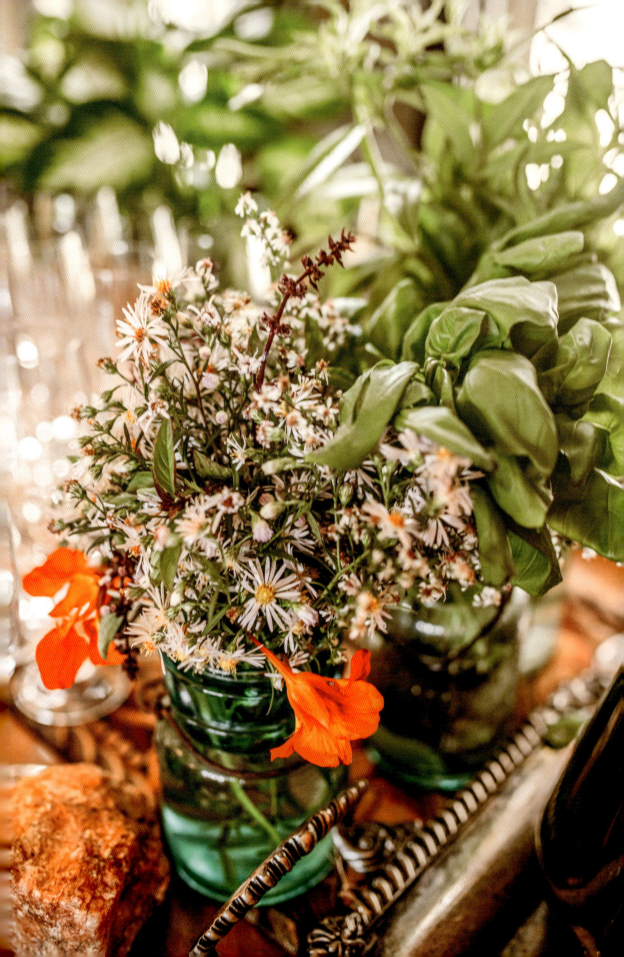

CHAPTER 8

Plant Monographs

Some of you may be asking: What is a monograph?

A monograph is a text dedicated to a single subject; in this case the subject is a plant. This chapter is an ode to the classical herbal pharmacopeias and the materia medica of history.

The purpose of these plant profiles is to help you get acquainted. A monograph is a good place to start when you're learning a new plant personality. I hope they will give you the resources you need to go deeper than first impressions, because true knowledge comes from experience. These monographs are your introduction, but the relationship will only bloom when you touch, smell, taste, and spend time with these plants in a garden, in the woods and fields, and in your kitchen or behind the bar.

Each monograph covers several topics: habitat and cultivation; taste and energetics; actions and uses; constituents and chemistry; preparation.

Habitat and Cultivation: In this section of each monograph, you'll find information on what the plant looks like and what its native range is. You'll also get some gardener's advice on how to grow your new friend— how it behaves in the garden and what conditions it prefers to thrive.

Taste and Energetics: In many ways taste is the gateway to understanding herbal energetics, as discussed in chapter 3. For this reason, I recommend tasting each new botanical you encounter, either by nibbling directly on the plant or by making a tea or single extract with just one ingredient. This taste-it-plain-first approach is how you develop your palate, learn to build formulations, and develop a good concept of flavor pairing.

Actions and Uses: In many ways actions *are* uses. Herbalists categorize herbs based on their actions; each monograph elaborates on some of them. Refer back to chapter 3 to refresh your memory on herbal actions as needed.

Constituents and Chemistry: This section of each monograph is your gateway to deciding how to extract a plant properly and which kitchen preparations are suitable for it. Knowing the important chemical constituents in a plant is also the key for conducting your own research. For my nerdy friends, I suggest visiting the PubMed website, a resource for navigating all the scientific studies and current research. Type in the botanical name of the herb and one of its constituents to see what kind of discoveries are being made about the plant's healing potential.

Preparation: In this section I focus on my favorite ways to process and preserve a plant based on my ten years' experience as both herbalist and mixologist. My criteria include taste and ease of use as well as what a plant's phytochemistry indicates about the best choice of solvent.

Caution: It is important to note that there are safety concerns around some plants. For example, some are not safe to consume when raw, and some cause photosensitivity. I highly recommend consuming a very small amount of any new substance at first, because some people have idiosyncratic allergies. Every body is different. Another important thing to note is that some herbs are not pregnancy-safe. I have noted these where applicable.

Angelica

Angelica archangelica
APIACEAE

Her Majesty rises in the second year, taking up most of the garden, reaching toward the sun and sky. Hollow stems make better conduits for angelic frequencies. She sometimes wears the royal colors, purple over garden green. All the winged come to visit. Seeds form, harden, then scatter. The first-year roots are delightfully spicy and bitter. Angelica is a traditional European folk remedy for "blood purification" and protection against all infectious diseases. Historically, it was known to be protective against dark magic and spells—quite popular in olden times! There are two explanations for the name *archangel*. One story says the name was revealed in a dream by an archangel as a cure for the plague. Some also say *archangel* refers to angelica's tendency to come into bloom on the day of Michael the Archangel (May 8).

Habitat and Cultivation

Angelica archangelica is a biennial medicinal herb that is functional as well as stunningly bold and beautiful. In the first year of growth, the plant produces a clump of compound leaves close to the ground and establishes big, sprawling roots. In the second year, a thick, hollow, ridged stem rises to 6 feet (1.8 m) tall and bears large, ornamental, globular flower umbels that are loved by many pollinators. All parts of angelica exude a pleasant spicy aroma.

Angelica likes to grow in deep, fertile, and moist soil, ideally near running water, and thrives in full sun to part shade. If given the desired conditions, she spreads enthusiastically and self-seeds readily!

Taste and Energetics
warming • bitter • aromatic • pungent

Actions and Uses
alterative • analgesic • antidepressant • anti-inflammatory • antibacterial • antimicrobial • antiviral • antiseptic • antispasmodic • aromatic • astringent • bitter • carminative • circulatory stimulant • diaphoretic • emmenagogue • expectorant • mild nervine • sialagogue

---

Angelica increases blood circulation, stimulates the appetite, and promotes digestion through warming, carminative, and bitter actions. It increases secretion of bile from the liver and enzymes from the pancreas.

The parts used are the dried roots, stems, leaves, and seeds. Roots are dug in the fall of the first year of growth. The root has been used as a purification agent in many Native American cultures and is also considered a "bear medicine" within several tribes, where it is customary to associate the energetic healing quality of plants with the symbolic medicine of animal totems.

The stems and seeds have traditional use in confections. Angelica is a popular and historical flavoring agent for liqueurs such as Bénédictine and Chartreuse. With its earthy fragrance and flavor, it's also commonly used as a botanical ingredient in the distillation of gin.

Angelica is energizing to the respiratory system, promoting rejuvenation of tissue, and it has been used as an ally in the cessation of smoking, both to curb cravings and to help the airways recover.

Angelica moves the blood and "waters of the body," increasing circulation to the extremities, and thus can help with arthritis, gout, and Raynaud's syndrome. It can relieve swelling, inflammation, and pain by helping provide fresh blood to the tissues.

Research studies indicate that angelica may have antimutagenic and antitumor effects as well as hepatoprotective actions and anti-anxiety effects.

Purple-stemmed angelica (*A. atropurpurea*), which is native to North America, is remarkably similar to *A. archangelica* and can be used interchangeably. *A. sinensis* is a species used in Traditional Chinese Medicine as a warming bitter with circulatory-stimulating effects as well as additional blood-building effects.

Constituents and Chemistry
coumarins, furanocoumarins • flavonoids • polyphenols, phenolic acids, fatty acids, phytosterols • silica, sugar, tannins • terpenes

Preparations
My favorite way to use angelica is to add the dried root to bitters. Candied angelica is delicious as a garnish. This plant also makes a beautiful flower essence.

Caution
Be cautious about touching live angelica plants. All plants in the genus *Angelica* contain furanocoumarins, which are medicinal phenols that increase skin sensitivity and can cause allergic dermatitis in some people.

Do not forage for angelica in the wild unless you have experience with identifying it properly. It is unlikely that you would find *A. archangelica* in the wild in North America, and there are some deadly poisonous species in this plant family. Both poison hemlock (*Conium maculatum*) and poison parsnip (*Heracleum* spp.) can be mistaken for angelica. It is best to find a nice damp spot on your property and grow your own!

Other precautions for this herb:

- People with diabetes should avoid excess consumption of angelica, because it can increase blood sugar levels in the urine.
- It is active on liver enzyme pathways that affect drug metabolization; consult with a doctor before using angelica if you are taking any pharmaceutical drugs.
- Avoid during pregnancy.

Plant Monographs

Artichoke

Cynara cardunculus var. *scolymus*
ASTERACEAE

In Greek mythology, Kynara was a beautiful mortal woman whom Zeus captured for a seat next to him on the throne. But she would sometimes sneak off to her old home, and the vengeful god turned her into an artichoke out of jealousy and spite.

Habitat and Cultivation

The artichoke is native to the Mediterranean region and loves heat and sandy, well-drained, fertile soil. It persists from year to year as a perennial in USDA Zones 9 or warmer but is treated as an annual in colder climates. To produce flower buds, the plants require a growing season of at least eighty-five days. Fortunately, a shorter growing season is fine for growing leaves, which is the plant part desired for its use as a bitter remedy. In Maine we sow artichoke seeds indoors eight to twelve weeks before the planned date for outdoor planting, and we raise them under grow lights (among many other crops). The seeds require cold treatment (vernalization) to stimulate germination.

Taste and Energetics

bitter • cold (leaves)

Actions and Uses

Artichoke leaf is an indispensable resource for its bitter taste and can be used as a substitute for wild gentian (*Gentiana lutea*), which is the source of flavor in many commercially produced bitters. Wild gentian grows only in the Alpine valleys of Central and Southern Europe, such as the Italian Alps, and thus its use on a commercial scale is unsustainable. (This plant can be grown in the garden, but with limited success.) It is slow growing, and harvesting the roots kills the plant.

Artichoke leaf is a replenishing source of bitter and can be grown organically. It is a better option for both home garden and commercial herb growers.

Constituents and Chemistry

bitter sesquiterpenes • polyphenols • phenolic acids

Preparation

Use fresh or dried artichoke leaves as a quarter to a third of a bitters blend. To "warm up" the bitters, add angelica or cinnamon.

Birch

Betula spp.
BETULACEAE

Birch is "the lady of the woods," according to English poet Samuel Taylor Coleridge. I agree that birch is a beautiful, enchanting muse, but it's also a hard worker: a gift for boatbuilders, a balm for your pain, shelter from the rain (roof), a place for your expressive heart (paper). The name _birch_ is thought to have come from the Sanskrit word _bhurja_, meaning "tree whose bark is used for writing on." The bark is shimmering metallic pink-and-gold mystery historically used for baskets and witch's brooms. The druids used birch for ceremonies, particularly at Beltane and Samhain, for igniting the new as well as cleansing the old: grace, renewal, and purification. Paper birch is one of the first species to colonize an area after a fire.

Habitat and Cultivation

Birch species grow throughout the woodlands of the Northeast, along edges and in wetlands, and are often considered a pioneer species. Eleven species are found in New England, in slightly differing microclimates and ecosystems. Paper birch (_B. papyrifera_) prefers northern and alpine climates, whereas yellow birch (_B. alleghaniensis_) likes cool ravines and swampy areas. They like to grow in small groups (groves) together.

Taste and Energetics

astringent • bitter • pungent • cooling

Actions and Uses

alterative • analgesic • anti-cancer • anti-inflammatory • antimicrobial • antitumor • astringent • diuretic • nutritive • styptic • tissue tonic

---

I include birch in these monographs because birch sap and birch soda are so delicious, but this plant has much medicinal merit as well. The minty smell and taste are telltale sign of its use: That odor is evocative of salicylates, the natural compounds (also found in willow and teaberry) that are the main active ingredient in aspirin, produced by plants for their own protection but offering potent anti-inflammatory and pain-relieving effects in humans.

Birch bark has also been studied for its anti-inflammatory and specific anti-cancer and antitumor uses. It has potential for complementary and integrative care for inflammatory cancers, but its use can also be preventive.

Constituents and Chemistry

polyphenols • salicylic acid (phenolic acid) • tannins • triterpenes • botulin • betulinic acid

Preparation

Birch syrup is made by tapping a tree and boiling the sap—the same process as is used to make maple syrup (see "Maple" on page 257). However, it takes 100 gallons of birch sap to make 1 gallon of birch syrup.

Birch tea infusion: To make a birch tea infusion, cut small pieces of birch twigs and simmer in water on medium heat for 30 minutes, covered. Use about 1 tablespoon chopped twigs per 8 ounces (240 ml) water.

Blueberry

Vaccinium angustifolium
ERICACEAE

I never pick wild blueberries without thinking about my neighbors the black bears, who can eat as many as thirty thousand berries a day. Bell-shaped blueberry flowers are some of the first that native bumblebees visit in the Maine forests to harvest pollen. Although the blooms are a wonderful garnish, do not take too many of them—remember the bees! Blueberries love growing underneath pine trees, and their crimson fall foliage is striking.

Habitat and Cultivation

Blueberries abound here in Maine, as they love acidic soils. They prefer mildly acidic soil but can tolerate a very low pH, which is why both lowbush and highbush types grow wild on the edge of swamps and lakes as well as on the tops of small mountains. On blueberry barrens in Maine as well as in the Midwest, it is traditional (first an indigenous practice) to operate controlled burns in the late fall to prune, maintain the open space, and promote new growth. Blueberries are a wonderful plant for home landscapes, too, where you can prune them rather than burning them.

Taste and Energetics

cooling • nutritive

Actions and Uses
Anti-cancer • anti-inflammatory • cardioprotective • DNA-preserving • immune tonic

---

Blueberries are the quintessential tonic, where food meets medicine. They are a powerhouse for preventive healthcare. Wild blueberries have a high antioxidant capacity. Unlike many other fruits, blueberries are low glycemic and consuming them does not raise blood sugar levels. Studies indicate that blueberries may help prevent against Type 2 diabetes as well as inflammation-caused cognitive decline such as Alzheimer's and dementia.

Constituents and Chemistry
polyphenols (many types) • tannins • nutrients: carotenoids, potassium, manganese, copper, iron, zinc

Preparation
Simmer fresh or frozen berries in water as a base for syrups. Use a 1:2 ratio of berries to water.

They are also excellent in oxymels and shrubs, paired with aromatic herbs like lavender or tulsi. The leaves have higher antioxidant levels than the berries and make an excellent, mildly fruity, astringent tea. Try combining blueberry leaves with other leafy tea herbs or in fruit-based preparations.

Butterfly Pea
Clitoria ternatea
FABACEAE

The Latin name *Clitoria* comes from this plant's flowers, which resemble the vulva (clitoris) in shape. This flower is an aphrodisiac and a nervine. It will dye liquid alcohol and water a brilliant blue.

Habitat and Cultivation
Butterfly pea is native to the Indonesian island of Ternate, and it prefers to grow in humid conditions between 70 and 100°F (21–38°C). It has also been introduced to Australia, Africa, and the Americas. Fabaceae is the pea

family, and plants in this family are legumes, which means that their roots have a symbiotic relationship with the soil bacteria known as rhizobia. These bacteria process atmospheric nitrogen into a form that plants can absorb and use. Because of this quality, butterfly pea is grown as a revegetation species in former coal mines of Australia. This functional ornamental creeping vine is easy to grow in warm climates (it is hardy in USDA Zones 9 to 11), but it requires some structural support and can grow up to 10 feet (3 m) tall. In cooler zones, butterfly pea can be grown as a container plant indoors (mist it frequently) or in a heated greenhouse.

Taste and Energetics
slightly bitter • vegetal • cooling

Actions and Uses
analgesic • anthelmintic • anticonvulsant • antidepressant • antidiabetic • antifungal • anti-inflammatory • antimicrobial • antioxidant • antiproliferative • anxiolytic • aphrodisiac • diuretic • emmenagogue • febrifuge • hypnotic • insecticidal • nervine • nootropic

---

The roots and seeds are aperient and laxative.

The flowers are used to make a natural blue food dye used for cooking and traditional textiles in South Asia, where the flowers are known as pigeonwings. More recently, they have been adopted for their use in color-changing gins. This type of gin turns from a deep blue to an electric pink-violet when mixed with lemon juice or tonic water (the change occurs because of the drop in pH). Butterfly pea is featured in my Nootropical Paradise recipe on page 182.

Young pea pods and flowers are edible raw and have been used as animal fodder. The plant has also been employed traditionally for coughs, thyroid problems, and even for snakebites!

Butterfly pea is traditionally used in Ayurvedic medicine as a tonic agent for the nervous system: a memory-enhancing nootropic and mood booster as well as sedative. This is unusual—sedatives are not ordinarily applied to depressive states. The extract has a marked effect on the central nervous system and was proven to reduce the intensity of behavior mediated via serotonin and acetylcholine in stressed-out rats.[1]

Because the plant contains cyclotides, isolated constituents from butterfly pea plants and flowers are being studied for their application in biotech and pharmaceutical industries.

Constituents and Chemistry

amino acids • butelase (enzyme) • phytosterols • polyphenols, such as anthocyanins and kaempferol • tannins • triterpenoids, such as taraxerol and taraxerone

Preparation

Use butterfly pea flowers raw or dried as a water-soluble, natural food and drink coloring. Most of the studies on the plant's medicinal and tonic benefits used hydroethanolic extracts (tinctures) of the aerial parts including leaf and flower. For this reason, I suggest making your own tincture or brewing a simple "butterfly tea" with the dried flowers, which are readily available due to their trendiness in the food and beverage world.

Butterfly tea: Add 1 tablespoon each dried butterfly pea flowers and lavender flowers to 8 ounces (240 ml) hot water. Steep for 15 minutes. Strain and sweeten with honey to taste. You can make a syrup by adding equal parts honey to the strained tea.

The Shapeshifter: I also like to make butterfly tea lemonade, which I call The Shapeshifter because you can magically change the color of the liquid, just like that. Brew some butterfly tea and add organic sugar or honey in a 1:1 ratio while the tea is still warm. Pour 1 ounce (30 ml) of this syrup over ice with 6 ounces (180 ml) of water and an oversized lemon wedge. You can watch the colors change. Great for kids!

Cacao

Theobroma cacao
MALVACEAE

Cacao's botanical name, *Theobroma*, was bestowed by Linnaeus (the founder of modern taxonomy) in 1725. The name means "food of the gods" and reflects the belief of Aztecs and Mayans that chocolate was a gift from the goods. In ancient Mexico the seeds were valuable enough to be used as coins. This sacred bean has been a facilitator of ritual and ceremony to open the heart and communicate with the divine for thousands of years.

Habitat and Cultivation

A tropical understory tree, cacao grows in lush rain forests in Central and South America. The typical harvesttimes for the fruit are June and December, although the trees produce some fruit year-round. The traditional method of processing is to cut open the fruit, allow the pulp to ferment off the beans, and then allow the beans to dry in the sun. *Theobroma cacao* is the most common species used in trade, but historically the beans of *T. bicolor* (the jaguar tree) were also cultivated (and the fruits were also eaten).

Taste and Energetics

bitter • sour • astringent • moist

Actions and Uses

antidepressant • anti-inflammatory • antiseptic • aphrodisiac • bronchodilator • cardioprotective • circulatory stimulant • diuretic • emollient (cacao butter) • entheogen • euphoric • hypolipidemic • hypotensive • nervine • nutritive • psychotropic

Constituents and Chemistry

alkaloids (such as theobromine) • anandamide • polyphenols • tryptophan • protein, fat

Preparation

Many of the commercial preparations for chocolate and cocoa powder remove some of the fat. I prefer to use the most intact and least processed version: cacao paste.

Xocolatl or Aztec Hot Chocolate: My favorite way to prepare cacao paste is to chop or shave small pieces of cacao paste from a block into warmed or steamed milk. It's traditional to sweeten this lightly with honey, but it's also good unsweetened. I add vanilla, allspice, or cinnamon (not traditional) and a small pinch of cayenne. I also love to add a few dropperfuls of rose petal glycerite or rose water for synergistic heart-opening effects. The Aztecs also sometimes included cornmeal or native dried flowers. Blend until frothy! Very yummy spiked with Mezcal.

Chamomile
Matricaria chamomilla
ASTERACEAE

Folk traditions include wearing chamomile for good luck, fortune, and to attract a lover. Symbolizing purity and innocence, these sweet little flowers that some say smell like apples have long been associated with the sun and its energy, from the Egyptian sun god Ra to the Greek sun god Helios.

Habitat and Cultivation

Chamomile enjoys full sun in well-drained soil and is a self-seeding annual. In Maine, chamomile reaches peak flowering typically around the end of June, the same time as strawberries! Use your whole hand with fingers spread out to create a rake for pulling the blossoms from the plant and into your harvest basket.

Taste and Energetics

bitter • sweet • aromatic • pungent

Actions and Uses

anodyne • anti-inflammatory • carminative • emmenagogue • nervine

---

Chamomile is a gentle but very powerful remedy! It serves as a calming nervine as well as a carminative and stimulant to the appetite. And it's a potent anti-inflammatory, particularly for the digestive system. But it's also gentle enough to give to babies and the elderly. Primary traditional uses have been for neuromuscular tension, fever, and digestive problems.

Constituents and Chemistry

amino acids • fatty acids • flavonoids • mucilage • phenolic acids • sesquiterpene lactones • tannins • terpenes (such as azulene, which is blue in color)

Preparation

Chamomile combines well with fennel, licorice root, and turmeric for digestion-inspired tonics. Combine it with lavender or ashwagandha for nervine relaxant tonics. See "Ginger" on page 245 for a ginger-chamomile tea.

Chamomile tea: Use 2 tablespoons dried chamomile blossoms per 8 ounces (240 ml) hot water. Steep, covered, for 15 minutes or more and then strain.

Cinchona

Cinchona spp.
RUBIACEAE

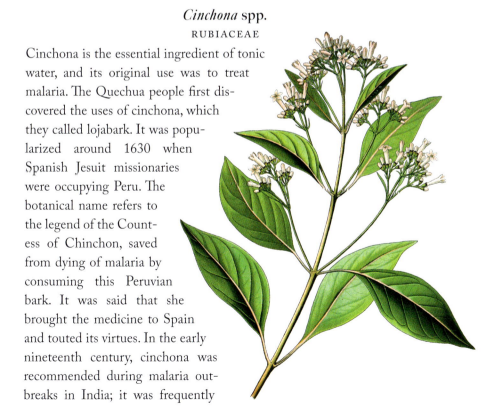

Cinchona is the essential ingredient of tonic water, and its original use was to treat malaria. The Quechua people first discovered the uses of cinchona, which they called lojabark. It was popularized around 1630 when Spanish Jesuit missionaries were occupying Peru. The botanical name refers to the legend of the Countess of Chinchon, saved from dying of malaria by consuming this Peruvian bark. It was said that she brought the medicine to Spain and touted its virtues. In the early nineteenth century, cinchona was recommended during malaria outbreaks in India; it was frequently mixed with soda water and sugar to help mask the bitter taste. The first commercial tonic water was produced in 1858.

Habitat and Cultivation

Native to the western Andes, cinchona is a small tropical tree growing at elevations up to 9,800 feet (3,000 m). For commercial production, it is grown like a shrub, with its height limited by a technique called coppicing.

Taste and Energetics

bitter • astringent

Actions and Uses

antimalarial • antimicrobial • antipyretic

In the United States the FDA limits the amount of quinine in tonic water to 83 mg per liter, which is far less than a medicinal dose for malaria (500–1,000 mg/day) but still enough to be used as a bitter digestive tonic. Cinchona bark has also been used in treatment of babesiosis (a tick-borne disease), neuralgia, rheumatic complaints, and heart palpitations.

Constituents and Chemistry

alkaloids (including quinine) • flavonoids • sterols • tannins • terpenes

Preparation

To make your own tonic water, start by making a cinchona bark extract. Add up to 15 drops per 8 ounces (240 ml) club soda and sweeten as desired.

DIY cinchona bark extract: Fill a small glass jar a quarter of the way full with dried bark and cover with a neutral spirit such as 40 to 50 percent vodka. Label and let macerate for at least 4 weeks, shaking occasionally. Strain and funnel into a tincture dropper bottle.

Caution

Overdose of the key alkaloidal constituent quinine can cause cinchonism, whose symptoms include headache, nausea, skin eruptions, and tinnitus, as well as far more serious neurological and cardiac symptoms. The toxic dose is between 1 and 4 grams pure quinine, which is present in the dried root at 1 to 4 percent. Traditional medicinal uses call for a dose of approximately 1 gram for an adult, distributed throughout the day, for about 6 days. It is traditionally consumed as a decoction. It is inadvisable to use cinchona bark as medicine without a doctor's supervision.

Cinnamon

Cinnamomum spp.
LAURACEAE

Your plants are an orchard of pomegranates
With pleasant fruits,
Fragrant henna with spikenard,
Spikenard and saffron,
Calamus and cinnamon,
With all trees of frankincense,
Myrrh and aloes,
With all the chief spices...
—FROM SONG OF SOLOMON

Habitat and Cultivation

Native to East Asia, India, and Sri Lanka but also widely cultivated throughout the tropics, cinnamon is an evergreen tree that can grow 20 to 30 feet (6–9 m) tall. It grows from sea level up to 3,000 feet (914 m) in elevation. The part used is the dried inner bark of the shoots. Cinnamon grows best in almost pure sand, sheltered by the constant rain and heat of a tropical forest.

Taste and Energetics

pungent and warm, but neutral moisture because it contains both demulcent mucilage and astringent tannins that balance

Actions and Uses

antidiabetic • antifungal • antimicrobial • antioxidant • antiseptic • antispasmodic • aromatic • astringent • carminative • circulatory stimulant • tissue tonic

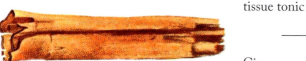

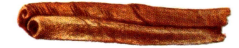

Cinnamon is mentioned as medicine in the Bible as well as in Egyptian texts and is used in Ayurvedic medicine as well as Traditional Chinese Medicine. TCM employs *Cinnamomum cassia*, which is widely cultivated in South Asia and Southeast Asia. It is similar to Ceylon or true cinnamon (*C. verum*) but harder, spicier, and higher in coumarin content.

Cinnamon is a digestion-aiding spice that promotes circulation, regulates gut dysbiosis, stops vomiting and diarrhea, and relieves nausea and flatulence. It also helps regulate blood sugar, which makes it the perfect spice in sweets!

Cinnamon can reduce high blood pressure and may slightly lower cholesterol; is a menses amphoteric; and is excellent in cold and flu formulations, as well as for oral health and hygiene.

Constituents and Chemistry
flavonoids • mucilage • phenolic acid • tannin • terpenes

Preparation
You likely won't be able to grow and harvest your own cinnamon bark, but I like to use this spice in an adaptogenic tea.

Adaptogenic chai tea: Combine 1 tablespoon each of Ceylon cinnamon chips, cardamom pods, crushed (dried) gingerroot, codonopsis root, and astragalus root with 1 teaspoon of whole cloves and 1 teaspoon of licorice root. Simmer the spices in 20 ounces (600 ml) of water for about 15 minutes. Toward the end of decocting, add 8 ounces (240 ml) of your favorite full-fat milk. Gently warm for several more minutes. Strain and froth if desired. I like to transfer the strained tea into a high-performance blender and pulse at high speed for 1 minute or until adequately frothed.

Caution
Cassia cinnamon has a much higher coumarin content than Ceylon cinnamon. Coumarin has been linked to liver and kidney damage in high doses. Ceylon cinnamon contains only trace amounts and is entirely safe to consume in large tonic doses in food and teas.

Coriander
Coriandrum sativum
APIACEAE

The word *coriander* is derived from the Greek word *koris* (meaning "stinking bug"), so named because the leaf of the plant was thought to smell like crushed bedbugs. Despite that impression, coriander is one of the spices with a long history of cultivation in many parts of the world, from ancient Greece to Israel. Coriander seeds were found in the tomb of Tutankhamun (King Tut), an Egyptian pharaoh who reigned around 1330 BCE. The leaves of this plant are the popular culinary herb called cilantro.

Habitat and Cultivation

This is a fast-growing annual hardy to USDA Zone 2. Cultivating coriander requires successive seeding every four weeks during the summer to ensure a continuous harvest. Sow seeds in bands in fertile, well-drained soil. The plant will be ready to harvest in 120 to 150 days; you can also harvest the seeds while they're green (still ripening).

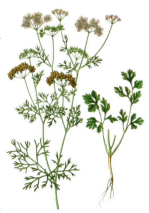

Frequent cutting prevents premature bolting (going to seed). If coriander is allowed to develop ripe seeds, it will self-seed in the garden. It is an insectary plant and attracts beneficial insects.

Taste and Energetics

leaves: some say soapy, slightly bitter, cooling • seeds: lemony, bright, spicy, pungent, warm, dispersive

Actions and Uses

anticonvulsant • antimicrobial • antioxidant • anxiolytic • carminative • hypolipidemic

---

From pickles to curries and to Belgian wheat beers, coriander seeds as well as cilantro leaves are deeply intermeshed in culinary practices, bridging many cultures. Coriander has a special penchant for beverages and is even included as one of the ingredients in the secret syrup formula of Coca-Cola. And although it is not a required ingredient (like juniper), lemony aromatic seeds are commonly used to flavor and infuse gin.

In addition to being a flavoring agent, coriander is an aromatic digestive tonic. Its potential for removal of heavy metals from the body has been studied but requires more research; other herbs may be more promising for this purpose.

Constituents and Chemistry

flavonoids • phenolic acids • sterols • terpenes

Preparation

My favorite way to use coriander is to prepare it as a digestive tonic and a gentle calming remedy that is safe for kids.

Cassandra's Three C's Calming Colic Tonic: Fill a jar three-quarters of the way full with equal parts crushed fresh coriander seeds, chopped chamomile flowers, and catnip flowers. Cover with food-grade vegetable glycerin and let macerate for 6 weeks. Then strain and bottle. Use 1 to 3 dropperfuls in mixed drinks or water.

Dandelion

Taraxacum officinale
ASTERACEAE

Dandelions are happiness rebels, heroic symbols of the wild abundance available for all, carrying the wishes of the next generation.

Habitat and Cultivation

Believe it or not, some of us cultivate, rather than weed out, dandelions—even though they can grow just about anywhere in a temperate climate, including through asphalt! An opportunistic individual's success can always be controversial. But is the plant really a weed when it is so medicinal and nutritious?

Dandelions are fast-growing biennials that like well-drained fertile (rich in potassium and nitrogen) garden soil. They will grow single taproots more readily when they are not constantly being pulled out by their lion's tooth (*dent de lion*). After what seems like a season, a hollow straw filled with milky white latex arises from the rosette of jagged leaves to produce a fluffy flower the color of May sunshine. Bees frolic among the pollen-rich blooms, which mature to those infamous orbs of fluffy seeds. These seed parachutes hold a record for the most effective wind-dispersed seeds: They can travel over 60 miles (100 km). The vortex technology invented by the dandelion is being studied to improve drone technology.

Taste and Energetics

bitter • cooling

Actions and Uses

anti-inflammatory • antimutagenic • bitter digestive tonic •

chemoprotective • cholagogue • choleretic • diuretic • hepatic • hypolipidemic • laxative (mild) • prebiotic

---

The bitter flavor of this tonic helps the liver, our chief organ of detox, help itself in clearing out toxins as well as in the production of bile, which is essential for good digestion. The bitterness also stimulates the pancreas to produce enzymes and the stomach to generate adequate HCl, which helps the body prepare for optimal digestion and boosts the absorption of fat-soluble vitamins.

Bitters help lower sugar cravings, regulate blood sugar, and boost appetite while also helping the body reach satiety. All of these actions can lessen potential digestive afflictions such as bloating, gas, and heartburn, as well as systemic inflammation caused by poor digestion.

Constituents and Chemistry

enzymes • flavonoids • phenolic acids • sterols • terpenes • polysaccharides

Preparation

Tooth of the Lion Bitters: In the springtime, close to the new moon, dig up a few dandelion plants. Place the plants, roots and all, in a 5-gallon bucket filled with water. Rinse the plants well in the bucket (it's best to do this outdoors to avoid mess). Chop up enough washed roots and leaves to fill a glass jar three-quarters of the way full. Cover the plant matter completely with a high-quality neutral base spirit. Cover and label. Let macerate for 4 to 8 weeks, shaking occasionally. Strain, press, and bottle. If you have any chopped dandelions left from your preparation, eat them for dinner!

Elderberry

Sambucus canadensis
CAPRIFOLIACEAE

Elderberry is laced with the lore and mystery of Hyldemoer, the Elder mother, a dryad or tree spirit who was the gatekeeper for harvest and the faerie realm. It was common superstition in England and Scandinavian countries that this spirit would haunt or punish those who did not ask permission prior to harvesting and using elderberry wood.

Elderberry juice was a common adulterant of port wine in the mid-1700s; vintners added its color to fake the aging process of this fortified wine. The cultivation of elderberry was thus forbidden in Portugal at this time.

Habitat and Cultivation

Elderberry is a fast-growing, deciduous shrub native to North America and Europe, hardy in USDA Zones 5 through 10. The shrubs have large woody stalks and a compound leaf structure. They produce creamy white umbels of lace-like flowers in very late spring. Elderberry likes nitrogen-rich soils and grows well with "wet feet" in ditches, along forest edges and clearings, in hedgerows, and near running water. It's very easy to propagate by taking cuttings. It can be a challenge beating the birds to the berries!

Taste and Energetics

cooling • drying

Actions and Uses

alterative • antirheumatic • antiviral • aperient • astringent • demulcent • diaphoretic • expectorant • immune tonic • laxative

———————

The parts most used are the ripe berry (cooked) and flowers (distilled as a hydrosol or dried for tea). The flowers are traditionally used as a gentle diaphoretic for breaking fevers and an expectorant for bronchial afflictions, often combined with peppermint. The darkly pigmented berries have been studied extensively for their antiviral properties, particularly for preventing and reducing the length of the common flu. Elderflower water can be used in tonic beverages but was a mainstay of cosmetics several generations ago; women used it to keep their skin fair.

Constituents and Chemistry

alkaloid • flavonoids • phenolic acids • polysaccharides • tannins • terpenes • nutrients: phosphorous, potassium, carotenoids, vitamin C, B vitamins

Preparation

Separate your harvest of fresh berries into two equal parts: one part to freeze for later use in a water-based syrup, and the other part to make a tincture.

Elderberry tincture: Place berries in a blender and just cover with overproof rum. Blend, then transfer to a glass jar, covering with more spirit if necessary. Cover the jar. Let macerate for 4 weeks, shaking occasionally. Then strain.

Elderberry syrup (water-based): Place 1 part of frozen berries in a small pot with 3 parts of water. Add a handful of spices (such as a few slices of fresh ginger and a cinnamon stick) if desired. Simmer on medium heat for 20 to 30 minutes. Strain. Add an equal amount of honey as the strained liquid.

Combine the syrup and tincture together in equal proportions. Sip in a cordial glass or add to elixir recipes. Half an ounce (15 ml) is a good starting dose for mixing.

Caution

The leaves and other uncooked parts of this plant contain sambunigrin, a toxic cyanogenic glycoside. The fresh leaves and root also contain sambucine, an alkaloid that is in deadly concentrations in the root. It is recommended that you use only the ripe berries or flowers, and that you cook or dry them.

Ginger

Zingiber officinale
ZINGIBERACEAE

Fresh ginger rhizome is known as Sheng Jiang in Traditional Chinese Medicine, and has been used in TCM for five thousand years. It was one of the first spices conveyed by the spice trade routes and was also used as food and medicine by ancient Rome and Greece.

Habitat and Cultivation

Likely native to Asia, ginger is a tropical, heat loving perennial plant that thrives in USDA Zones 8 to 12. The rhizomes (underground stems) can be grown in colder zones as an annual in greenhouses for personal use or as a novelty, and some small-scale market gardeners are experimenting with it in greenhouses as well.

Taste and Energetics

hot, dry • spicy • stimulating

Actions and Uses

antibiotic • anti-cancer • antidiabetic • anti-inflammatory • anti-nausea • antioxidant • aphrodisiac • circulatory enhancer • digestive •

hepatoprotective • hypoglycemic • hypolipidemic
• neuroprotective • stimulant

In herbal formulas, particularly in TCM, ginger is often used as a catalyst or spark to help activate and carry other ingredients. It is one of the most effective circulatory enhancers available in our kitchen cabinets. Its stimulating properties help improve digestion and warm up the body, particularly moving circulation to achy and arthritic joints. Bioactive gingerols are flavonoids that have been demonstrated to reduce inflammation-creating chemicals such as prostaglandins and leukotrienes.

Preparations of gingerroot are also well known as treatments to relieve or prevent motion sickness and morning sickness.

Constituents and Chemistry

fatty acids • flavonoids (such as gingerol) • terpenes • polysaccharides

Preparation

Ginger-chamomile tea: To make a soothing ginger-chamomile tea, cut and mince fresh gingerroots and combine about 1 tablespoon minced roots and 12 ounces (360 ml) water in a small pot. Simmer on medium-high heat for about 15 minutes, adding more water if necessary. Then add 1 tablespoon dried chamomile and cover to steep for about 10 minutes. Strain and sweeten with honey as desired; serve with a small squeeze of lemon.

Green Tea

Camellia sinensis
THEACEAE

The Japanese culture of tea, including the Japanese tea ceremony, involves tea drinking as a transformative practice. It reflects a Zen Buddhist worldview accepting transience and imperfection. One of my favorite Zen Buddhist writers, Thich Nhat Hanh, instructs to "Drink your tea slowly and reverently," encouraging presence and mindfulness, "as if it is the axis on which the whole earth revolves—slowly, evenly, without rushing toward the future."

Tea is consumed worldwide, second only to water in importance as a beverage. This plant has had a significant influence on political history as well as religious ceremony and culture. Best known is the Tea Act of 1773 in Great Britain, which catalyzed a series of events, including the dumping of 10,000 pounds of tea into the harbor during the Boston Tea Party, that led to the Revolutionary War.

Habitat and Cultivation

Tea is an evergreen shrub or small tree native to Southeast Asia and India that is cultivated for its leaves. Much of its traditional use and development was in Burma, Tibet, Japan, and China. Plants grown at higher elevations, up to 7,200 feet (2,200 m), are esteemed for their superior flavor. The plants prefer a little bit of shade. Tea plants can survive and thrive in the proper conditions in USDA Zones 7 through 9.

Taste and Energetics

cold • astringent

Actions and Uses

antiaging • anti-cancer • antidepressant • anti-inflammatory • antimicrobial • antioxidant • astringent • cardiovascular tonic • diuretic • hyperlipidemic • nootropic • osteoprotective • stimulant • styptic • tissue tonic

---

Tea is a stimulating, circulatory-enhancing agent that increases mental clarity and prevents the inflammation that typically causes brain fog, improving focus.

Green tea is an excellent ally for healthy weight loss as an energizing stimulant, but it has also been shown to inhibit fat absorption and suppress adipose cell proliferation.[2]

The combination of these effects and studies showing that green tea catechins help maintain the strength of bone architecture and prevent bone loss make it an excellent lifelong tonic for athletic individuals![3]

Constituents and Chemistry

alkaloids: caffeine, theobromine • flavonoids: epicatechin gallate and other catechins • tannins

Preparation

Tea can be processed in several ways. Green tea is the least processed form, and the most medicinal. Techniques used in tea production include oxidation, fermentation, and steaming. Tea oxidation is a phytochemical process that causes the leaf to turn brown after harvest. The leaves are rolled or bruised, breaking the cell walls and exposing enzymes in the leaf to oxygen. This process affects the look, taste, and aroma of finished teas. Traditionally much of this process was done in the field, drying in the sun, but higher-tech processes with supplied heat, conveyers, and machine rollers are now employed.

For use in tonic elixirs, you can simply brew green tea, or you can make a matcha latte. Matcha is a traditional Japanese tea made from minimally processed ground green tea leaves.

Matcha latte: To prepare matcha traditionally, you will need a large teacup or bowl, a small strainer, and a bamboo whisk. The traditional ingredients are matcha powder and hot water prepared in cast iron or copper. I like to whiz up my matcha lattes in a blender, and my ingredients list is a bit of a cultural hybrid: 1 cup (240 ml) warm water, 1 tablespoon ghee (clarified butter), 2 teaspoons matcha, 1 teaspoon vanilla extract, 3 dropperfuls wild rose glycerite, and 1 tablespoon raw honey.

Hawthorn

Crataegus spp.
ROSACEAE

A fairy tree and the harbinger of spring, blossoming in May, hawthorn is a gatekeeper of death as well as life. Thorns that can cut deep line the stems, and the flowers have been described as smelling like the plague. Hawthorn flowers contain trimethylamine, a substance that is also released from decaying bodies. Perhaps not the wisest choice for perfume. Historically, before this chemical was discovered, folks believed that carrying these blooms into a house would bring about a death.

Habitat and Cultivation

Hawthorn is a shrub or small tree, growing up to 30 feet (9 m) tall, depending on the species, and hardy in Zones 4 through 8. Many species can be used medicinally and as food. It is also an excellent contender for a hedgerow or wildlife corridor. Deer, rabbits, and bears as well as many species of bird browse on the twigs and berries. Hawthorn can grow in a variety of soils, in full sun or a woodland edge. It can tolerate drought but prefers moist, slightly acidic soils. Named cultivars are available as landscape plants, but I recommend planting wild varieties.

Taste and Energetics
sweet, sour • astringent, cooling • nutritive

Actions and Uses
antiarrhythmic • anti-inflammatory • anti-ischemic • antioxidant • cardio-protective • cardiotonic • diuretic • hypolipidemic • hypotensive • positive inotrope

---

Hawthorn belongs to the same plant family as roses and apples. It is very safe to use as a food-like daily tonic. Ripe hawthorn berries are rich in flavonoids and are the essential cardiac tonic of Western herbal medicine. The flowers and leaves have even higher levels of these active constituents. The flavonoids help prevent inflammatory damage to the lining of the cardiovascular system caused by oxidative stress. This plant can help promote healthy circulation, blood vessels, capillary function, heart rhythm, and cholesterol balance.

Constituents and Chemistry
alkaloids (such as crataegin) • amygdalin (a cyanide precursor present in the seeds) • flavonoids • phenolic acids • terpenes

Preparation
If you have the good fortune to harvest fresh hawthorn berries, tincture them in brandy to make a hawthorn berry cordial: Add enough brandy to cover the berries, macerate for 6 to 8 weeks, strain, and add honey to sweeten as desired.

You can also make a hawthorn honey syrup—see the recipes on page 128 and 207.

Hibiscus

Hibiscus sabdariffa
MALVACEAE

Hibiscus is a significant flower of Hinduism. It is associated with Kali, the goddess of destruction and primordial root energy, as well as the elephant-headed Hindu deity Ganesha, symbolizing good luck, the removal of obstacles, and new beginnings. The flowers are used in their rituals of worship.

Habitat and Cultivation

Hibiscus is a tropical plant native to Africa; it thrives in Zones 9 through 12. It grows in disturbed soil and can reach a height of 9 feet (2.7 m). In cooler climates, cultivate the beautifully pigmented roselle hibiscus as an annual in pots, overwintering inside.

Taste and Energetics

aromatic • astringent • demulcent • refrigerant (very cooling)

Actions and Uses

anti-inflammatory • antioxidant • antiscorbutic • blood building • cardiotonic • cellular tonic • demulcent • diuretic • hepatoprotective • hypotensive • nephroprotective • nutritive • UV-protective

---

In places where hibiscus grows naturally, the whole plant is eaten as food and used as medicine. The flower is soft and demulcent and can be eaten or used for tea, but the most popular plant part is the deeply pigmented calyxes (the outer portion that surrounds the flower petals).

Hibiscus is used in traditional Ayurvedic medicine as well as in the Middle East. It is one of the best tonics to consume in summer drinks for beating the heat. The flowers are high in vitamin C, and the pigments contain flavonoids that can help protect the cardiovascular system maintain healthy blood pressure levels. Hibiscus has also been studied as a treatment for dry mouth and weight loss. It is helpful in anemia because vitamin C assists with the absorption of iron. It has also been traditionally used for cosmetic purposes, for healthy skin and hair, and as a restorative for the kidneys.

Constituents and Chemistry

pectin, vitamin C • anthocyanidin • hibiscus (a glycoside) • malic and citric acids

Preparation

I like a sweetened chilled hibiscus flower tea called Agua de Jamaica, a type of "aguas frescas" served in Latin American countries, particularly Mexico.

Agua de Jamaica: Steep ½ cup (17 g) of dried roselles per quart (liter) of hot but not boiling water (too much heat destroys vitamin C). Sweeten with sugar to taste while the tea is still warm. Chill before serving.

Caution

Hibiscus is often intercropped with peanuts in commercial cultivation, so use caution sourcing hibiscus for those with severe peanut allergies.

Hops

Humulus lupulus
CANNABIDACEAE

Hops and cannabis are the only two plants in the family Cannabidaceae. The first recorded use of hops in brewing dates to ninth-century monks, who capitalized on its antibacterial properties to preserve beer.

Habitat and Cultivation

Hops is a perennial vine that can climb up to 20 feet (6 m) high! Hops can grow in full sun but prefers dappled shade or a garden edge. It will need a sturdy support to climb. I once planted a very successful hops vine on an east-facing outer barn wall underneath an old metal ladder. After a couple of years, the vine had made its way to the roof, and it is still growing happily there. It grows well in Zones 5 through 8 and can grow at elevations up to 7,000 feet (2,134 m). It prefers humus-rich soil. Plants are either male or female, so you must grow both if you wish to harvest seeds. The seeds contain gamma-linoleic acid, which is highly nutritive and not often found in plant sources. The cone of the female flower is the plant part typically used for flavoring and preserving beer, and for medicine. Plants are propagated through root division, cuttings, and cloning. Large-scale production can be challenging.

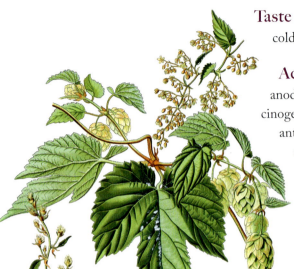

Taste and Energetics
cold • very bitter

Actions and Uses
anodyne • antibacterial • anticarcinogenic • anti-inflammatory • antioxidant • antispasmodic • anxiolytic • bitter tonic • cholagogue • choleretic • estrogenic • hepatic • hypnotic • nervine • psychoactive sedative

Constituents and Chemistry
flavonoids (including prenylnaringenin—the most potent phytoestrogen known) • terpenes (such as bitter alpha acids) • phenolic acids

Preparation
Hop and grapefruit bitter: You'll need about 1 cup (120 g) fresh hop stobiles (cones), the peel from 1 grapefruit, and 10 cardamom pods. Pour high-quality overproof over the botanicals in a pint jar. Ensure that all the plant matter is full covered, even after shaking. Add more spirit if needed. Label and infuse for 2 to 4 weeks, shaking occasionally, then strain and bottle.

Caution
Handling this plant causes dermatitis in some people. It is not safe for use during pregnancy.

Juniper
Juniperus communis
CUPRESSACEAE

A juniper is a wise old soul. Individual plants can live for hundreds of years, snaking around and hugging a rock. Juniper is cleansing to the mind, body, and spirit, energetically and physically. Juniper smoke and aroma purify spiritually, while ingestion is antimicrobial for the digestive system, urinary tract, and kidneys. This plant's tropism for the kidneys makes me wonder about its connection to water. Perhaps juniper has evolved to use water intelligently because the places where it thrives are arid. Good psychic boundaries (not having infectious diseases plus prickliness) equals freedom (the places it grows).

Habitat and Cultivation

I love the transporting aroma of crushed juniper berries and the open, desert-like places where it grows: the mountaintop expanses, the granite scrabble, and the winding edges of forest rock walls nostalgic for a time when humans were more industrious and lived closer to the earth's seasonal rhythms.

In the wild, juniper grows on chalk downs in southern England and in the northeastern United States. Plant in a well-drained spot in full sun, on a ledge or surrounded by rocks.

Taste and Energetics

hot, dry, diffusive • pungent, camphorous, sweet

Actions and Uses

alterative • antibacterial • antidiabetic • antifungal • antihyperlipidemic • anti-inflammatory • antimicrobial • antioxidant • antirheumatic • antitumor • carminative • circulatory stimulant • diaphoretic • diuretic • emmenagogue • hepatoprotective • nootropic

---

Juniper has a long history of traditional use for kidney and bladder infections, but it is of medicinal strength; overly large doses or overlong use can cause renal damage.

A small piece of dried juniper stem burning on top of a beverage evokes a deep history of using plant aromatics via smoke to carry our prayers and cleanse or move energy.

To legally have the moniker of *gin*, the spirit must contain the aromatics and flavor of juniper, giving its characteristic pine-tree taste.

Gotlandsdricka, or Drikka, is a juniper beer made in Sweden, where it is a medicinal tonic. The potion is traditionally made by women on the island of Gotland.

Both the green berries and ripe purple berries (cones) have culinary uses, but the latter is the plant part usually used for medicine and gin. Juniper is likely a part of the 4 Thieves formula—the legendary plant-infused vinegar that saved four thieves from dying of the plague in medieval times.

Constituents and Chemistry

acids: acetic, malic, formic • flavonoids, such as juniperin • terpenes • trace nutrients: protein, vitamin C

Preparation

Juniper berries dry and store well for later use. If you are picking many of them, wear gloves to protect your hands from the spiky foliage. I like to use a strong juniper berry tea or a hydrosol as a substitute for gin in non-alcoholic recipes. I like to crush the berries first, using a mortar and pestle, then measure 1 tablespoon per 8 ounces (240 ml) of hot water. Steep, covered, for 20 minutes.

Lavender

Lavandula spp.
LAMIACEAE

In the Greek herbal of Dioscorides, he instructs us to make medicinal wine by infusing *Lavandula stoechas* (Spanish or French lavender) in wine. Dioscorides states: "It dissolves thick fluids, gaseousness, pains of the side and the nerves, and extreme cold. It is effectively given with pyrethrum and sagapenum for epilepsy."

Habitat and Cultivation

Native to the Mediterranean, lavender is a woody perennial that likes warm and well-drained sandy, chalky soils. Plants should be mulched well with straw or leaves for the winter in areas with harsh cold. Species used include *Lavandula angustifolia* and *L. stoechas*. The plant prefers neutral to slightly alkaline soils; test your soil pH and amend accordingly before planting if needed. Plant seedlings 18 to 24 inches (46–61 cm) apart; lavender looks best planted in masses, and it's traditional to plant it along walkways. Lavender is best propagated by taking cuttings. It's drought-tolerant once established. Prune older woody plants in the spring by cutting back stems by a third.

Taste and Energetics
pungent • sweet • acrid • bitter • diffusive • cooling

Actions and Uses
antiseptic • antispasmodic • aromatic • carminative • cholagogue • diuretic • nervine • perfume • sedative • stimulant • vermifuge

---

The Complete German Commission E Monographs, a therapeutic guide to herbal medicine, approves *Lavandula angustifolia* for loss of appetite, nervousness and insomnia, circulatory disorders, and dyspeptic complaints. One nickname for lavender is palsy drops, as it was used for relieving tension headaches.

The Latin name comes from *lavare*, meaning "to wash." Lavender has been used as an antiseptic agent and added to baths and soap for thousands of years.

Lavender is a relaxing remedy with a long history of use for anxiety and sleep, affirmed by modern research. It is especially useful for those with a high degree of neuromuscular tension that may negatively impact digestion and peripheral circulation. It is also beneficial for hyperactivity disorders and those who need to relax to focus, such as those with ADHD.

The essential oil of *L. stoechas* is being studied for its potential ability to protect the liver and renal function.

Constituents and Chemistry
flavonoids • phenolic acids • terpenes

Preparation
Lavender dries well when the stems are tied in bunches and hung upside down. It is a great ingredient for winter tea blends (aka syrups!) as well as a prime candidate for hydrosol distillation. It's delicious in glycerite blends and infused honeys or oxymels.

Lemon Balm
Melissa officinalis
LAMIACEAE

Klosterfrau Melisana is one of the oldest and most popular medicinal remedies of Europe, made in Germany by a company founded by a nun. It was a mainstay of medicine cabinets for more than a century and is still in production today.

Habitat and Cultivation

Lemon balm is native to Southern Europe and naturalized in the Americas and in most of England. This little garden cutie that smells and tastes like the sun is incredibly easy to grow. I direct-seed it , but it can also be transplanted. It's a perennial that will spread, but not aggressively. Plant in full sun or dappled shade in Zones 4 through 8 in moderately well-drained soil. Lemon balm has a special affinity for the bees. If you are a beekeeper, plant it by your hives! Lemon balm produces a higher volatile oil content in hotter and dry places. Try planting it under or around hollyhocks.

Taste and Energetics

warm, dry • sour, cooling

Actions and Uses

antibacterial • antidepressant • antiviral • anxiolytic • carminative • diaphoretic • emmenagogue • febrifuge • nervine

---

Paracelsus used lemon balm as an "elixir of life." It has a long history of use to promote emotional well-being; it's a gentle sedative commonly used for nervous irritability, hyperthyroidism, and heart palpitations. Avicenna wrote that lemon balm made the heart merry.

A hydrosol distilled by Carmelite nuns in the seventeenth century combined lemon balm with lemon peel, nutmeg, coriander, and angelica. It was used for treating neuralgic complaints.

Lemon balm has also been studied and used for prevention and treatment of herpes lesions.

Constituents and Chemistry

flavonoids • phenolic acids • tannins • terpenes • volatile oils

Preparation

I like to combine lemon balm with other bright and sunshiny ingredients like lemons or watermelon. Combining it with lemon juice for extra lemon taste provides some added nervine benefit. It's a prime candidate for amaro, vermouths, and aperitifs. Harvest when the weather is warm and dry and the plant is flowering.

Lemon balm tincture: Fill a glass jar with finely chopped fresh plant material. Remember to inhale the lemony aroma as you work! Cover with high-quality overproof liquor at a 1:2 ratio and label. Macerate for 4 weeks; strain and bottle.

Maple
Acer spp.
SAPINDACEAE

Maple is a cornerstone of both ecosystems and the economy in parts of the United States and Canada. Early-spring maple flowers provide food for native bees. The annual monetary value of maple syrup production in Maine is nearly $18 million, which is only 17 percent of US production. In Canada it is $616 million! Canada exported more than 11,000 gallons (42,000 liters) of syrup in 2022.

Habitat and Cultivation
Maples like to be cold. They are forest trees that grow in light woodland and can adapt to slightly alkaline or slightly acid soils. There are over two hundred species in the genus *Acer*, and all of them reside in the North. Sugar maple (*A. saccharum*) is one of the most shade-tolerant trees. It was a popular tree to plant roadside about two hundred years ago, and there are many impressive, wise old maple trees in New England.

Taste and Energetics
sweet

Actions and Uses
anti-inflammatory • antiseptic • astringent • diuretic • expectorant • nutritive

---

Maple sap can be drunk in season much like the commercialized coconut water; it is high in trace minerals and electrolytes.

Native Americans used decoctions made from the inner bark to allay coughs and colds. Tea from the leaves has been used as a wash for wounds.

The boiled syrup has a lower glycemic index than sugar. Indigenous people of New England tapped maple trees for sap to make maple syrup long before European colonists came to North America. The process was a communal activity that involved the entire tribe. Offerings were made in gratitude to the tree for providing for the people, especially through the harsh winter months. Europeans, upon learning of this practice, traded iron kettles with the Native Americans, who boiled sap by dropping hot stones into buckets made of elm wood. Tribes of Maine include Abenaki, Wabanaki, Passamaquoddy, and Penobscot.

Maple wood is used to make bowling pins, pool cue shafts, bows for archery, and musical instruments. Native Americans utilized the leaves to produce a purple dye.

Constituents and Chemistry

vitamin B_2 • calcium • copper • iron • magnesium • manganese (1 tablespoon of maple syrup contains about 33 percent of the recommended daily intake) • potassium • zinc

Preparation

Maples bear edible flowers in the spring, if you can reach them!

If you live in a climate where sugar maples grow, I highly suggest you tap a tree in late February or early March. It's one more way to stay intimate with nature. Tapping occurs when nighttime temperatures are below freezing and daytime temperatures are above. It is easy to do with fairly minimal equipment. I like to use traditional equipment and boil the sap over a wood fire. It takes 40 gallons of sap to make 1 gallon of precious sugar syrup.

Milk Thistle

Silybum marianum
ASTERACEAE

The seeds of our prickly friend milk thistle are the ultimate hangover remedy. They help the liver with its two-phase detoxification process, making it more efficient, which helps reduce the inflammatory damage caused by the breakdown of alcohol. Use milk thistle anytime you have consumed more than one alcoholic beverage. Take standardized capsules that contain a milk thistle extract (with plenty of water) after overindulging, before you go to bed. Sometimes I follow this up by including ground milk thistle seeds in my diet the following day. Studies show that milk thistle consumption may increase the body's production of glutathione, an endogenous antioxidant synthesized in the liver.

Habitat and Cultivation

Milk thistle is native to the Mediterranean, and its name refers to the white speckles on the thorny leaves. It has also been called Mary's Thistle, a biblical reference to breast milk. Because milk thistle seeds are dispersed by wind, it has become invasive in Washington State and in some European countries in places where it is field-cultivated in large plantings.

Grow milk thistle in full sun with arable soil, away from places where people might accidentally brush into it (ow!). It is a biennial but often grown as an annual. Seeds require a period of exposure to cold to stimulate germination, as well as light. Wear very thick gloves when harvesting milk thistle seed.

Taste and Energetics

bitter • oily

Actions and Uses

anti-cancer • antihyperglycemic • anti-inflammatory • antioxidant • cholagogue • diuretic • galactagogue • hepatoprotective • immunomodulant • nutritive

---

The seeds can be eaten as food, as can the young leaves and shoots (de-spined). The flowers can be eaten like artichokes.

Milk thistle is the most researched plant in the treatment of liver disease. Studies show its effectiveness in cases of chemical injury, viral hepatitis, alcohol cirrhosis, and fatty liver. It has also been used to treat gallstones (assisting movement by the production of bile) and is useful in cases of GI dyspepsia, stagnation, inflammation, and cancers. It may help improve elimination of toxins that happen in cases of cancer and also is helpful in liver damage caused by chemotherapy.

It is traditionally indicated for liver-related ailments such as "liver headaches" (pressure behind the eyes) as well as for skin complaints including topical-presenting allergies.

Constituents and Chemistry

fatty acids • flavonoids • flavonolignans (such as silymarin) • protein

Preparation

I make a breakfast remedy to relieve hangover symptoms; I call it About Last Night.

About Last Night: You can grind milk thistle seeds in a coffee grinder or use a mortar and pestle. To make this remedy, you'll need about 4 tablespoons ground milk thistle seeds. Put them in a blender with 2 cups (480 ml) full-fat raw milk, ¼ cup (33 g) blueberries, half a beet (raw), a banana, a tablespoon sunflower seed butter, and a teaspoon each ground cinnamon and vanilla extract. Blend until smooth. Sweeten lightly with maple syrup.

Caution

Because milk thistle affects liver metabolism, consult with your doctor prior to combining it with pharmaceutical drugs; milk thistle is contraindicated with some drugs. Conversely, though, taking milk thistle with certain medications *is* advised, because it can help to buffer some potentially toxic effects of the pharmaceuticals on the liver.

Mint

Mentha spp.
LAMIACEAE

"Relax to focus." This is the gift of mint.

Mentha is a nymph in Greek mythology, a noble beauty and the mistress of Hades, god of the underworld. Trampled by the jealousy of another goddess, Mentha was resurrected as a plant.

Habitat and Cultivation

Among the noteworthy species of mint are wild mint (*Mentha canadensis*), peppermint (*M. piperita*), spearmint (*M. spicata*), apple or woolly mint (*M. suaveolens*), ginger mint (*M. arvensis*), and water mint (*M. aquatica*). Peppermint and spearmint are commonly used in beverages, and chocolate mint is a variety of peppermint. The mint family contains more than two hundred genera including *Salvia* (sage), *Scutellaria* (skullcap), *Ocimum* (basil), and *Thymus* (thyme). There are over seven thousand species in this family, which includes many common kitchen herbs. Some common features of plants in Lamiaceae include square stems, opposite leaves, and blossoms with four stamens.

Mint is quite opportunistic, so plant where you do not mind it spreading. Otherwise, plant in a container or within edging. Avoid planting mint varieties together—this can alter their aromatic profile. They prefer moist soil and succeed in part shade. Many kinds of mint like water so well they can grow directly in it! Harvest directly prior to flowering for the highest content of aromatics.

Taste and Energetics
cooling • pungent • dispersive

Actions and Uses
analgesic • antioxidant • antiseptic • antispasmodic • aromatic • carminative • diaphoretic • nootropic • relaxant • stimulant

---

Key uses include both a stimulating and a relaxing digestive tonic. The volatile oils in mint help to relax the smooth muscles of the body, including those on the outside of major organs: heart, lung, vasculature, and intestines. Plants high in aromatic compounds have been shown to improve heart rate variability, as discussed in chapter 3. The antioxidants in mint have been studied for therapeutic usage in cognitive decline caused by inflammation.

Constituents and Chemistry
flavonoids • phenolic acids • terpenes (such as menthol)

Preparation
Spearmint is a classic ingredient for mojitos, but all mints are delicious in drinks and botanical waters! Mints are an excellent choice as a clapped garnish. The bruising of the foliage releases their aroma to entice the nose and transcend reality. A fresh mint garnish is the perfect touch for a classic Grasshopper (crème de menthe, white crème de cacao, and heavy cream or half-and-half).

After-dinner mint cordial: Chop up an abundance of fresh mint clippings to fill a glass jar three-quarters of the way full. Cover with overproof rum and a lid. Macerate for several weeks, shaking occasionally. Strain and sweeten with honey to taste. Store at high proof, but add water to taste upon serving.

Peppermint Tea-Tini: Brew a strong peppermint tea by pouring 8 ounces (240 ml) hot water over 1 tablespoon dried peppermint. Steep, covered, for 30 minutes. Strain and add 4 tablespoons raw unfiltered honey per cup of strained tea. Let cool. Shake the sweet tea vigorously with ice and strain into a coupe glass. The honey will foam. Optional: Add a squeeze of lime and several drops of liquid chlorophyll. Cheers! (Here's a good tip: This Tea-Tini can be created using any kind of aromatic tea.)

Mugwort
Artemisia vulgaris
ASTERACEAE

Mugwort is an *oneirogen*: When placed under the pillow, it is said to enhance dreams. The genus name comes from the wild goddess Artemis, a virgin huntress ruled by the moon. This archetype is a master in the realm of dreams and visions.

Silvery like the moon, sharp like the arrow, mugwort is a bitter aromatic: It's first grounding, then transcending. It's no surprise that mugwort, with its lunar influence, also has ties to the ocean. It was sacred to the Aztec goddess of salt. Also known as sailor's tobacco, mugwort was used by sailors when they ran out of tobacco at sea. And in both Europe and China/Japan, it was believed that mermaids were the original purveyors of the knowledge of mugwort's supernatural powers.

Habitat and Cultivation

I often see these plants growing along roadsides (the highways of our imagination). She is a weedy (strong and successful) plant, considered invasive in many parts of the United States and Canada. Take care where you plant her. She thrives in places where soil has been disturbed. If her rhizomes are chopped, each small piece becomes its own new plant. Mugwort likes full sun and edge habitats. It is appropriate to plant her on the woodland border of a yard, ideally south facing, or along the edge of a driveway.

Taste and Energetics

bitter • pungent • diffusive

Actions and Uses

anthelmintic • anti-cancer • antimalarial • antimicrobial • antioxidant • antispasmodic • antitumor • bitter tonic • carminative • diaphoretic • emmenagogue • hepatoprotective • hyperlipidemic • oneirogen • stimulant • uterine tonic

———

Mugwort has been used in ritual and ceremony for protection and purification in the form of incense and in smudging practices. It is the primary herb used for moxibustion practices of TCM. Mugwort is used in Asian cooking.

As a uterine tonic, it promotes gentle contractions, and has been used to regulate menstrual cycles as well as induce labor. It promotes appetite and digestion as an aromatic bitter tonic, thus improving assimilation of nutrients.

Mugwort was once one of the predominant bittering agents in beer. It is also made into an absinthe-like spirit with medicinal origin in Mexico, infused with tequila called Yolixpa (meaning "medicine of the heart" in Nauhuatl).

A sister plant, *Artemisia annua*, has become renowned for its use as an antimalarial drug with its important constituent artemisin. Mugwort has slightly higher levels. It is also closely related to grand wormwood, *A. absinthium*.

Constituents and Chemistry

flavonoids • phenolic acids • terpenes (sesquiterpene lactones such as artemisin)

Preparation

I believe the most interesting way to introduce yourself to this plant is place a fresh leafy stem underneath your pillow. Mugwort is one of my favorite ingredients in bitters. See the "Are You a Dreamer?" Bitters recipe on page 128.

Mugwort-infused oil: This oil is wonderful for dropping into your Martinis or rubbing on your temples prior to sleep. Put a few tablespoons of dried flowering mugwort in a jar and cover with about a cup (240 ml) of raw cold-pressed virgin olive oil. Place it in a sunny spot to infuse for 1 to 2 weeks. Or you can place the sealed jar in a Crock-Pot filled with water and heat on the lowest setting for several days. Either way, when the infusion is ready, strain and bottle. Store in a cool dark place.

Mushrooms

Mycology presents a kingdom of myceliated and medicinal majesty. The fungal realm is still being discovered, with an estimated species count ranging from two to four million, many of which are not yet described or understood. Of the approximately 148,000 known species of fungi, 8,000 are known to be harmful to plants and 300 harmful to humans and animals. Many others, however, are friends that have a wide range of applications, including medicine, health support, bioremediation, filtration, and insulation, not to mention their indispensable place in the environment as the primary decomposers of organic matter. In this act of breakdown, they make nutrients available to many.

We celebrate the discovery of fungi that have beneficially reciprocal relationships with trees, their web-like mycelium weaving in and out with tree roots. The trees share some of the sugars they produce via photosynthesis with the fungi in exchange for the nutrients and moisture the fungi can mine from the soil beyond the reach of the tree roots. There is much research suggesting that fungi can convert pesticides into more innocuous compounds and remove heavy metals from the environment, and they even have been shown to break down plastic!

Habitat and Cultivation

Mushrooms grow in a wide range of natural environments in North America, but identifying edible and useful mushrooms in the wild is a skill to acquire before you try collecting any. I recommend learning from an experienced mycologist. Always double- and triple-check the ID of a specimen across multiple sources before ingesting it.

I highly recommend cultivating shiitake mushrooms on oak logs and wine cap mushrooms in hardwood chips in your garden paths. Both techniques are easy to learn. Boomr Bags available from North Spore in Maine (shown on page 188) make mushroom cultivation available on the kitchen countertop for reishi mushrooms and many other species.

Taste and Energetics

often bitter • sometimes acrid, usually a sweet component as well from the beta-glucan polysaccharides (long-chain sugars)

Actions and Use

The actions and uses of mushrooms differs among species, but many of the tonic mushrooms have immunomodulant or tonic actions as well as antimutagenic and antitumor actions against active cancer as well as in the prevention of cancer. Broadly speaking, mushrooms contain constituents that encourage the body to exercise the immune response and more adaptive or specific immunity. Mushrooms and other fungi often also have nutritional or nootropic effects.

Mushroom polysaccharides are thought to be tonic because the body perceives them as invaders, and thus they tonify many aspects of the immune response. Mushrooms contain sterols and trace elements as well. Nucleic acids in mushrooms have antiviral as well as nutritional-boosting effects that enhance metabolism, aid muscle recovery, improve digestion, and reduce the harmful effects of oxidative stress. Mushrooms all contain ergosterols, which can be converted into vitamin D in the human body.

Birch polypore (*Piptoporus betulinus*) grows on dying birch trees. The mushroom has a rubbery texture, like many of the medicinal polypores. It is common wherever *Betula* species are found in a forest. I often collect these in November or December in Maine, but sometimes also early spring. It is not edible, but medicinal as an immunomodulant and anti-inflammatory agent. It's best prepared as a decoction or a dual extraction and taken as a tonic. I like to combine it with birch bark in recipes.

Lion's mane (*Hericium erinaceus*) isn't easy to find when foraging, but it's one of the most prized tonics. This toothed mushroom also grows on trees. Beech trees are its preferred host, but it also grows on maples and birches. This species and other closed related species caught widespread attention due to the discovery of the constituent, erinacine E, a diterpenoid compound, which is a potent stimulator of nerve growth factor synthesis. This presents the potential for lion's mane to serve as an indispensable ally in the event of neurodegenerative inflammatory disorders such as Alzheimer's disease. These are delicious and choice edibles when young, with a fabulous texture and a taste and texture that many liken to seafood.

Reishi mushroom (*Ganoderma lucidum*, *G. tsugae*, *G. curtisii*) species can be used interchangeably, but *G. lucidum* is the species used for thousands of years in Traditional Chinese Medicine. Highly revered as the mushroom of immortality, this gorgeous deep-red lacquered polypore offers many health benefits. One of its specific uses is as a heart or Shen "spirit" tonic in TCM known as Ling Zhi. Pharmacologically speaking, reishi has specific indication for those dealing with allergies or a hypersensitivity response due to its antihistamine action accompanying anti-inflammatory and immunomodulating actions.

I often find the hemlock reishi (*G. tsugae*) in deep, damp forests on fallen or standing dead eastern hemlocks, usually around the time of the first thunderstorms of summer.

Turkey tail (*Trametes versicolor*) mushrooms are my personal favorite, due to their abundance within the ecosystem around me. I love understated but powerful remedies! This is not a choice edible species, but is usually extracted into immune tonics in the form of decoctions, broths, and double extracts.

Constituents and Chemistry

Birch polypore: triterpenes • beta-glucans • piptamine (natural antibiotic)
Lion's mane: erinacines
Reishi: steroids • polysaccharides • triterpenes • triterpenoids
Turkey tail: polysaccharides (these are being investigated for their potential as antimutagenic agents in cancer therapy and as antivirals that may have activity against human papillomavirus and hepatitis C virus)

Preparation

A double extraction is usually needed to obtain all benefits from mushrooms and for the most potent tonic, but many benefits can be obtained from water-based decoctions.

Nutmeg

Myristica fragrans
MYRISTICACEAE

This mystical spice was one of the most valuable in the historical spice trade. It was used as incense by ancient Romans and as currency after the violent Dutch conquest of the Banda Islands, where they enforced a monopoly on the trade of nutmeg. Later, during the peak of the spice trade, the Dutch traded their claim to what is now Manhattan to the British for control of the Banda Islands in Indonesia, which was the only producer of this expensive seed.

Habitat and Cultivation

Nutmeg is a tropical tree that grows up to about 65 feet (20 m) tall in Zones 10 and 11. The dried kernel of the seed is the part used. The tree begins producing flowers and the fruit about nine years into its growth cycle but will continue producing without much maintenance, offering multiple harvests per year. Production is greatest when trees are fully mature at twenty years. The seed covering, called the *aril*, is separated from the seed and sold as the spice called mace. Nutmeg is traditionally dried with a combination of solar exposure and a slow-low charcoal fire.

Taste and Energetics
pungent • warming

Actions and Uses
analgesic • anticonvulsant • anti-nausea • antihypertensive • anti-inflammatory • antimicrobial • antioxidant • antiparasitic • antispasmodic • aphrodisiac • aromatic stimulant • carminative • hepatoprotective • orexigenic (appetite stimulant) • psychoactive • relaxant

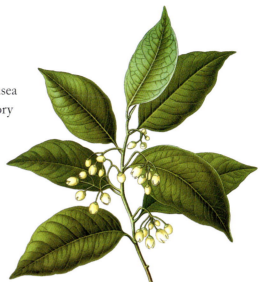

———————

Nutmeg is known as Jatiphala in Ayurveda and has been traditionally used to promote *agni* (digestive fire) as well as to treat pain. It is also used in TCM for digestion and circulating qi (life force). It can be a remedy for anxiety, to calm the nerves and promote relaxation, and for headaches. It is an aphrodisiac for men. Surprisingly, nutmeg has also been used to tonify the voice.

Constituents and Chemistry
alkaloids • flavonoids • lignans • oxalates • tannins • terpenes (such as myristicin)

Preparation
Although the easiest way to grate whole nutmeg seeds is with a nutmeg rasp, it is entirely feasible to do so with a knife. I do recommend the long slender nutmeg grater for garnishing cocktails. In addition to familiar uses of nutmeg such as in muffins and eggnog, I like to put it in creamy tropical drinks.

Passionflower
Passiflora incarnata
PASSIFLORACEAE

Wildly intricate and electrifying, passionflower blossoms are an exquisite example of the fascinating concept of the doctrine of signatures, which postulates that plant structures that resemble a part of the human body can be used to treat that part of the body. With their spiral clasping tendrils on the vines, passionflowers are said to look like the wild minds of the passionate, tightly wound people they're prescribed for.

Habitat and Cultivation

Hardy in Zones 7 through 11, these enthusiastic climbers, are quite delightful and easy to grow. *Passiflora incarnata* is native to the southeastern United States, from Florida, reaching west to eastern Texas and as far north as Pennsylvania. Passionflower prefers moisture and full sun. Plants are male or female, and pollen is spread by carpenter bees and honeybees. Passionflower can be overwintered in a protected microclimate in Zones 5 or 6, or by blanketing the roots with mulch. Grown as houseplants, they require a lot of water. Some varieties of passionflower require more than one plant for cross-pollination and fruit production.

P. caerulea is used in Traditional Chinese Medicine. Indigenous people in Argentina use *P. edulis*.

Taste and Energetics

fruit: sweet, cooling • leaf and flower: bitter, aromatic, cooling

Actions and Uses

anodyne • antinociceptive • antioxidant • antispasmodic • gabanergic • hydrating • hypnotic • narcotic • nervine • nutritive • tranquilizing • sedative • vasodilator

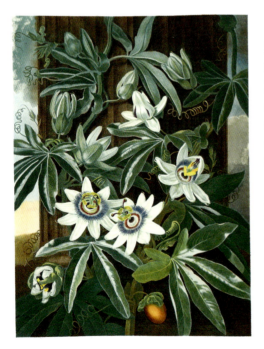

Maypop has a long history of medicinal use by indigenous peoples in North America. They used it as a sedative and a topical preparation of the roots for inflammation. Other traditional uses include treating epilepsy and preventing seizures.

Passiflora is specifically indicated for insomnia, particularly in individuals experiencing manic circular thoughts, and for all types of tension symptoms such as irritability, PMS, neuralgia, spasmodic asthma, and irritable bowel syndrome. It is a spinal cord depressant and has potential for use in treating ADHD.

It has been studied to attenuate morphine withdrawal as well as alcohol withdrawal in rats.

It has been used as an ayahuasca alternative called prairiehuasca, combined with the root bark of Illinois bundleflower (*Desmanthus illinoensis*).

Constituents and Chemistry

alkaloids, such as harmine, which is a monoamine oxidase inhibitor • cyanogenic glycosides • flavonoids • phytosterols • fruits contain polyphenols, fatty acids, vitamin C, vitamin B_3, niacin, iron, phosphorus

Preparation

I like to make a drink I call Temple of the Goddess, which is a very effective (and sexy) nonalcoholic version of the classic Porn Star Martini with a strongly brewed passionflower tea moonlighting as the alcohol. To brew the strong tea, steep 1 tablespoon dried leaf and flower in 8 ounces (240 ml) hot water, covered, for 20 minutes prior to straining.

Caution

The roots of some *Passiflora* species have toxic levels of narcotic constituents. Use caution overall with *Passiflora* extracts, because they can potentiate the effects of alcohol. Doubling up on agents with sedative effects is ill advised.

Pine

Pinus spp.
PINACEAE

The white pine (*Pinus strobus*) is the state tree of my great forested homeland, Maine. The sticky pine pitch on children's clothes and the abundant yellow pollen covering everything in June is a part of our life's memories here. Pine is survival food, lumber, medicine, kindling, shelter, wildlife habitat, and—when allowed the space to grow—a wonderful climbing tree.

Habitat and Cultivation

Maine is known as the Pine Tree State, and the eastern white pine (*Pinus strobus*) is our sovereign tree. A forest of pines looks like a canopy of paintbrushes touching the sky. Where pine trees are planted individually, they retain their lower branches and make for great climbing trees.

The genus *Pinus* comprises more than 120 species that span the entire Northern Hemisphere. All are edible and many share similar uses. Pines

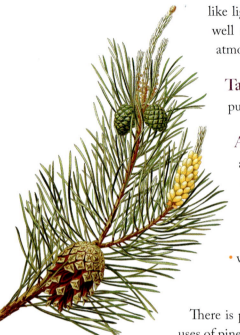

like light soil and can tolerate poor soils as well as drought, but they do not tolerate atmospheric pollution.

Taste and Energetics
pungent • sour • warming • dispersive

Actions and Uses
anti-aging • anti-inflammatory • antioxidant • antiseptic • antiscorbutic • antitumor • antiviral • cardioprotective • carminative • expectorant • immune tonic • respiratory tonic • vermifuge

---

There is plenty of active research on medicinal uses of pine due to intense interest in Pycnogenol, which is the trademarked name of an extract from maritime pine (*Pinus pinaster*).

Most of the research on pine relates to its potential benefits to cardiovascular and heart health—it enhances circulation and offers antioxidant and photoprotective properties. There is also research on use of pine in treating metabolic syndrome as well as corresponding disorders such as obesity, dyslipidemia, diabetes, and hypertension. The natural polyphenols in pine may improve erectile function as well as cholesterol balance in men.

Pine pollen is sold as a supplement for boosting testosterone in men.

The needles are high in vitamin C, the content far exceeding common cultivated sources.

Pine with all its uses has a rich ethnobotanical history. Native Americans would eat the inner bark when other food sources were scarce; they also used it to treat wounds.

Constituents and Chemistry
flavonoids • terpenes (particularly pinene) • phytosterols • vitamin C

Pine pollen contains testosterone and other male hormones; it is also known as a natural micronutrient bank because it contains many enzymes, lipids, proteins, vitamins, and minerals.

Preparation

Use whole pine sprigs to make a festive winter garnish. I like to instruct the drinkers to nibble on the pine needles for the vitamin C benefits. Use scissors to chop the needles as confetti to decorate chocolate and other confections. Fresh is best—heating destroys vitamin C.

One of the methods for collecting pine pollen is to place a large, clean tarp under a tree just prior to the release of the spores. My favorite way to use the pollen cones, however, is to collect them in clusters and freeze for use in smoothies and performance shakes. (Testosterone and nutrients help build muscle for workouts!) I do this around the first week of June. They break off easily from the tips of the branches. Pine pollen is also delightful as a bright-yellow garnish sprinkled atop egg white cocktails or spread on the side of a glass.

Pine resin honey: Pine resin honey is useful for making pine-infused beverages and for keeping in a first-aid kit. In springtime scrape off exuding resin from freshly cut pine branches or trunks and mix it with raw honey. Both substances have preservative qualities, so mix them in about a 50:50 ratio. This is often an opportunistic harvest—watch for trees that have been cut or that fell during storms of the previous winter. Avoid freshly cut logs under utility lines, because these areas are often sprayed with herbicides and also accumulate roadside salt. If you do not live in a place where chopped pines are readily available, you can cut some branches and scrape them using a draw knife to collect the resin. The result will be messy but effective.

Rose

Rosa spp.
ROSACEAE

A love affair must always begin and end with rose. She is the queen of hearts, inviting us to open our hearts, trusting that the thorn is there to protect us from any real danger. Rose is beauty medicine, symbolically and practically.

Habitat and Cultivation

Many roses are dense shrubs, but some have vining habits. Stems are sometimes thorny, sometimes bristly, and the leaves are compound with five to nine toothed leaflets; flower colors range from white to red depending on species. Each flower is surrounded by five erect sepals that often form a star shape. Flowers mature to orangey-red, sometimes fleshy hips that contain seeds.

Most roses like to grow in well-drained soil. *Rosa rugosa* and some other species tolerate and prefer sandy maritime locations. Others prefer woodland edge or hedgerow with dappled shade. The swamp rose (*R. palustris*) likes to grow on the edge of wetlands or wet field edges, in acidic soil.

I avoid growing hybrid roses in my garden, because many hybrid varieties do not have the glorious rose aroma. If you are collecting roses from others to use for garnish or preparations, be sure to ask whether they have been sprayed, and do not use any roses from plants that have been treated with pesticides.

The hips of *R. virginiana* and *R. palustris* are dry and persist on the plant well into the winter, making them a valuable foraging treat.

Taste and Energetics
astringent • cooling

Actions and Uses
anti-aging • anti-edemic • antimicrobial • antioxidant • antiscorbutic • antispasmodic • aromatic nervine • astringent • cardiovascular tonic • cosmetic • immune tonic (rose hips) • love potion • mucous membrane tonic • nutritive

---

Rose is a traditional remedy for the emotional heart and is used in love potions, for grief, and for anxiety and depression. It is used energetically to promote balanced emotional boundaries and the opening of the heart.

A wash prepared from rose petals, fresh or dried, is useful for irritated eyes. Drink rose hip tea for relief of upper respiratory distress.

Rose hips are a connective tissue tonic that can be employed in diabetes or metabolic syndrome and for those suffering from chronic Lyme disease. The petals are astringent and antioxidant, qualities that are employed for cosmetic uses, with rose stem cells (cells found in the meristem of the plant) having extra antioxidant capacity and rose hip seed oil contains protective and emollient fatty acids.

Constituents and Chemistry

flavonoids • phenolic acids • polysaccharides • sterols • tannins • terpenes • nutrients: omega-3 fatty acids (seeds), vitamin C, carotenoids, lycopene; vitamins B_3, E, and K (in rose hips)

Preparation

You can prepare rose in many ways: a water-soluble infusion, a tea, and foams; infused in spirits, mead, honey-based syrups, or glycerin; in confections; distilled in hydrosol or essential oil; and in a syrup (rose hips).

It's possible to grind whole dried hips to include the nutritious seeds (although some people complain of the hairs being irritating).

Fresh roses are beautiful as aromatic garnishes.

Rose water: Rose water is a hydrosol, and it is wonderful for misting over the surface of cocktails. To prepare rose water, you will need a large pot with a lid and two bowls—one that can be placed upside down in the bottom of the pot and another placed on top of the first bowl, face up. When the setup is complete, fill the pot with water to the level where the two bowls meet.

Place fresh roses in the water in the pot. Put the pot on the stovetop and set the lid on the pot upside down; fill the lid with ice. Heat on high until the water in the pot starts to boil, then reduce to medium-high. The rose-infused steam inside the pot will rise, make contact with the cold lid, condense back into liquid, and rain down into the empty bowl. Transfer the collected rose water into an atomizer for misting.

Rosemary

Rosmarinus spp.
LAMIACEAE

Hark! Rosemary is for Remembrance, as Shakespeare wrote in the tragic drama *Hamlet*. But did you know that rosemary has long been regarded as a sacred plant and also a symbol of fidelity, loyalty, and everlasting love? Bringing decorated rosemary to weddings in the bride's bouquet as well as gifts for guests is a long-standing tradition. In ancient Egypt rosemary was used to remember the dead. It was also sometimes burned as incense, further evidence of its connection past the veils of mortality.

Habitat and Cultivation

Evergreen rosemary prefers to grow on dry, rocky places near the sea in Zones 6 through 11. It is native to the Mediterranean and grows up to 6 feet (1.8 m) tall and 4 feet (1.2 m) wide. Its Latin name means "dew of the sea." Plant rosemary in slightly alkaline and well-drained soil in full bright sun. Mix in a small amount of lime if necessary to alkalize the soil in your bed or container to mimic the calcareous soils of its native habitat. Rosemary requires only medium to low fertility. It is susceptible to root rot if the soil is kept too moist. These plants prefer temperatures between 55 and 80°F (13–27°C) with good air circulation. A plant can live as long as thirty-five years.

Taste and Energetics
pungent • warming bitter • diffusive

Actions and Uses
anti-cancer • antidepressant • anti-inflammatory • antimicrobial • antioxidant • bitter tonic • carminative • circulatory stimulant • diaphoretic • nootropic • rubefacient • serotonergic

---

As a warming bitter tonic, rosemary helps promote digestion, move liver congestion, and regulate blood sugar.

As a circulatory stimulant, it helps improve blood flow, innervating all tissues, muscles, and nerves as well as opening peripheral circulation. It can help relieve muscular skeletal tension, particularly headaches, and increase oxygenation to the brain. In ancient Greece and Rome, it was used as a nootropic or cerebral enhancing agent—students in ancient Greece placed rosemary behind their ears to enhance concentration. Because of its two-pronged action of enhancing circulation as well as being a potent antioxidant, rosemary is a prime tonic for preventing cognitive decline caused by inflammation as well as for enhancing focus and memory.

It is also used as a stimulant topically in shampoos to promote hair growth and prevent baldness.

Rosemary has been traditionally taken for neurological disorders including anxiety, depression, and insomnia. It has the potential to improve these conditions for the reasons mentioned as well as by decreasing cortisol levels.

Constituents and Chemistry

flavonoids • phenolic acids (such as rosmarinic acid) • tannins • terpenes

Preparation

My favorite preparations and preservations for rosemary include hydrosol, infused sea salt, and powder. It is a good ingredient for all aperitifs—vermouths, bitters, and amaros; fresh sprigs are best. It can be used as a bittering agent for beer.

Schisandra

Schisandra chinensis
SCHISANDRACEAE

Known as magnolia vine or Wu Wei Zi in Traditional Chinese Medicine, schisandra is also called the five-flavor fruit because of its ability to elicit all five tastes: sweet, salty, pungent, bitter, and sour. It is said the first taste you experience on your palate is the one needed for healing.

Habitat and Cultivation

Schisandra is a perennial vine, hardy in Zones 4 through 8 and requiring part to full shade. It is native to woodland areas in East Asia. This plant requires a strong, tall trellis (it climbs up to 30 feet / 9 m tall) plus patience, because they can take seven years to fruit. Male and female plants are necessary for fruit production. Ample moisture is essential.

Bay starvine (*Schisandra glabra*) is the only species native to the United States (found in the Southeast). Little is known about its traditional usage (if any), but the constituent analysis is similar to that of *S. chinensis*. *S. glabra* would be of interest for cultivation, but wild harvest is not recommended as it is considered a threatened species.

Taste and Energetics
All five tastes. The profile differs slightly between fresh and dried berries. Warming, astringent.

Actions and Uses
adaptogen • antidepressant • antimicrobial • antioxidant • antitumor • antitussive • aphrodisiac • cardioprotective • cosmetic • emmenagogue • expectorant • hepatoprotective • hypotensive • immunomodulant • nephroprotective • nootropic • respiratory tonic • stimulant • tissue tonic • trophorestorative nervine • vulnerary

---

Knowledge of use is rooted in TCM, where schisandra is known to "astringe the jing." (*Jing* can be defined as "essence," and it refers to the source of life and vitality that is stored in the kidneys.) Schisandra tonifies both yin and yang energies.

Modern clinical trials have shown the efficiency of schisandra in helping to improve several types of neuralgic and psychiatric disorders. It is specifically indicated in deficient conditions such as neurasthenia or insomnia and night sweats caused from deficiency. As an adaptogen, it helps mitigate the effects of stress and can help prevent immune weakness as well as increasing endurance, physical ability, precision, mental acuity, and working capacity.

As a cardiovascular tonic, it is vasodilative and can help relax blood vessels, decrease arterial pressure, strengthen and normalize capillaries, decrease bleeding, and decrease stress-induced palpitations.

Schisandra is hepatoprotective and can help improve detox function and metabolism. It can also protect the liver from the inflammation caused by excess toxins, such as in cases of cirrhosis or hepatitis.

In the respiratory system, schisandra can be used as an immune stimulant; this is helpful in some types of disease as well as asthma, chronic coughs, wheezing, and lung weakness.

As an immunomodulant and anti-inflammatory, it can be useful in the treatment of cancer both by regulating the body's immune response and preventing chemo-induced immune suppression. Additionally, it helps to improve wound healing both inside the body (say, ulcers) and outside (skin issues, including allergic dermatitis).

Constituents and Chemistry
flavonoids • lignans (such as schisandrins) • terpenes • phenolic acids • plant acids: tartaric, malic, citric • polysaccharides • tannins • nutrients: vitamins A, C, and E; minerals, including phosphorous, manganese, silicon; pectin

Preparation

Making a tincture or oxymel with fresh schisandra berries is the best choice, but fresh berries are difficult to source.

Schisandra oxymel: The medicinal tonic berries of Wu Wei Zi are traditionally processed with vinegar, possibly to enhance its hepatic tropism or perhaps due to solubility. Either way, the results are shown to produce more potent medicine. Using a vinegar solvent no doubt assists in extracting some of the minerals as well. Fill a glass pint jar one-quarter of the way full of fresh or dried schisandra berries. If you're using dry, cover this with 2 tablespoons boiling water first to activate and rehydrate. Then cover the berries with a mixture of 2 parts rice vinegar and 1 part raw unfiltered honey to fill the jar. Shake vigorously to dissolve the honey. Transfer to a blender to quickly blend before replacing it in the jar. Cover with a noncorrosive lid or place a small piece of fabric between a metal lid and the jar rim when closing to avoid having the vinegar corrode the metal lid. Label and allow to macerate for 2 to 4 weeks before straining.

Caution

Schisandra is contraindicated for those with epilepsy as well as those suffering from mania, particularly individuals who run warm. Do not take schisandra if you have taken any medications that are metabolized by human gene locus CYP3A or ABCB1.

Skullcap

Scutellaria lateriflora
LAMIACEAE

Ever feel like your senses are being assaulted from all directions? Too loud, bright? Too stimulated, and your nerves are raw? Look to skullcap for relief. Skullcap is like having an insulator from the overwhelm—a magic hat that relaxes you and leaves you replete.

Habitat and Cultivation

Skullcap is a perennial herb that grows along streams in much of North America. It's very easy to grow in the garden and readily self-seeds. It will also bloom multiple times in one summer, offering continual harvest of the bright-blue flowering tops. *Scutelaria galericulata* (marsh skullcap) is used more or less interchangeably, but it is wild-harvested. Choose *S. lateriflora* for the garden.

Taste and Energetics
bitter • cooling

Actions and Uses
anticonvulsant • anti-inflammatory • antimicrobial • antioxidant • antispasmodic • anxiolytic • bitter tonic • diuretic • emmenagogue • gabanergic • relaxant • trophorestorative • nervine

---

Skullcap is a powerful tonic, calming remedy with traditional use by the Eclectics (see chapter 1) for many types of neurological disorders and nervous conditions.

It can be useful for those in withdrawal from addictive substances, particularly opiates and alcohol. And it can help you sleep off symptoms of delirium tremens.

Indigenous Americans including the Cherokee used skullcap in their medicine. It was known as mad dog skullcap in reference to its use in treating rabies. It was also traditionally drunk as a tea to relieve PMS and promote menstruation.

Baical skullcap (*Scutellaria baicalensis*) of TCM is also a neuroprotective agent and has similar chemistry but some different history of use.

Despite the seriousness of some of the conditions that skullcap can be used as a tonic for, it is considered a class 1 safety herb in the American Herbal Pharmacopoeia. Toxicity reported is due to the adulteration of products with the toxic species *Teucrium chamaedrys* (germander).

Constituents and Chemistry
flavonoids • terpenoids (bitter-tasting iridoids) • nutrients: amino acids and electrolytes: calcium, magnesium, potassium

Preparation
Skullcap tincture: Fill a glass jar three-quarters of the way full with finely chopped flowering skullcap. Cover with 100 proof or higher neutral grain spirits. Shake and let macerate for 2 to 4 weeks, shaking occasionally. Strain, press, and bottle.

"Calm Down, Psycho": This was one of our typical remarks in the 1990s when we were rude teenagers. This beverage hydrates, soothes, and relaxes. It is a blend of equal parts skullcap tea and a cold infusion of marshmallow root and tulsi, along with some apple cider or apple juice and a pinch of smoked sea salt. Optional: Adding several cloves as you brew the skullcap tea warms up this drink overall. To make the infusion, I combine 1 tablespoon marshmallow root powder and 8 ounces (240 ml) cold water in a jar and add as many fresh tulsi sprigs as will fit.

Caution

Skullcap may cause adverse drug interactions because it interacts with the CYP3A4 enzyme pathway in the liver. Consult with a doctor or clinically trained herbalist if you're combining it with pharmaceuticals.

Spilanthes
Acmella oleracea
ASTERACEAE

For those who like to embrace the full multisensory experience of craft, let a spilanthes flower enhance, activate, and tingle your taste buds. If you consume a lot of them, it will numb your lips and mouth.

Habitat and Cultivation

This eccentric plant—also known as jambu, buzz buttons, or electric daisy—is native to Brazil and Peru. It also grows in India. Plant it in full to part sun in moist, well-drained soil. It is hardy only in Zones 9 to 11, but will grow as an annual in colder zones.

Taste and Energetics

acrid • warming • astringent

———————

Warm and moist as it increases salivation and secretions, tingling the tongue and bringing circulation to tissues topically and internally.

Actions and Uses

analgesic • anesthetic • antifungal • anti-inflammatory • antimalarial • antimicrobial • antiparasitic • antipyretic • aphrodisiac • bioinsecticide • diuretic • insecticidal • gastroprotective • immunomodulator • sialagogue • vasorelaxant

———————

Spilanthes promotes salivation and stimulates appetite, helps boost immunity at the onset of illness, and can increase testosterone levels in animals.[4]

The leaves are used fresh and dry in Amazonian cooking. It's a traditional medicine in South America and Asia, where it has been used for gout (uric acid) and rheumatism.

It is often called the toothache plant, because of its trifecta of numbing, antimicrobial, and immune-stimulating qualities, useful for all dental conditions as well as sore throats. In addition to the circulation-enhancing and numbing anesthetic action, it assists with modulating pain and inflammation.

Use of spilanthes as a natural pesticide is being explored.

Constituents and Chemistry
alkaloids, including alkamide and spilanthol • flavonoids • tannins • terpenes

Preparation
Spilanthes tincture: Fill a small (4 to 8 ounce / 120 to 240 ml) glass jar with fresh spilanthes flowers. Cover with overproof alcohol. You can transfer the alcohol and flowers to a blender for a quick immersion before replacing in the jar. Let sit for 4 weeks before straining.

Spilanthes foam: In a whipped cream dispenser, combine 2 ounces (60 ml) lime juice, 6 ounces (180 ml) water, 1 ounce (30 ml) agave syrup, 2 teaspoons spilanthes tincture (made with tequila), 4 egg whites, and a couple pinches of sea salt. I use this foam to top off one of my creations, a very low alcohol-by-volume (ABV) margarita.

Sweetfern
Comptonia peregrina
MYRICACEAE

We are walking in each other's footsteps: I am intimate with this plant because it is abundant in the forests and fields where I frolic. To me it is the quintessential smell of August, especially when accompanied by the aroma of ripening pinecones. Walking in the winter woods of Maine, I have noticed that sweetfern is also a favorite food of the white-tailed deer during the cold seasons.

Habitat and Cultivation
Sweetfern is a large plant or shrub of dry, sandy habitats, often abundant in woodland clearings and fields as well as sandplains. The flowers are catkins, and the fruits are encased with

fuzzy green burrs. These as well as the funky zigzag leaves and buds are all aromatic. The plant is a great candidate for the edges of your property, as long as the soil conditions are favorable for it. Sweetfern is very drought-tolerant and has the ability to help supply nitrogen for itself and neighboring plants.

Taste and Energetics
pungent • astringent • warming • diffusive

Actions and Uses
anti-inflammatory • antimicrobial • antispasmodic • astringent • carminative

―――――

Many indigenous tribes have used this species as an antidote for poison ivy exposure and other minor skin conditions, helping to reduce inflammation and itching. The Chippewa drank a tea made from the leaves.

Constituents and Chemistry
flavonoids • phenolic acids • tannins • terpenes

Preparation
Sweetfern makes a tasty tea and an aromatic for aperitifs and bitters. Collect and use the leaves, flowers, and buds at all times in the year where it is native (be sure you have correctly identified the species before collecting, though). Use fresh or dry. It also makes an intriguing garnish with its unique zigzag leaves! See the Chocolate Sweetfern Bitters recipe on page 143.

Tulsi

Ocimum spp.
LAMIACEAE

In India, tulsi is called sacred basil, and it is revered by those who practice Hinduism. They keep it in special clay pots at the doorstep to connect those living there with the divine and to purify and protect the home and self. Tulsi is known as the elixir of life and the queen of herbs in Ayurvedic medicine. *Tulasi* means "the incomparable one" and is associated as a physical manifestation of Lakshmi, the goddess of wealth, prosperity, and success. The stem wood is used for making mala beads, which are used in meditation and prayer. The antimicrobial components of the plant can help "clean" water. Tulsi is known as a natural air purifier and is being studied for its potential to decrease atmospheric pollution.

Habitat and Cultivation

Useful species of *Ocimum* include Krishna tulsi (*O. tenuiflorum* syn. *sanctum*), Amrita tulsi (a subvariety of *O. tenuiflorum*), Vana tulsi (*O. gratissimum*), and temperate tulsi (*O. africanum*). Temperate tulsi is the best known species and the easiest to grow. It is a fast-growing annual in colder climates. Tulsi requires fertile and moist soil. Direct-seeding is recommended. Thin plants to 6 to 8 inches (15–20 cm) apart. This plant offers a very abundant and continual harvest throughout the growing season. If seeds are allowed to mature on the plants, they will sometimes self-sow.

Taste and Energetics

pungent, sweet • diffusive, warm, and neutral • clove-esque aromatic profile, although the aroma varies among species. Some think the temperate species tastes like bubblegum.

Actions and Uses

adaptogen • anti-asthmatic • anti-cancer • antidepressant • anti-inflammatory • antioxidant • antimicrobial • antiviral • aromatic nervine • carminative • expectorant • immune tonic • neuroprotective • radio-protective

---

Tulsi is traditionally used for regulating the mind-body-spirit spectrum, specifically mood, digestion, energy, and immunity as well as in cases of arthritis, diabetes, dementia, and heart disease. It has been used to mitigate and repair the detrimental cognitive effects caused by excessive cannabis use. The root has been used as an aphrodisiac. Tulsi is also a common ingredient in Thai cooking.

Constituents and Chemistry

alkaloids • flavonoids • phenolic acids • polysaccharides • tannins • terpenes • nutrients: vitamins A and C; calcium, iron, zinc

Preparation

The first time I ever tasted tulsi was in a gifted infused honey made by Avena Botanicals in Maine. Using honey is an incredible way to preserve the aromatics of this plant. My favorite way to use tulsi, however, is fresh. I cut the flowering tops and include them in infused waters, distill them into hydrosols, and add them into otherwise complete preparations fresh and unheated to infuse.

Plant Monographs

Vanilla

Vanilla planifolia
ORCHIDACEAE

It's a bit ironic that vanilla is not common, conventional, or ordinary. The fact that it's been used traditionally as an aphrodisiac is amusing, too. The slang use of this word is quite contrary to the truth: Vanilla is a highly specialized luxury; a rare breed. The flowers are estimated to have only 1 percent chance of being pollinated in the wild, partially due to the depletion of bee habitat. In cultivation, vanilla plants must be hand-pollinated. The complex flavor of vanilla is the result of a biological cocktail of over 250 compounds found in the seeds.

Habitat and Cultivation

Vanilla is native to Mexico and Central and South America in warm tropical rain forests. The plant is an epiphytic orchid and vine that climbs and clings to trees, enjoying the moist air at heights up to 50 feet (15 m). It is endangered in the wild.

In commercial production, flowers are hand-pollinated in the early morning. The plants are propagated easily through cuttings.

Vanilla pompona and *V. tahitensis* are also grown, but *V. planifolia* has the plumpest beans and most concentrated vanilla flavor. Tahitian vanilla has smaller beans but a more diverse aromatic profile, which some describe as a lighter floral with cherry and licorice notes.

The vanilla beans purchased in commerce are cured through a specialized process that requires controlled drying, steaming, and some fermentation. The raw, fresh pod has no aroma! It is a wonder how anyone figured it out.

A "vanilla crisis" has been reported! Vanilla is one of the most popular spices in the world despite its highly specialized production and limited, threatened habitat, including pollinator habitat. The fake vanilla flavor "vanillin" is produced during the breakdown of petrochemicals. Researchers have suggested exploring the cultivation of different vanilla species, of which there are 140 total. Reforestation and awareness surrounding conscious agricultural practices may help.

Taste and Energetics
sweet • pungent

Actions and Uses
antimicrobial • antioxidant • antispasmodic • aphrodisiac • aromatic nervine • carminative • emmenagogue • febrifuge

———

Vanilla has been traditionally used as and considered an aphrodisiac, particularly for women, based on implication via the doctrine of signatures (explained in the "Passiflora" monograph on page 267); modern research has yet to confirm this. The earliest reference to use of vanilla was in a cacao beverage made by the Aztecs.

Constituents and Chemistry
flavonoids • lignans • vanillin, a phenolic aldehyde, which makes up the largest percentage of the compounds thought to contribute to flavor • terpenes

Preparation
Homemade vanilla extract: Once you try making your own vanilla extract, you'll be hooked. Cut 12 beans in half lengthwise and put them in a pint jar. Cover with overproof rum. Let macerate for 1 to 2 months. When you're ready to strain it, shake it vigorously first. After straining, scrape the inside of the beans into your extract.

Yarrow
Achillea millefolium
ASTERACEAE

A materia medica of tonics would be remiss not to include yarrow, a tonic in the truest sense. Yarrow tones tissues with its tannins. The ancients called it knight's milfoil or military herb for what is arguably its most important use: to stanch bleeding and heal wounds. It was named after Achilles, the greatest of warriors in Greek mythology. The fossilized pollen of yarrow has been found in Neanderthal burial caves from as far back as sixty thousand years ago. Speaking of coevolution…

Habitat and Cultivation
Yarrow is wild and weedy, although you can plant it in the garden among strong companions. The flowers can be pink as well as neon yellow on

ornamental varieties that can also be incorporated as edible flowers. The leaves and flowers are both useful; the flowers are good for native pollinators and bloom midsummer here in Maine. *Achillea millefolium* is ubiquitous on roadsides and in fields. It's native throughout North America and Europe. The best way to introduce yarrow into your garden is to dig up a piece of a wild plant and transplant it, because yarrow seed can take as long as three months to germinate.

Taste and Energetics
bitter, astringent, pungent • diffusive

Actions and Uses
antimicrobial • cardiotonic • cholagogue • diaphoretic • emmenagogue • styptic • tissue tonic • urinary antiseptic • vasodilator • vulnerary

---

Yarrow has a history of metaphysical and magical use. Modern mystics used it for enhancing healthy boundaries and as divine protection. Yarrow stalks were traditionally used to cast the I Ching, the Chinese book of prophecy.

A powerful diaphoretic, a hot yarrow tea can help you sweat off a fever. As a cardiovascular tonic, it has been used for varicose veins and hemorrhoids. As mentioned above, it has been used to stop bleeding of wounds, and it helps to improve blood flow throughout the body.

Constituents and Chemistry
alkaloids, including achillein • flavonoids • phenolic acid • tannins • terpenes

Preparation
Yarrow is a good candidate for wild bitters blends. It is very easy to dry: I usually make a bundle of five to eight whole flowering stems, tie them near the base with jute, and hang in a breezy place out of direct sunlight. When they are fully dry, the stems and flowers should be brittle feeling. You can store them in a glass jar in a cool, dry place.

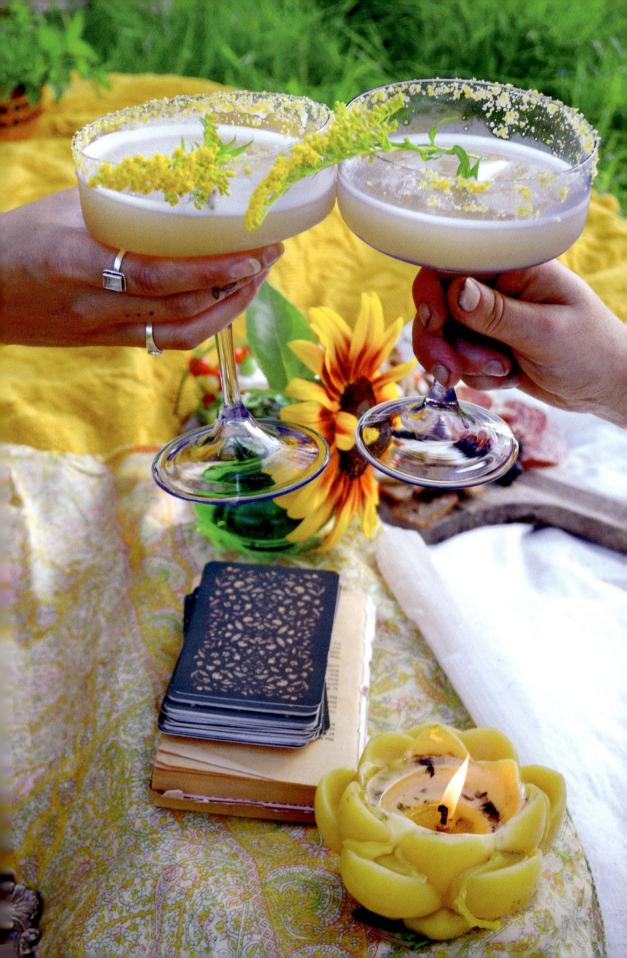

EPILOGUE
Three Generations at the Bar

I walk into a small-town pub in a quaint inn in rural Vermont. There are six bar seats and two guys with the same name. It's only about eight o'clock, but the face on the fellow beside me is quite red. He immediately zeroes in on me as a source of interesting conversation. He introduces me to the bartender. Upon hearing of my journey and its purpose, these two men collectively share the intel about local distilleries and tell me the stories of the founders. They are both local. My tippled older gentleman, probably in his mid-sixties but with a weathered face that indicates the reality of many more stories, asks questions with fervor. The nineteen-year-old bartender, obviously not drunk, is stoked to chat, too. He is the perfect bartender: perceptive and captivating, with curious, piercing eyes and a deep thirst for life. His whole life is laid out in front of him like a magic tapestry studded with sparkling gems of possibility. I hope he gets to be a rock star.

I always prefer people with character, but I am a curious sort. This is what it means when you tell people, "I'm a bar person." This is what you sign up for: swapping stories, philosophy, and favorite books, sharing the essence and beauty of the passion of your life with strangers.

I am on a journey, on a bridge between past and present, and these two men symbolize the opposite edges of time perception. I see myself in both characters, humanity, love, and comedy reflecting back at me.

As a bartender, this is an experience that I play host to all the time. People make new connections—friends and ideas. The bar is a place of freedom for people and culture, and by no means does it require lubrication to enjoy. I am getting less and less thirsty for alcohol as the years go on. But I find myself just as thirsty—no, even thirstier—for experience and sharing my humanity with other people. It is what improves us: the ability to be real and raw with each other. As the world becomes more and more impersonal, we crave deeply to be welcomed someplace where everyone knows our name.

Botanical Bar Craft

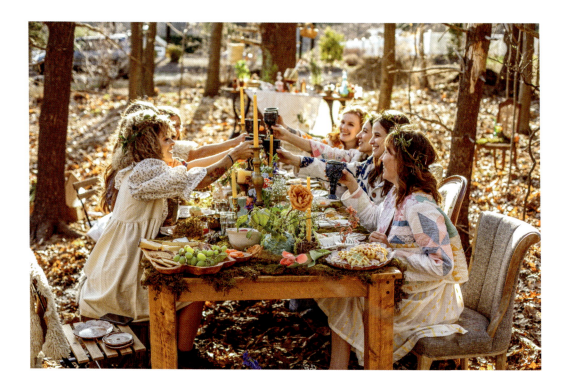

This is my humble invitation to continue caring about the simple things. Cocktail craft is an extension of the culinary and the inspiration is garden-to-glass, celebrating this exact moment in time and the way it tastes in nature. The process is love, just as food is love, imbued with heartfelt care and attention, beginning with a seed.

ACKNOWLEDGMENTS

Love is the foundation of everything. I would like to express deep gratitude for my fabulous family of enlightened rebels, who have been supportive in allowing and then assisting me in becoming the full expression of myself, fostering and encouraging both discipline and freedom, the development of my creativity and gifts, so that I have been able to share my inspiration, guided by the breath of nature, with you. Thank you for sharing your own dreams, lessons, and magic with me. It is a beautiful thing when your family become your best friends.

I am grateful for the beautiful tapestry of relationships and friendships, for all the good shiny souls with whom I get to share ideas and collaborate on fun projects. You know who you are, and I love you. Cheers to shared values. Conscious collaboration is the way of the future! Thank you for building the new world with me.

Thank you to my very first teachers, the green beings who called to me from the beginning to be their voice and champion, who continue to inspire curiosity and deep reverence.

I believe every experience and person is a teacher, in both a spiritual and practical sense, but there are some wonderful people who dedicate themselves to teaching others. I thank all my teachers who fanned my flames, offered criticism when necessary, and were patient with my boundless and sometimes erratic energy. I am so grateful to have had many mentors on this path, each offering and informing my heart. You know who you are.

Similarly, I thank all my bosses and mentors who helped to show me the way and provided space for my creativity. I've been so lucky to have so many great jobs!

I appreciate all my soulmate clients who have supported my work through hiring my business, the Remedy Cocktail Co., and all those who have written five-star reviews and spoken kindly of this business to friends and colleagues. Thank you for your generous support, and for hiring me again! Thank you to investors, benefactors, and my angels.

I would like to thank the White Barn Inn in Kennebunkport, Maine, for putting many of these recipes on their Forbes five-star menu!

Thank you to the distillers who made chapter 5 of this book possible. I had so much fun taking a deeper dive into the soul behind the spirit. Thank you to the companies that provided some of the materials and equipment I needed for recipes and photos: Culinary Solvent, Cocktail Kingdom, North Spore, Tepotztli, and Anima Mundi.

Fern and Chelsea Green Publishing were an absolute pleasure to collaborate with in the production of this book.

Thank you to all the photographers with whom I have had the pleasure of working; many of their images are featured in this book. A special thanks to Jenn Bakos, who has taken many beautiful photos for me over the years and also helped me with last-minute photos!

. . . and last but not least, a big basket of love to all of the farmers without whom I could not imagine and mix.

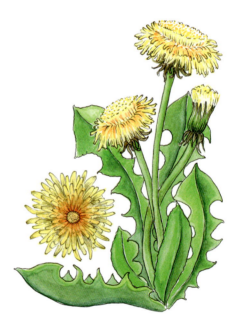

RESOURCES

Botanicals and Extracts

Beyond what you can garden and forage yourself, look to local herb farms for fresh and dried herbs and extracts. The list below includes several from my region of the Northeast United States. If the herb you seek is not available from a local producer, check a reputable wholesaler; I've also included some of the wholesale companies I know and trust in this list.

ANIMA MUNDI
https://animamundiherbals.com

AVENA BOTANICALS
https://www.avenabotanicals.com

EARTH SPIRAL APOTHECARY
https://earthspiralapothecary.com

FOSTER FARM BOTANICALS
https://fosterfarmbotanicals.com

FOUR ELEMENTS ORGANIC HERBALS
https://fourelementsherbals.com

FRONTIER CO-OP
https://www.frontiercoop.com/herbs-and-teas

HERBAL REVOLUTION
https://www.herbalrev.com

HERB PHARM
https://www.herb-pharm.com

MEETING HOUSE FARM
https://www.meetinghouse.farm

MOUNTAIN ROSE HERBS
https://mountainroseherbs.com

ROOTED HEART REMEDIES
https://www.rootedheartremedies.com

STARWEST BOTANICALS
https://www.starwest-botanicals.com

WILD FEW HERB FARM
https://wildfewherbfarm.com

ZACK WOODS HERB FARM
https://www.zackwoodsherbs.com

Medicine-Making Guides

Making Plant Medicine by Richo Cech (Herbal Reads, 2016)
Alchemy of Herbs by Rosalee de la Forêt (Hay House, 2017)
Herbal Constituents by Lisa Ganora (HerbalChem Press, 2009)
Herbal Recipes for Vibrant Health by Rosemary Gladstar (Storey Publishing, 2008)
The Herbal Medicine-Maker's Handbook by James Green (Crossing Press, 2000)

Body into Balance by Maria Noel Groves (Storey Publishing, 2016)
The Wild Medicine Solution by Guido Mase (Healing Arts Press, 2013)
The Modern Herbal Dispensatory: A Medicine Making Guide by Thomas Easley and Steven Horne (North Atlantic Books, 2016)

Gardening

Look for a Cooperative Extension Master Gardener program in your area at https://mastergardener.extension.org.

Many seed companies offer growing information on their websites. Johnny's Seeds here in Maine has an "Ask a Grower" feature on their website, https://www.johnnyseeds.com.

Connect with agricultural organizations that offer workshops and mentoring programs. Here in New England, we have the Northeast Organic Farming Association (NOFA) and the Maine Organic Farmers and Gardeners Association (MOFGA).

Go to your local agricultural fair. Introduce yourself to your neighbors who garden. They make great gardening friends and mentors that you can share some of the harvest with!

Here are some of my favorite and most-used gardening books:

The Organic Gardener's Handbook of Natural Pest and Disease Control edited by Fern Marshall Bradley, Barbara W. Ellis, and Deborah L. Martin (Rodale Books, 2010)
The Organic Medicinal Herb Farmer, revised edition, by Melanie and Jeff Carpenter (Chelsea Green Publishing, 2023)
The New Organic Grower, 3rd edition, by Eliot Coleman (Chelsea Green Publishing, 2018)
The Resilient Farm and Homestead, revised and expanded edition, by Ben Falk (Chelsea Green Publishing, 2024)
Gaia's Garden by Toby Hemenway (Chelsea Green Publishing, 2009)
Carrots Love Tomatoes by Louise Riotte (Storey Publishing, 1998)
The Vegetable Gardener's Bible by Edward C. Smith (Storey Publishing, 2009)
How to Move Like a Gardener by Deb Soule (Steiner Books, 2013)
Old Farmer's Almanac Vegetable Gardener's Handbook (Old Farmer's Almanac, 2019)

NOTES

Chapter 1. Ancestral Botanicals in Spirits and Medicine

1. Anabel Ford, Ann Williams, and Mattanjah S. de Vries, "New Light on the Use of *Theobroma cacao* by Late Classic Maya," *PNAS* 119, no. 40 (2022), https://doi.org/10.1073/pnas.2121821119.
2. W. Jeffrey Hurst et al., "Cacao Usage by the Earliest Maya Civilization," *Nature* 418 (2002): 289–90, https://doi.org/10.1038/418289a.
3. Tatiana V. Morozova, Trudy F. C. Mackay, and Robert R. H. Anholt, "Genetics and Genomics of Alcohol Sensitivity," *Molecular Genetics and Genomics* 289, no. 3 (2014), 253–69, https://doi.org/10.1007/s00438-013-0808-y.
4. Blaine Caslin et al., "Alcohol as Friend or Foe in Autoimmune Diseases: A Role for Gut Microbiome?" *Gut Microbes* 13, no. 1 (2021), https://doi.org/10.1080/19490976.2021.1916278.
5. J. Leigh Leasure et al., "Exercise and Alcohol Consumption: What We Know, What We Need to Know, and Why It Is Important." *Frontiers in Psychiatry* 6 (2015): 156, https://doi.org/10.3389/fpsyt.2015.00156.
6. Adrian F. Rogne, Willy Pedersen, and Tilmann Von Soest. "Intelligence, Alcohol Consumption, and Adverse Consequences. A Study of Young Norwegian Men," *Scandinavian Journal of Public Health* 49, no. 4 (2021): 411–18, https://doi.org/10.1177/1403494820944719.

Chapter 3. Herbal Actions and Tonics

1. Hui-Chen Lu and Ken Mackie, "An Introduction to the Endogenous Cannabinoid System," *Biological Psychiatry* 79, no. 7 (2016): 516–25, https://doi.org/10.1016/j.biopsych.2015.07.028.

Chapter 4. The Chemistry of Extraction

1. Christopher Weyh et al., "The Role of Minerals in the Optimal Functioning of the Immune System," *Nutrients* 14, no. 3 (2022): 644, https://doi.org/10.3390/nu14030644.

Chapter 6. The Garnish Garden

1. "Study Linking Beneficial Bacteria to Mental Health Makes Top 10 List for Brain Research," *CU Boulder Today*, January 5, 2017, https://

www.colorado.edu/today/2017/01/05/study-linking-beneficial-bacteria-mental-health-makes-top-10-list-brain-research.

Chapter 8. Plant Monographs

1. Neeti N. Jain et al., "*Clitoria ternatea* and the CNS," *Pharmacology, Biochemistry and Behavior* 75, no. 3 (2003): 529–36, https://doi.org/10.1016/S0091-3057(03)00130-8.
2. Mariangela Marrelli et al., "Effects of Saponins on Lipid Metabolism: A Review of Potential Health Benefits in the Treatment of Obesity," *Molecules (Basel, Switzerland)* 21, no. 10 (2016): 1404, https://doi.org/10.3390/molecules21101404.
3. Hsuan-Ti Huang, "Osteoprotective Roles of Green Tea Catechins," *Antioxidants (Basel, Switzerland)* 9, no. 11 (2020): 1136, https://doi.org/10.3390/antiox9111136.
4. Vikas Sharma et al., "*Spilanthes acmella* Ethanolic Flower Extract: LC-MS Alkylamide Profiling and Its Effects on Sexual Behavior in Male Rats," *Phytomedicine : International Journal of Phytotherapy and Phytopharmacology* 18, no. 13 (2011): 1161–69, https://doi.org/10.1016/j.phymed.2011.06.001.

SELECTED BIBLIOGRAPHY

Beinfield, Harriet, and Efrem Korngold. "Between Heaven and Earth: A Guide to Chinese Medicine." *Journal of Nurse-Midwifery* 36 (1991). https://doi.org/10.1016/0091-2182(91)90114-5.

Cech, Richo. *Making Plant Medicine.* Williams, OR: Horizon Herbals, 2000.

Ganora, Lisa. *Herbal Constituents: Foundations of Phytochemistry.* HerbalChem Press, 2009.

Grieve, Margaret. *A Modern Herbal: The Medicinal, Culinary, Cosmetic and Economic Properties, Cultivation and Folklore of Herbs, Grasses, Fungi, Shrubs and Trees with All Their Modern Scientific Uses*, volumes 1 and 2. New York: Dover Publishing, 1971.

Haines, Arthur. *Ancestral Plants: A Primitive Skills Guide to Important Edible, Medicinal, and Useful Plants of the Northeast.* Anaskimin, 2010.

Harvard Health. "Understanding the Stress Response," April 3, 2024. https://www.health.harvard.edu/staying-healthy/understanding-the-stress-response.

Johns Hopkins Medicine. "The Brain-Gut Connection," January 24, 2024. https://www.hopkinsmedicine.org/health/wellness-and-prevention/the-brain-gut-connection#:~:text=Hidden%20in%20the%20walls%20of,enteric%20nervous%20system%20(ENS).

Masé, Guido. *The Wild Medicine Solution: Healing with Aromatic, Bitter, and Tonic Plants.* Rochester, VT: Healing Arts Press, 2013.

McGovern, Patrick E. *Uncorking the Past: The Quest for Wine, Beer, and Other Alcoholic Beverages.* Oakland: University of California Press, 2009.

Mills, Simon, and Kerry Bone. *Principles and Practice of Phytotherapy: Modern Herbal Medicine.* Edinburgh: Churchill Livingston, 1999.

Pitchford, Paul. *Healing with Whole Foods: Asian Traditions and Modern Nutrition.* Berkeley, CA: North Atlantic Books, 1993.

Plants of the World Online. "Plants of the World Online | Kew Science," n.d. https://powo.science.kew.org/.

Schaal, Barbara. "Plants and People: Our Shared History and Future." *Plants, People, Planet* 1, no. 1 (December 4, 2018): 14–19. https://doi.org/10.1002/ppp3.12.

Winston, David, and Steven Maimes. *Adaptogens: Herbs for Strength, Stamina, and Stress Relief.* Rochester, VT: Healing Arts Press, 2007.

Wood, Matthew. *The Earthwise Herbal*, volume 1: *A Complete Guide to Old World Medicinal Plants.* Berkeley, CA: North Atlantic Books, 2008.

IMAGE CREDITS

Unless noted below, all images are from the collection of Cassandra Elizabeth Sears.

Images on pages iv and 224 by Emily Sawchuck Photography.

Image on page viii by Shannon Shipman.

Image on page x by Alexa Demsey.

Images on pages 3, 5, 9, 10, 23, 33, 35, 36, 42, 45, 52, 57, 74, 76, 101, 106, 108, 126, 151, 152, 162, 166, 179, 182, 188, 206, and 288 by Jenn Bakos.

Images on pages 6, 26, 48, 131, 144, 170, 173, 177, 185, 197, and 286 by Hannah Martin.

Image on page 43 by Johanna Sorrell.

Image on page 80 by Sarah Dellen.

Image on page 107 by Rhonda Evans.

Image on page 147 by Nick Eaton.

Image on page 183 by Rebecca Seger.

Image on page 193 by Antoinette Photography.

Image on page 209 by Jalin Ink Photography.

Illustrations on pages 123, 154, 176, and 198 by Isabella-Zoe Ciolfi.

Illustrations on pages 227, 229, 230, 232, 233, 235, 236, 237, 239, 241, 242, 244, 246, 247, 249, 250, 252, 253, 254, 256, 257, 259, 261, 262, 264, 267, 268, 270, 272, 274, 275, 277, 279, 280, 282, 283, and 285 used courtesy of the Biodiversity Heritage Library | www.biodiversitylibrary.org

INDEX

Note: Page numbers in **bold** indicate recipes, page numbers in *italics* indicate photographs and illustrations, and page numbers followed by *t* indicate tables.

A

About Last Night, **260**
açai berries, in Infused Pisco, 137
acetums (vinegar extracts), 32, 39, 83*t*. *See also* apple cider vinegar
adaptive immune response, 64
Adaptogenic Chai Tea, **240**
adaptogens, 54–55, 64
addiction to alcohol, 22, 24–25
After-Dinner Mint Cordial, **262**
agave nectar
   in Hibiscus Agave, 185
   in Sea-Salted Agave Caramel, 211
agave syrup
   in Embrace the Dragon, 155
   in Euphoria, 211
   in Juice of Life, 180
   in Spiced Chocolate Syrup, 220
   in Spilanthes Foam, 280
Agua de Jamaica, **251**
Al-Ambiq copper stills, 104, *105*
alchemy, 17–18
alcohol abuse, 22, 24–25
alcohol consumption, risks and benefits of, 20–25
alcohol solvents, quick reference guide, 83*t*, 85
Alexander-style drinks, 50
alkaloids, extraction of, 78
alkylamides, 81
allspice dram liqueur, 222
Altar & Intent, **183**, *183*
alteratives, overview, 55
altered consciousness
   early practices of, 11
   risks and benefits of alcohol consumption, 20–25

amaro
   summary of preparation, 31
   Winter Amaro, 140, 142, 169
Ambrosia, **222**, *222*
American ginseng (*Panax quinquefolius*), as adaptogen, 55
amino acids, extraction of, 82
anandamide, 69
ancestral cocktails, overview, 47
Ancho Reyes Ancho Chili Liqueur, 220
ancient Egypt
   alchemy practice in, 17
   use of the blue lotus, 11–12
ancient Greece
   alchemy practice in, 17
   plant-based medicine in, 16
   winemaking in, 12–13
angelica (*Angelica archangelica*), *227*
   in "Are You a Dreamer?" Bitters, 128
   bitter qualities of, 59
   monograph on, 226–28
Angel's Envy bourbon, 142
Anima Mundi Herbals, 124, 125, 182, 291
anise hyssop (*Agastache foeniculum*)
   in Anise Hyssop & Blueberry Leaf Tea, 212
   aromatic qualities, 58
   growing, 112
Anise Hyssop & Blueberry Leaf Tea, **212**
anti-inflammatory herbs, 55
aperitifs
   about, 157
   Bitter Orange Cordial, 148
   Bitters & Soda, 158
   bitters for, 58

   Everyday Aperitif, 156
   Secret Grove, 130
aphrodisiacs, overview, 56
apple cider
   in Ambrosia, 222
   in Apple Cider Caramel, 169
   in Ginger-Cinnamon Cider, 210
   in Harvest Gold, 209
   in Sultry Look, 210
Apple Cider Caramel, **169**
apple cider vinegar
   in Digestivo Oxymel, 156
   in Red Raspberry Leaf & Stinging Nettle Tea, 167
   in Seafarer's Oxymel, 213
   in Spring Tonic Oxymel, 160
   in Wormwood Vinegar Bitters, 159
aqua vitae (water of life), 17
aralia (*Aralia nudicaulis*)
   in Aralia Root & Ginger Tea, 160
   in Winter Amaro, 140
Aralia Root & Ginger Tea, **160**
"Are You a Dreamer?" Bitters, 127, **128**
aromatics
   in nonalcoholic spirits, 104
   overview, 56, 58
artichoke (*Cynara cardunculus* var. *scolymus*), 229
   bitter qualities of, 59
   in Digestivo Oxymel, 156
   monograph on, 229
ashwagandha (*Withania somnifera*)
   as adaptogen, 55
   as alkaloid, *78*

ashwagandha (*continued*)
    in Ashwagandha Decoction, 202
    as nervine trophorestorative, 62
Ashwagandha Decoction, **202**
astragalus (*Astragalus membranaceus*)
    as adaptogen, 55
    in Adaptogenic Chai Tea, 240
    in Chai-Spiced Elderberry Syrup, 146
    in Harvest Gold, 209
astringents, overview, 58
Atlantic Sea Farms, 90
atomizers, 44, *45*
autumn
    in Five Element Theory, 72–73
    qualities of, 198
Avicenna, 16, 256

B

Babe in the Woods, **178**, *179*
bachelor buttons (*Centaurea cyanus*), *33*
    in flower confetti, 221
    growing, 112
bacopa (*Bacopa monnieri*), as nootropic, 62
bad liquor (fusel), 92
balsam fir and pine hydrosol
    in Everyday Aperitif, 156
    in Secret Grove, 130
balsam fir tips, in Forest Green Juice, 163
Barr Hill, *98*
    gin from, 170, 171, 172, 187
    profile of, 98–100
    vodka from, 141
bar spoons, *40*, 41
beach bay (*Myrica pensylvanica*), 213
bee balm (*Monarda* spp.)
    aromatic qualities, 58
    in Ruby Throat Sunset, 177
bee pollen
    in Cheshire Cat, 170
    nutritional chemistry of, 80
Bee's Knees sour, 98–99

beet (*Beta vulgaris*)
    in Beet Kvass, 213
    in Bitter Orange Cordial, 148
    in Wildfire Hearts, 184
Beet Kvass, 212, **213**
Betts, Briana, *177*
Bhumi Farms, 97
binomial nomenclature, 54
birch (*Betula* spp.), *230*
    anti-inflammatory qualities, 55
    in Birch Bark Syrup, 145
    bourbon infused with, 146
    monograph on, 230–31
    in Winter Amaro, 140
Birch Bark Syrup, **145**
birch polypore mushroom (*Piptoporus betulinus*)
    in Birch Bark Syrup, 145
    monograph on, 265, 266
Bitter Orange Cordial, **148**
bitters
    defined, 31
    in Five Element Theory, 72
    herbal actions of, 58–59
    summary of preparation, 31–33
Bitters & Soda, **158**
blackberry (*Rubus* spp.)
    as cardioprotective, 60
    in Fields of Gold Mead, 190
    in "Fields of Gold" Mead Spritzer, 192
black tea (*Camellia* spp.)
    as astringent, 58
    as nervine stimulant, 61
Black Trumpet & Butter-Washed Bourbon, **214**
black trumpet mushroom (*Craterellus cornucopioides*), 214
black walnut (*Juglans nigra*), 223
Black Walnut Bitters, 222, **223**
blenders, 44
Bloody Botanist, **152**, *152*
Bloody Mary mix, 152, **153**
Bloody Mary-style drinks, 51
Blue Barren Distillery, 89–90
blueberry (*Vaccinium angustifolium*), *57*, *232*
    in Altar & Intent, 183

    in Anise Hyssop & Blueberry Leaf Tea, 212
    as aphrodisiac, 56
    in Blue Barren Distillery, 89–90
    in Blueberry-Chaga Elixir, 178
    in Blueberry Jamboree, 126
    as cardioprotective, 60
    in Fields of Gold Mead, 190
    in Gates of Immortality, 188
    monograph on, 231–32
    in Pregnancy Punch, 167
    in Seafarer's Oxymel, 213
Blueberry-Chaga Elixir, **178**
Blueberry Jamboree, **126**, *126*
blue lotus (*Nymphaea caerulea*)
    ancient use of, 11–12, *12*
    in Blue Lotus Wine Spritzer, 13
    in Opening Doors, 131
Blue Lotus Wine Spritzer, **13**
bluet (*Houstonia caerulea*), 173
blue vervain (*Verbena officinalis*), 59
Boles's Dirty Gardener Martini, **150**, *151*
book resources, 291–92
Boomr Bags, *188*, 264
borage, growing, 112
Boston shakers, 40
botanical names, 54
bottles and jars, 42–43, *43*
Bottoms Up (Saucier), 14
bourbon
    in Black Trumpet & Butter-Washed Bourbon, 214
    in Gates of Immortality, 188
    in Savant or Savage? 142
    in Wisdom of Old, 146
Brandy Alexander, 50
buck-style drinks, 49
building cocktails, 29–30
bull thistle (*Cirsium vulgare*), 59
Bully Boy Rum Cooperative Volume 2, 134, 219
burdock (*Arctium lappa*)
    as alterative, 55
    in Embrace the Dragon, 154
    in Spring Tonic Oxymel, 160
butane torches, 46

Index

butterfly pea (*Clitoria ternatea*), *233*
   in Butterfly Tea, 234
   in Dreamer's Tea, 200
   monograph on, 232–34
   in Nootropical Paradise, 182
Butterfly Tea, **234**

C

cacao (*Theobroma cacao*), *235*
   ancient use of, 12
   as aphrodisiac, 56
   in Chocolate Sweetfern Bitters, 143
   in Heart of Venus, 164
   in Kava Cacao Flip, 127
   in Like Bunny Rabbits, 165
   in Lovers' Tequila, 211
   monograph on, 234–36
   as nervine stimulant, 61
   in Quantum Entanglement, 136
   in Sexy Hot Chocolate, 132
   in Spiced Chocolate Syrup, 220
   in Xocolatl, 220
calendula (*Calendula officinalis*), *116*
   in Altar & Intent, 183
   in Calendula & Gotu Kola Honey Tea Syrup, 124
   in flower confetti, 221
Calendula & Gotu Kola Honey Tea Syrup, **124**
California poppy (*Eschscholzia californica*)
   in Dreamer's Tea, 200
   as nervine relaxant, 62
"Calm Down, Psycho," **278–79**
cannabinoids
   CBD, 200, 202
   endogenous, 68–69
cardamom (*Elettaria cardamomum*)
   in Adaptogenic Chai Tea, 240
   aromatic qualities, 58
   in Cardamom Bitters, 159
   in Cardamom-Orange Bitters, 223
   in Cardamom-Rose Sea Salt, 181
   in Chai-Spice Bitters, 147
   in Digestivo Oxymel, 156
   in Harvest Gold, 209
   in Maca Chai Syrup, 137
   in "Rum-Spiced" Molasses, 167
   in Spicy Pink Salt, 187
Cardamom Bitters, 158, **159**, 211
Cardamom-Orange Bitters, 222, **223**
Cardamom-Rose Sea Salt, 180, **181**
cardioprotectives, overview, 59–60
cardiovascular tonics, 56, *57*
Carol's Elderflower Champagne, **194**
Carthusian monks, 13–14
Cassandra's Three C's Calming Colic Tonic, **241–42**
cayenne (*Capsicum annuum*)
   as aphrodisiac, 56
   in Aztec Hot Chocolate, 236
   in Homemade Bloody Mary Mix, 153
   in Like Bunny Rabbits, 165
   in Sexy Hot Chocolate, 132
   in Spicy Pink Salt, 187
CBD (cannabidiol)
   in Dreaming with Morpheus, 200
   in The Queen's Fortress, 202
Cerebrum Tonic, 182
chaga mushroom (*Inonotus obliquus*), in Blueberry-Chaga Elixir, 178
Chai-Spice Bitters, 146, **147**
Chai-Spiced Elderberry Syrup, **146**, 149, 199
Chai-Spiced Syrup, **175**
chamomile (*Matricaria chamomilla*), *236*
   in Cassandra's Three C's Calming Colic Tonic, 242
   in Chamomile Glycerite, 219
   in Chamomile Tea, 237
   in Digestivo Oxymel, 156
   in DIY Dry Vermouth, 150
   in Ginger-Chamomile Tea, 246
   monograph on, 236–37
   as nervine relaxant, 62
   in Victory Garden, 173
Chamomile Glycerite, **219**
Chamomile Tea, **237**
Champagne, Carol's Elderflower, **194**
Chartreuse (liqueur), 13–14
A Chartreuse Trendsetter, **14**
cherry (*Prunus* spp.)
   in Altar & Intent, 183
   in Gates of Immortality, 188
   preserves of, 175
   in Very Cherry, Thorns & Flowers Syrup, 174
cherry tomato (*Solanum lycopersicum*), growing, 112
Cheshire Cat, **170**, *170*
chia seed (*Salvia hispanica*), 60
chickweed (*Stellaria media*)
   in Forest Green Juice, 163
   in The Mosscat, 162
chinoises (sieves), 42
chocolate. *See* cacao (*Theobroma cacao*)
Chocolate Sweetfern Bitters, **143**, 145
Christiansen, Ryan, 98, 99
chronic inflammation, 64–65
cinchona (*Cinchona* spp.), *237*
   in Bitter Orange Cordial, 148
   monograph on, 237–38
   in Tonic & Tonic, 135
cinnamon (*Cinnamomum* spp.), *239*
   in Adaptogenic Chai Tea, 240
   in Ambrosia, 222
   in Birch Bark Syrup, 145
   in Chai-Spice Bitters, 147
   in Chai-Spiced Elderberry Syrup, 146
   in Cinnamon Girl, 145
   in Cinnamon Marshmallows, 133
   in Cinnamon-Vanilla Honey Syrup, 201
   in The Common Sage, 205
   as demulcent, 60
   in Ginger-Cinnamon Cider, 210
   in Golden Touch, 134

cinnamon (*continued*)
   in Harvest Gold, 209
   in Kava Cacao Flip, 127
   in Kava Hula Girl, 193
   in Maca Chai Syrup, 137
   monograph on, 239–240
   in Opening Doors, 131
   in Pear & Cinnamon Stick Infused Calvados, 223
   in Pregnancy Punch, 167
   in The Queen's Fortress, 202
   in "Rum-Spiced" Molasses, 167
   in Sexy Hot Chocolate, 132
   in Spiced Chocolate Syrup, 220
   in Vision of Adonis, 129
Cinnamon Girl, *144*, **145**
Cinnamon Marshmallows, 132, **133**
Cinnamon-Vanilla Honey Syrup, 200, **201**
classic cocktail recipes, 47–51
cloves (*Syzygium aromaticum*)
   in Adaptogenic Chai Tea, 240
   in Chai-Spice Bitters, 147
   in Ginger-Clove Syrup, 130
   in Maca Chai Syrup, 137
   in Opening Doors, 131
   in "Rum-Spiced" Molasses, 167
cobbler-style drinks, 51
cobbler-style shakers, 40
Cocktail Kingdom, 40, 41, 42
coconut cream
   in Kava Cacao Flip, 127
   in Nootropical Paradise, 182
   in Sexy Hot Chocolate, 132
   in Transcendental Lilac, 172
coconut milk, in Kava Hula Girl, 193
coconut oil, for fat washing, 34
coconut water, in Mojito Popsicles, 195
Cold River Vodka, 196
collins-style drinks, 48–49
column stills, 96
The Common Sage, *204*, **205**
Complete Herbal (Culpeper), 18
constituents, of plants, 225–26
constitutional energetics, 70–71
copper alembic stills, 104, *105*

cordials
   After-Dinner Mint Cordial, 262
   Altar & Intent, 183
   Bitter Orange Cordial, 148
   Golden Touch, 134
   from hawthorn, 249
   overview, 33
coriander (*Coriandrum sativum*), 241
   in Bitter Orange Cordial, 148
   in Cassandra's Three C's Calming Colic Tonic, 241
   in DIY Dry Vermouth, 150
   in Maple Coriander Syrup, 219
   monograph on, 240–42
coumarins, 77, 240
Craddock, Harry, 50
cranberry (*Vaccinium macrocarpon*)
   as cardioprotective, 60
   in Cranberry, Rose Hip & Ginger Syrup, 138
   in The Gypsy and the Monk, 138
   in Juicy, 206
   in Tonic & Tonic, 135
Cranberry, Rose Hip & Ginger Syrup, **138**
Crew Supply Co., 42
Crimes of Passion, *196*, *197*
cucumber
   in Cucumber Infused Gin, 171
   growing, 112
Cucumber Infused Gin, **171**
Culinary Crystals Unflavored Popping Candy, 196
Culpeper, Nicholas, 18

D

dahlia (*Dahlia* spp.), growing, 112
daisy-style drinks, 48–49
damiana (*Turnera diffusa*)
   as aphrodisiac, 56
   in Like Bunny Rabbits, 165
   in Lovers' Tequila, 211
   as nervine relaxant, 62
   in Sexy Hot Chocolate, 132

dandelion (*Taraxacum officinale*), 242
   as alterative, 55
   bitter qualities of, 59
   in Heart of Venus, 164
   monograph on, 242–43
   in The Mosscat, 162
   in Spring Tonic Oxymel, 160
   in Street Smarts Tincture, 168
   in Tooth of the Lion Bitters, 243
Dandelion Hypothesis, 1
Darthia Farm, 2
dasher bottles, *40*, 43
decoctions, 32, 38–39
Dellner, Allison, 103–5, *104*
De Materia Medica (Dioscorides), 16
demulcents, 60, 82
Digestivo Oxymel, 156
dilution of drinks, 30–31
Dionysus (god of winemaking), 12–13
Dioscorides, Pedanius, 16, 254
distillation
   bad liquor, 92
   column stills, 96
   copper alembic stills, 104, *105*
   craft approach to, 87–89
   cutting heads and tails after, 88, 91
   defined, 88
   development of, 17
   mash bills, 93
   pot stills, 92, *93*
distilleries
   Barr Hill, 98–100, *98*
   Blue Barren Distillery, 89–90
   Matchbook Distilling, 95–98, *95*, *97*
   New England Distilling, 92–94, *93*, *94*
   Sherwood Distillery, 94
   Tamworth Distilling, 100–102, *100*, *101*
   WhistlePig, 102–3, *103*
   Wiggly Bridge Distillery, 90–92, *91*
   Wild Sings the Bird, 103–5, *104*, *105*, 124

Index

distiller's beer, 94
diuretics, defined, 55
DIY Cinchona Bark Extract, **238**
DIY Dry Vermouth, **150**
DIY Wild Transforming Vermouth, 142, *142*, **143**
DMG Designs, 40, 41
Doctor's Orders, **149**
dose-response relationship, 79
double-straining, 42
Dreamer's Tea, **200**
Dreaming with Morpheus, **200**
drugs, development and regulation of, 19–20
dry curaçao, 21, 46, 138
drying herbs, 118
duo-style cocktails, 50

E

earthing, health benefits of, 69
Earth Spiral Apothecary, 183, 291
Eclectics, 19
Eden Acres, 213
edible flowers. *See also* garnish gardens
    in flower confetti, 220, 221, *221*
    ice cubes with, 46–47
    overview, 33
effervescence, 192
egg nog, 50
egg white sours, 48
eighteen twenty wines, 173
elderberry (*Sambucus canadensis*), *244*
    in Chai-Spiced Elderberry Syrup, 146
    in Doctor's Orders, 149
    in Elderberry Syrup, 245
    in Elderberry Tincture, 245
    in Harvest Gold, 209
    monograph on, 243–45
    in Tonic & Tonic, 135
"Elderberry Sour," **199**, *199*
Elderberry Syrup, **245**
Elderberry Tincture, **245**
elderflower (*Sambucus canadensis*)
    in Carol's Elderflower Champagne, 194
    in Elderflower Collins, 194
    in Gates of Immortality, 188
    in Mojito Popsicles, 195
Elderflower Collins, **194**
electuaries, overview, 37
élevage (bringing up), 95
elixirs, overview, 33
Embrace the Dragon, *28*, **155**
emulsifiers, 84
emulsions, 84
endocannabinoid system, 68–69
energetic herbalism, 53, 70–73, 225
energy, in extraction, 85
The English Physician (Culpeper), 18
enteric nervous system, 67–68
Ephemeral Beauty, **163**
equipment, 27, *28*, 29–30, 40–47
essentials of botanical bar craft, 27–51
    building cocktails, 29–30
    classic cocktail recipes, 47–51
    dilution of drinks, 30–31
    equipment, 27, *28*, 29–30, 40–47
    fresh ingredients, 27, 28–29
    overview, 27–28
    preparation methods, 31–39
Euphoria, *48*, **211**
Everyday Aperitif, **156**
extraction, 75–85
    of alkaloids, 78
    of amino acids, 82
    chemistry of, 75–77
    defined, 32
    of lipids, 81–82
    of minerals, 81
    nomenclature of, 32
    of phytosterols, 83
    plant monograph information on, 225–26
    of polyphenols, 77
    of polysaccharides, 82
    quick reference guide, 83–85, 83*t*
    of sulfur-containing compounds, 79–81
    summary of preparation, 31–33
    of tannins, 82
    of terpenoids, 78–79

F

fats
    extraction of, 81–82
    role in nutrition, 66–67
    sources of fatty acids, 60
fat washing, 34, 214
fennel (*Foeniculum vulgare*)
    in Digestivo Oxymel, 156
    in DIY Dry Vermouth, 150
    in Fennel Honey Syrup, 159
Fennel Honey Syrup, 158, **159**
fermented beverages, overview, 34
Fields Fields Blueberries, 212
Fields of Gold Mead, **190**, *191*, 192
"Fields of Gold" Mead Spritzer, **192**
Five Element Theory, 15, 70–73
Five-Plum Syrup, **216**
fizzes, overview, 48–49
flavonoids, 59, 77
flip-style drinks, 50
flower confetti, 220, 221, *221*
flower essences, 34, 189
food mills, 42
Forest Green Juice, **163**
Foster Farm Botanicals, 291
four elements, 18
four humors/four temperaments, 15
free radicals, 64–65
Free the Qi, **124**, *125*
French shakers, 40
fusel (bad liquor), 92

G

GABA (gamma-amino-butyric acid), 62
Galen of Pergamon, 16
Garden Honey Tea Syrup, 170, **171**
gardening. *See also* garnish gardens
    plant monograph information on, 225
    resources for, 292
garnishes
    atomizers for, 46
    oversized ice cubes, *30*
    overview, 33

garnish gardens, 107–19
   bed preparation and planting, 114–15
   design and layout, 113–14
   harvesting and drying plants, 118, *119*
   maintenance tasks, 115–18
   overview, 107–8
   plant choices, 111–13
   site selection, 108–9
   soil, 109–11
   tools, 109
gastrointestinal system, inflammation effects on, 67–68
Gates of Immortality, 188
gentian (*Gentiana lutea*)
   in Bitter Orange Cordial, 148
   bitter qualities of, 59, 229
gin
   color-changing, 233
   infused, 187, 216
   juniper in, *96*, 99, 253
gin botanical apothecary (Matchbook Distilling), 97, *97*
ginger (*Zingiber officinale*), *246*
   in Adaptogenic Chai Tea, 240
   anti-inflammatory qualities, 55
   aphrodisiac qualities, 56
   in Aralia Root & Ginger Tea, 160
   in Birch Bark Syrup, 145
   in Chai-Spice Bitters, 147
   in Chai-Spiced Elderberry Syrup, 146
   in Cranberry, Rose Hip & Ginger Syrup, 138
   in Doctor's Orders, 149
   in Everyday Aperitif, 156
   in Free the Qi, 124
   in Ginger Beer, 208
   in Ginger-Chamomile Tea, 246
   in Ginger-Cinnamon Cider, 210
   in Ginger-Clove Syrup, 130
   gin infused with, 216
   in Golden Touch, 134
   in Harvest Gold, 209
   in Maca Chai Syrup, 137
   monograph on, 245–46

   in The Mosscat, 162
   in Pregnancy Punch, 167
   in Quantum Entanglement, 136
   in Savant or Savage? 142
   in Sexy Hot Chocolate, 132
   in Vanilla Ginger Honey Syrup, 186
   in Vision of Adonis, 129
Ginger Beer, 158, **208**
Ginger-Chamomile Tea, **246**
Ginger-Cinnamon Cider, **210**
Ginger-Clove Syrup, **130**
ginkgo (*Ginkgo biloba*)
   as nootropic, 62
   in Street Smarts Tincture, 168
glasses and serving vessels, 27, *28*, 43, *43*
glucosinolates, extraction of, 80–81
glycerin, as menstruum, 34, 83*t*
glycerites, overview, 34
golden milk, 134
goldenrod (*Solidago canadensis*)
   in Fields of Gold Mead, 190
   in "Fields of Gold" Mead Spritzer, 192
Golden Touch, **134**
gotu kola (*Centella asiatica*)
   in Calendula & Gotu Kola Honey Tea Syrup, 124
   as nervine and nootropic, 62
   in Raspberry Leaf & Gotu Kola Tea, 207
grain neutral spirits, 87
grapefruit (*Citrus paradisi*)
   bitter qualities of, 59
   in Bitters & Soda, 158
   in Digestivo Oxymel, 156
   in DIY Dry Vermouth, 150
   in Everyday Aperitif, 156
   in Poets & Outlaws, 174
   in Wildfire Hearts, 184
grape leaves, in Opening Doors, 131
Grasse, Steven, 100, 101–2
Greek mythology, winemaking in, 12–13
Green Coffee Tincture, 196, **197**

green tea (*Camellia sinensis*), *247*
   as astringent, 58
   as cardioprotective, 60
   monograph on, 246–48
   as nervine stimulant, 61
   as nootropic, 62
grinders, spice, 46
grounding, health benefits of, 69
The Gypsy and the Monk, **138**

H

habitat
   in garnish gardens, 107–8, *107*, 109, 115–16
   plant monographs on, 225
Happiness Tonic, 124, *125*
Hardie, Todd, 98
Harvest Gold, **209**, *209*
hawthorn (*Crataegus* spp.), *249*
   as cardioprotective, 60
   in Harvest Gold, 209
   in Hawthorn & Bitters Honey Syrup, 217
   in Hawthorn Flower Essence, 189
   in Hawthorn Honey Syrup, 128
   in Hawthorn Rose Hip Honey, 207
   monograph on, 248–49
   in Very Cherry, Thorns & Flowers Syrup, 174
Hawthorn & Bitters Honey Syrup, **217**
Hawthorne strainers, *40*, 42, *42*
Hawthorn Flower Essence, 188, **189**
Hawthorn Honey Syrup, **128**, *129*
Hawthorn Rose Hip Honey, 206, **207**
heads, from the distillation process, 88, 91
Healing with Whole Foods (Pitchford), 72
Heart of Venus, **164**
heart rate variability, 68
herbal actions, 53–73
   defined, 53
   energetics of, 53, 70–73, 225

Index

inflammation and stress
 response reduction by, 63–65
 nervous system balancing by,
  65–70
 overview, 53–54
 plant monograph information
  on, 225
 recipe notations, 122
 types of, 54–62
herbal medicine
 author's experience in, 2–3
 history of, 14–20
 intersection with craft
  cocktails, 7–9
 preparations in, 28–29, 31–39,
  122, 226
hermeticism, 17–18
hibiscus (*Hibiscus sabdariffa*),
  38, *250*
 in Hibiscus Agave, 185
 monograph on, 250–51
 in Street Smarts Decoction,
  168
 in Wildfire Hearts, 184
Hibiscus Agave, 184, **185**, *185*
Hildegard von Bingen, 17
Hippocrates, 14–15
Hippocratic Corpus, 15
history of spiritual and medical
 use of botanicals, 11–25
 alchemy, 17–18
 ancient medical applications,
  14–17
 risks and benefits of alcohol
  consumption, 20–25
 ritual and resurrection applications, 11–14, *12*
 shift to modern medicine,
  18–20
Homemade Bloody Mary Mix,
  152, **153**
Homemade Vanilla Extract, **284**
honey
 Barr Hill use of, 98, 99
 nutritional chemistry of, 80, *80*
 in simple syrups, 37
honey syrups
 Cinnamon-Vanilla Honey
  Syrup, 201

Fennel Honey Syrup, 159
 in Gates of Immortality, 188
 Hawthorn & Bitters Honey
  Syrup, 217
 Hawthorn Honey Syrup, 128
 Sweetfern Honey Syrup, 172
 in Tuscan Garden, 141
 Vanilla Ginger Honey
  Syrup, 186
honey tea syrups
 Calendula & Gotu Kola
  Honey Tea Syrup, 124
 Garden Honey Tea Syrup, 171
 Lavender Sage Honey Tea
  Syrup, 205
 overview, 37
Hop and Grapefruit Bitter, **252**
hops (*Humulus lupulus*), *252*
 monograph on, 251–52
 as nervine relaxant, 62
hormesis, 79
Horrigan, Dan, 98
Horse's Neck, 49
hot drinks, overview, 51
Howard, Jeremy, 89
How to Mix Drinks (Thomas), 49
humoral theory of medicine,
  15, 18
husk cherry (*Physalis* spp.),
  growing, 112
hydroethanolic extracts, 39
hydrosols
 nonalcoholic spirits from,
  103–4
 overview, 35
 by Wild Sings the Bird, 103–5
hyssop (*Hyssopus officinalis*)
 bourbon infused with, 146
 in "Elderberry Sour," 199
 in Hyssop & Teaberry Infused
  Rye Whiskey, 149
Hyssop & Teaberry Infused Rye
 Whiskey, **149**

I

ice, 31, 46–47
immune response, 63, 64
inflammation
 anti-inflammatories for, 55

overview, 63–65
Infused Pisco, 136, **137**
infusions, 32, 35, 39
innate immune response, 63, 64
ionic activity, health benefits
 of, 69
Ireland, Meghan, 102, 103
Irish moss (*Chondrus crispus*),
  60, 213

J

Japanese knotweed
 (*Reynoutria* spp.)
 polyphenols in, 60
 in Street Smarts Decoction,
  168
jiggers, *40*, 41, *41*
Juice of Life, **180**
juicers and juicing, 35, *35*, *40*, 46
Juicy, **206**, *206*
julep strainers, *40*, 42
julep-style drinks, 50
juniper (*Juniperus communis*), *253*
 in Blueberry Jamboree, 126
 in The Common Sage, 205
 gin from, *98*, 99, 253
 monograph on, 252–54
 in Opening Doors, 131
 in Tonic & Tonic, 135
 in Winter Amaro, 140

K

kava (*Piper methysticum*)
 in Kava Cacao Flip, 127
 in Kava Hula Girl, 193
Kava Cacao Flip, **127**
Kava Hula Girl, **193**, *193*
Ki Ceramics, 155

L

labeling of preparations, 44, *44*
landcrafted, as term, 100
Late Embers spirits, 96–97
lavender (*Lavandula* spp.), *254*
 in Altar & Intent, 183
 in "Are You a Dreamer?" Bitters, 128
 aromatic qualities, 58
 in Blueberry Jamboree, 126

lavender (*continued*)
   in Blue Lotus Wine
      Spritzer, 13
   in Butterfly Tea, 234
   in Dreamer's Tea, 200
   in Free the Qi, 124
   in Garden Honey Tea
      Syrup, 171
   in Lavender Sage Honey
      Tea Syrup, 205
   monograph on, 254–55
   as nervine relaxant, *61*, 62
   in Opening Doors, 131
Lavender Sage Honey Tea
   Syrup, **205**
lecithin, 193
lemon balm (*Melissa officinalis*),
   256
   aromatic qualities, 58
   in Blueberry Jamboree, 126
   monograph on, 255–57
   in Saving the Sun, 216
   tincture of, 257
Lemon Balm Tincture, **257**
lemon verbena (*Aloysia citrodora*)
   in Five-Plum syrup, 216
   growing, 112
lettuce. *See* wild lettuce
   (*Lactuca virosa*)
licorice (*Glycyrrhiza glabra*)
   as adaptogen, 55
   in Adaptogenic Chai Tea, 240
   in Doctor's Orders, 149
   in The Queen's Fortress, 202
life cycles, of plants, 117
Like Bunny Rabbits, **165**, *165*
like dissolves like principle,
   84, 85
lilac (*Syringa* spp.)
   in Street Smarts, 168
   in Transcendental Lilac, 172
limbic system, overview, 68
lion's mane mushroom (*Hericium
   erinaceus*), 62, 265, 266
lipids, extraction of, 81–82
local sources, benefits of, 3, 87–88
lovage (*Levisticum officinale*),
   growing, 112
Lovers' Tequila, **211**

low-alcohol cocktails, 44
lymphatics, defined, 55

M

maca (*Lepidium meyenii*)
   as adaptogen, 55
   as aphrodisiac, 56
   in Maca Chai Syrup, 137
   in Vision of Adonis, 129
Maca Chai Syrup, 136, **137**
macerating, defined, 32
Maillard reaction, 92
maple (*Acer* spp.) and maple
   syrup, 257
   in Birch Bark Syrup, 145
   in Blueberry Chaga Elixir, 178
   in DIY Wild Transforming
      Vermouth, 143
   in Heart of Venus, 164
   in Kava Cacao Flip, 127
   in Kava Hula Girl, 193
   in Maple Coriander Syrup, 219
   monograph on, 257–58
   production of, 257, 258
   in Pumpkin Seed Milk, 128
   in The Queen's Fortress, 202
   in Sugar on Snow, 169
   in Sultry Look, 210
Maple Coriander Syrup, **219**
marshmallow (*Althaea officinalis*)
   in "Calm Down, Psycho," 278
   as demulcent, 60
   in Heart of Venus, 164
   in Kava Cacao Flip, 127
Marshmallows, Cinnamon,
   132, **133**
Mary-style drinks, 51
mash bills and mashing, 93
Matcha Latte, **248**
Matchbook Distilling, 95–98,
   95, *97*
meads
   Fields of Gold Mead, 190
   "Fields of Gold" Mead
      Spritzer, 192
measuring cups, 47
Meeting House Farm, *119*, 291
menstruum, as term, 29, 32.
   See also solvents

Merinoff-Kwasnieski, Leslie,
   95–98, *95*
microplanes, 44
milk thistle (*Silybum marianum*),
   259
   in About Last Night, 260
   bitter qualities of, 59
   monograph on, 258–260
milky oat seed (*Avena sativa*)
   in Milky Oat Tincture, 203
   as nervine trophorestorative, 62
Milky Oat Tincture
   in Quantum Entanglement,
      136
   in The Queen's Fortress, 202
   recipe for, **203**
   in Vision of Adonis, 129
minerals, extraction of, 81
mint (*Mentha* spp.), 261
   in After-Dinner Mint
      Cordial, 262
   in Elderflower Collins, 194
   in Mojito Popsicles, 195
   monograph on, 260–62
   in Peppermint Tea-Tini, 262
misting, atomizers for, 44, *45*
mithridatism, 79
Mixed Fruit Purée, **196**
mixing vessels and shakers,
   29–30, 40–41, *40*, *42*
Mojito Popsicles, **195**
monophenols, 77
mortars and pestles, *40*, 46
Moscow Mule, 49
The Mosscat, **162**, *162*
muddleables, 33
muddlers, 41
mugwort (*Artemisia vulgaris*), 262
   in "Are You a Dreamer?"
      Bitters, 128
   bitter qualities of, 59
   in Dreamer's Tea, 200
   in Hawthorn & Bitters
      Honey Syrup, 217
   monograph on, 262–63
   in Mugwort Infused Gin, 187
   in Mugwort Infused Oil, 263
   in Opening Doors, 131
   in Street Smarts Tincture, 168

Index

Mugwort Infused Gin, 186, **187**
Mugwort Infused Oil, **263**
mule-style drinks, 49
mushroom, monograph on, 264–66, *264*. *See also specific types*

N

names, botanical, 54
nasturtium (*Tropaeolum* spp.), growing, 112
Natural History (Pliny the Elder), 15–16
Nei Ching (ancient Chinese text), 15
Nellis, Sam, 99, 100
nervines, overview, 60–62
nervous system, balancing through herbal actions, 65–70
nettle (*Urtica dioica*)
 as alterative, 55
 in Forest Green Juice, 163
 in Red Raspberry Leaf & Stinging Nettle Tea, 167
 in Spring Tonic Oxymel, 160
 in Vision of Adonis, 129
New England Distilling, 92–94, *93*, *94*
nogs, overview, 50
nonalcoholic spirits, from hydrosols, 104
Nootropical Paradise, **182**, *182*
nootropics, overview, 62
North Spore, 188, 264
"nose" of cocktails, 44
nutmeg (*Myristica fragrans*), *267*
 in Ambrosia, 222
 in The Common Sage, 205
 in Golden Touch, 134
 in Kava Hula Girl, 193
 monograph on, 266–67
 as nervine relaxant, 62
 in The Queen's Fortress, 202

O

oak (*Quercus* spp.)
 as astringent, 58
 in Oak Extract, 181
Oak Extract, 180, **181**

oat (*Avena sativa*)
 in Milky Oat Tincture, 203
 as nervine trophorestorative, 62
oils
 for fat washing, 34
 as solvent, 83*t*, 85
omega-3 and omega-6 fatty acids, 67
Opening Doors, **131**, *131*
orange (*Citrus sinensis*)
 in Bitter Orange Cordial, 148
 bitter qualities of, 59
 flower water of, 196, 200
overproof spirits, 31–32
oxidative stress, 64–65
oxymels
 Digestivo Oxymel, 156
 overview, 29, 37
 Schisandra Oxymel, 277
 Seafarer's Oxymel, 212, 213
 Spring Tonic Oxymel, 160

P

Paracelsus, 18, 79, 256
passionflower (*Passiflora incarnata*), *268*
 in Crimes of Passion, 196
 monograph on, 267–69
 as nervine relaxant, 62
 in The Queen's Fortress, 202
 in Temple of the Goddess, 269
peach (*Prunus persica*)
 syrup of, 36
 in The Visionkeeper, 186
Pear & Cinnamon Stick Infused Calvados, 222, **223**
peppermint (*Mentha piperita*)
 in Altar & Intent, 183
 aromatic qualities, 58
 in Gates of Immortality, 188
 monograph on, 260–62
 in Peppermint Tea-Tini, 262
Peppermint Tea-Tini, **262**
performance-enhancing herbal actions, 69–70
philosophy of botanical cocktails, 1–9, 287–88
Phyllis (still), *98*
Physica (Hildegard von Bingen), 17

phytosterols, extraction of, 83
pine (*Pinus* spp.), *270*
 hydrosol of, 130, 156
 monograph on, 269–271
 pollen of, 129
 resin of, 271
 in Winter Amaro, 140
 in Wisdom of Old, 146
Pitchford, Paul, 72
plant monographs, overview, 225–26. *See also specific plants*
plant names, 54
Pliny the Elder, 15–16
plum (*Prunus* spp.),
 in Five-Plum Syrup, 216
Poets & Outlaws, **174**
polarity, in extraction, 76, 77
pollinator habitat, in garnish gardens, 107–8, *107*, 109, 115–16
polyphenols
 as adaptogen, 55
 as cardioprotective, 59–60
 extraction of, 77
polysaccharides, extraction of, 82
pomegranate (*Punica granatum*)
 grenadine from, 21
 in Pregnancy Punch, 167
 in Secret Grove, 130
popping candy, 196
Popsicles, Mojito, **195**
pot stills, 92, *93*
pousse-cafés, 49
powders, herbal, 37
Power, Matt, *100*
Pregnancy Punch, *166*, **167**
preparations, herbal
 overview, 28–29
 plant monograph information on, 226
 recipe notations, 122
 summary of methods, 31–39
Preserved Cocktail Cherries, **175**
preserves, overview, 37
pressing and straining, defined, 32
prickly pear (*Opuntia* spp.), in Juice of Life, 180
Primitivo, **217**
pumpkin seed (*Cucurbita maxima*), 56, 128

305

Pumpkin Seed Milk, **128**, 129
pungent tastes, in Five Element Theory, 72–73

Q

Quantum Entanglement, **136**, *136*
The Queen's Fortress, **202**, *203*
quick reference extraction guide, 83–85, 83*t*

R

raspberry (*Rubus* spp.)
    aphrodisiac qualities, 56
    as astringent, 58
    as cardioprotective, 60
    in Euphoria, 211
    in Gates of Immortality, 188
    in Infused Pisco, 137
    in Opening Doors, 131
    in Quantum Entanglement, 136
    in Raspberry Leaf & Gotu Kola Tea, 207
    in Red Raspberry Leaf & Stinging Nettle Tea, 167
    in Ruby Throat Sunset, 177
Raspberry Leaf & Gotu Kola Tea, 206, **207**
ratios, in tinctures, 84–85
reamers, for citrus juicing, *40*, 46
red clover (*Trifolium pratense*), 28–29, 55
Red Raspberry Leaf & Stinging Nettle Tea, **167**
reishi mushroom (*Ganoderma* spp.), 66
    as adaptogen, 55
    growing, *188*
    monograph on, 265, 266
    in Reishi Tincture, *44*, 164, 188, 189
Reishi Tincture, *44*, 164, 188, **189**
Remedy Cocktail Co., 3, 101
resources, 291–92
rhodiola (*Rhodiola rosea*)
    as adaptogen, 55
    in The Common Sage, 205
    as nervine stimulant, 61

rickeys, overview, 48–49
ritual and resurrection use of botanicals, 11–14, *12*
Ritual Brand spirits, 152
Roederer Estate, 173
Rogers Farm, 96
rolling, of cocktails, 29–30
Rooted Heart Remedies, *108*, 200, 291
rose (*Rosa* spp.), *272*
    in Altar & Intent, 183
    as aphrodisiac, 56
    as astringent, 58
    in Cardamom-Rose Sea Salt, 181
    in Cranberry, Rose Hip & Ginger Syrup, 138
    in DIY Dry Vermouth, 150
    in flower confetti, 221
    in Hawthorn Rose Hip Honey, 207
    in Heart of Venus, 164
    in Kava Cacao Flip, 127
    monograph on, 271–72
    preparations from, 76
    in Spicy Pink Salt, 187
    in Street Smarts Decoction, 168
    in Wildfire Hearts, 184
    in Wild Rose Elixir, 139
    in Winter Amaro, 140
rosemary (*Rosmarinus officinalis*), *274*
    aromatic qualities, 58
    in Digestivo Oxymel, 156
    in Garden Honey Tea Syrup, 171
    hydrosol of, 124
    monograph on, 273–75
    as nootropic, 62
    in Rosemary Bitters, 139
    in Rosemary Infused Olive Oil, 141
    in Tuscan Garden, 141
Rosemary Bitters, 138, **139**
Rosemary Infused Olive Oil, **141**
rose water
    in Heart of Venus, 164
    in Juice of Life, 180

    in Juicy, 206
    in Kava Hula Girl, 193
    in Pregnancy Punch, 167
    preparation of, 273
    in Ruby Throat Sunset, 177
Ruby Throat Sunset, **177**, *177*
rum
    in After-Dinner Mint Cordial, 262
    Bully Boy Rum Cooperative Volume 2, 134, 219
    in Elderberry Tincture, 245
    in Golden Touch, 134
    in Green Coffee Tincture, 197
    in Homemade Vanilla Extract, 284
    in Poets & Outlaws, 174
    in Sweetened by Frost, 219
    Wray and Nephew white overproof rum, 140
"Rum-Spiced" Molasses, 167, 208
Runamok Maple, 102
rye whiskey
    from Barr Hill, 100
    in Hyssop & Teaberry Infused Rye Whiskey, 149
    in The Scofflaw, 21
    from WhistlePig, 102–3

S

safety considerations, 121, 226
sage (*Salvia officinalis*)
    in "Elderberry Sour," 199
    in Lavender Sage Honey Tea Syrup, 205
sake
    in Primitivo, 217
    in Saving the Sun, 216
salt
    Cardamom-Rose Sea Salt, 180, 181
    in Five Element Theory, 71
    in hermeticism, 18
    for preserving herbs, 38
    Spicy Pink Salt, 186, 187
saponins, extraction of, 78–79
Saucier, Ted, 14
Savant or Savage?, **142**, *142*
Saving the Sun, **216**

Index

savory drinks, overview, 51
The Savoy Cocktail Book (Craddock), 50
schisandra (*Schisandra chinensis*), 275
    as adaptogen, 55
    monograph on, 275–77
    oxymel of, 277
    tincture of, 206, 207
Schisandra Oxymel, **277**
Schisandra Tincture, 206, **207**
The Scofflaw, **21**
sea buckthorn purée, 196
Seafarer's Oxymel, 212, **213**
Sea-Salted Agave Caramel, **211**
secondary metabolites, 53–54
Secret Grove, **130**
seed planting, 111, 113
serotonin, 67
Sexy Hot Chocolate, **132**, *132*
shakers and mixing vessels, 29–30, 40–41, *40*, *42*
shaking
    of cocktails, 30
    in extraction, 85
The Shapeshifter, **234**
Sherwood Distillery, 94
shrubs, overview, 37
simple syrups, overview, 37. *See also* syrups
Siren Call, *30*, **212**
skullcap (*Scutellaria lateriflora*), 277
    in "Calm Down, Psycho," 278
    monograph on, 277–79
    as nervine trophorestorative, 62
    in Skullcap Glycerite, 203
    tincture of, 278
Skullcap Glycerite, 202, **203**
smashes, overview, 50–51
Smithline, Kylie, 155
soil, for garnish gardens, 109–11, *110*
solubility, in extraction, 76
solvents
    for bitters, 31–32
    menstruum, as term, 29, 32
    quick reference guide, 83–85, 83*t*

sours
    in Five Element Theory, 71–72
    overview, 47–49
spagyrics, 18
spearmint (*Mentha spicata*)
    in Mojito Popsicles, 195
    monograph on, 260–62
Spiced Chocolate Syrup, **220**
spice grinders, 46
Spicy Pink Salt, 186, **187**
spicy tastes, in Five Element Theory, 72–73
spilanthes (*Acmella oleracea*), *81*, *119*, 279
    in Cheshire Cat, 170
    monograph on, 279–280
    tincture of, 280
Spilanthes Foam, **280**
spirit-forward cocktails, overview, 47
spoons, *40*, *41*
spring
    in Five Element Theory, 71–72
    qualities of, 154
Spring Tonic #1, **160**
Spring Tonic Oxymel, **160**
star anise (*Illicium verum*)
    in Harvest Gold, 209
    in Siren Call, *30*, 212
Starwest Botanicals, 291
steam distillation, 35, *105*
Steiner, Rudolf, 19
Stewart, Andrew, 89
stinging nettle. *See* nettle (*Urtica dioica*)
stirring
    of cocktails, 30
    in extraction, 85
    vessels for, 29–30, 40
St. John's wort (*Hypericum perforatum*)
    as nervine trophorestorative, 62
    in Ruby Throat Sunset, 177
strainers, 30, *40*, *42*
straining and pressing, defined, 32
strawberry (*Fragaria* spp.)
    in Juice of Life, 180
    in Like Bunny Rabbits, 165
    in Victory Garden, 173

Street Smarts, **168**
Street Smarts Decoction, **168**
Street Smarts Tincture, **168**
stress responses, 1, 63–65
stripping runs, 88
sugar
    cardiovascular concerns from, 60, 67
    for preserving herbs, 38
Sugar on Snow, **169**
Sugar Snap Pea Juice, 170, **171**
sulfur-containing compounds
    extraction of, 79–81
    in hermeticism, 18
Sultry Look, **210**
summer
    in Five Element Theory, 72
    qualities of, 176
sunflower (*Helianthus annuus*), *108*
    growing, 112
    in Kava Hula Girl, 193
Sunsoil, 200
sweet Annie (*Artemisia annua*)
    in Altar & Intent, 183
    in Babe in the Woods, 178
    in Sweetened by Frost, 219
Sweetened by Frost, 218, **219**
sweetfern (*Comptonia peregrina*), 280
    in Chocolate Sweetfern Bitters, 143
    in Fields of Gold Mead, 190
    monograph on, 280–81
    in Sweetfern Honey Syrup, 172
    in Winter Amaro, 140
Sweetfern Honey Syrup, **172**
sweetness, in Five Element Theory, 72
swizzling cocktails, 29–30
syrups. *See also* agave syrup; maple (*Acer* spp.) and maple syrup
    Birch Bark Syrup, 145
    Chai-Spiced Elderberry Syrup, 146
    Chai-Spiced Syrup, 175
    Cranberry, Rose Hip & Ginger Syrup, 138
    Elderberry Syrup, 245
    Fennel Honey Syrup, 159

syrups (*continued*)
   Five-Plum Syrup, 216
   Garden Honey Tea Syrup, 170, 171
   Ginger-Clove Syrup, 130
   Hawthorn & Bitters Honey Syrup, 217
   Hawthorn Honey Syrup, 128
   honey syrup, 141
   Maca Chai Syrup, 137
   simple syrups overview, 37
   Spiced Chocolate Syrup, 220
   Sweetfern Honey Syrup, 172
   Vanilla Ginger Honey Syrup, 186
   Very Cherry, Thorns & Flowers Syrup, 174

T

tails, from the distillation process, 88, 91
Tamworth Distilling, 100–102, *100*, *101*
tannins, extraction of, 82
teaberry (*Gaultheria procumbens*)
   in Hyssop & Teaberry Infused Rye Whiskey, 149
   in Underground Matrix, 214, *215*
teas, overview, 38–39
Temple of the Goddess, **269**
tequila
   in Lovers' Tequila, 211
   in Wild Rose Tequila, 184
   in Xocolatl, 220
terpenes, as adaptogen, 55
terpenoids, extraction of, 78–79
Thayer, Cynthia, 2
Thomas, Jerry, 49
thumpers, 92, *93*
thyme (*Thymus* spp.)
   in Doctor's Orders, 149
   in Garden Honey Tea Syrup, 171
   in Homemade Bloody Mary Mix, 153
tiki-style drinks, 49–50
tinctures
   overview, 39
   for preparation of bitters, 32
Tonic & Tonic, **135**, *135*
tonics, definitions of, 5–6, 53
tonic water, 5, 237–38
Tooth of the Lion Bitters, **243**
traditional and complementary medicine, as term, 14. *See also* herbal medicine
Traditional Chinese Medicine
   bitters in, 59
   Five Element Theory in, 15, 70–73
   history of, 15
Transcendental Lilac, **172**
trillium flower essence, in Ephemeral Beauty, 163
trios, overview, 50
tropical-style drinks, 49–50
tulsi (*Ocimum* spp.), *282*
   aromatic qualities, 58
   bourbon infused with, 146
   in "Calm Down, Psycho," 278
   in "Elderberry Sour," 199
   monograph on, 281–82
   in The Queen's Fortress, 202
   in Tulsi Glycerite, 196
   in The Visionkeeper, 186
Tulsi Glycerite, 130, **196**
turkey tail mushroom (*Coriolus versicolor*)
   in Chai-Spiced Elderberry Syrup, 146
   in Harvest Gold, 209
   monograph on, 266
   in Winter Amaro, 140
turmeric (*Curcuma longa*)
   anti-inflammatory qualities, 55
   in Golden Touch, 134
   in Mixed Fruit Purée, 196
Tuscan Garden, **141**

U

Underground Matrix, **214**, *215*
Upside-Down Storm, **208**

V

vagus nerve, 68
vanilla (*Vanilla planifolia*), *283*
   aromatic qualities, 58
   in Cinnamon Marshmallows, 133
   in Cinnamon-Vanilla Honey Syrup, 201
   in Crimes of Passion, 196
   in Golden Touch, 134
   homemade extract of, 284
   in Kava Cacao Flip, 127
   in Like Bunny Rabbits, 165
   in Maca Chai Syrup, 137
   monograph on, 283–84
   in Pumpkin Seed Milk, 128
   in "Rum-Spiced" Molasses, 167
   in Sexy Hot Chocolate, 132
   in Spiced Chocolate Syrup, 220
   in Sultry Look, 210
   in Vanilla Ginger Honey Syrup, 186
Vanilla Ginger Honey Syrup, **186**
Vena's Fizz House, 155
Vendome, 101
Vermont Center for Integrative Herbalism, 3, 103
Vermont Marshmallow Company, 132
vermouth
   DIY Dry Vermouth, 150
   DIY Wild Transforming Vermouth, 142, *142*, 143
   overview, 39
   in The Scofflaw, 21
Very Cherry, Thorns & Flowers Syrup, **174**
Victory Garden, **173**, *173*
vinegar extracts (acetums), 32, 39, 83*t*. *See also* apple cider vinegar
violet (*Viola* spp.), *161*
   as demulcent, 60
   in Ephemeral Beauty, 163
   in The Mosscat, 162
   in Spring Tonic #1, 160
viriditas, as term, 17
The Visionkeeper, **186**
Vision of Adonis, **129**
vodka
   in Bloody Botanist, 152
   in The Gypsy and the Monk, 138
   kelp-infused, 90

Index

W

water
  choice of, 30–31
  for dilution of drinks, 30
  in Five Element Theory, 71
  for garnish gardens, 108–9, 116–17
  as solvent, 83*t*, 85
whiskey. *See also* rye whiskey
  in Cinnamon Girl, 145
  in Whiskey Garden Smash, 51
Whiskey Garden Smash, **51**
WhistlePig, 102–3, *103*
Wiggly Bridge Distillery, 90–92, *91*, 146
Wight, Ned, 92–94
Wild Few Herb Farm, 291
Wildfire Hearts, **184**
wild lettuce (*Lactuca virosa*)
  bitter qualities of, 59
  as nervine relaxant, 62
  in Wild Lettuce Tincture, 201
Wild Lettuce Tincture, 200, **201**
wild rose. *See* rose (*Rosa* spp.)
Wild Rose Elixir
  in The Gypsy and the Monk, 138
  in Heart of Venus, 164
  in Pregnancy Punch, 167
  in The Queen's Fortress, 202
  recipe for, **139**
  in Sexy Hot Chocolate, 132
Wild Rose Tequila, **184**
Wild Sings the Bird, 103–5, *104*, *105*, 124, 156
wild yeasts, 191
winter
  in Five Element Theory, 71
  qualities of, 123
Winter Amaro, **140**, 142, 169
wintergreen (*Gaultheria procumbens*)
  anti-inflammatory qualities, 55
  in Winter Amaro, 140
Winter Woods hydrosol, 130, 156
Wisdom of Old, **146**, *147*
Woods, David, Sr., 90–92, *91*
Woods, David, Jr., 90–92, *91*
wormwood (*Artemisia absinthium*), 159
Wormwood Vinegar Bitters, 158, **159**
Wray and Nephew white overproof rum, 140

X

Xocolatl, **220**, *221*
Xocolatl or Aztec Hot Chocolate, **235–36**

Y

yarrow (*Achillea millefolium*), *285*
  as astringent, 58
  in Hawthorn & Bitters Honey Syrup, 217
  in Juicy, 206
  monograph on, 284–85
yeasts, wild, 191
yin tonics, 70

Z

Zack Woods Herb Farm, 291

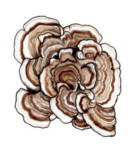

ABOUT THE AUTHOR

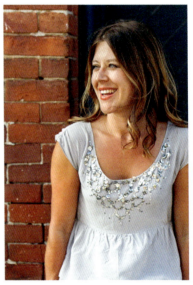

Cassandra Sears is an apothecary bartender, gardener, and herbalist. She has been studying herbal medicine for sixteen years, growing lush gardens while working as an organic gardener and playing in the wild while mixing drinks inspired by nature. She enjoys the dynamic intersection of the hospitality industry, wilderness, and organic agriculture in her native state of Maine. You can find her behind the bar part-time at the White Barn Inn in Kennebunkport. The rest of the time, you can find her elevating private events and teaching botanical cocktail classes in her role as proprietor of the Remedy Cocktail Co., for which she grows her own ingredients and works closely with local small farmers. She enjoys creative collaborations and brand ambassador work with like-minded businesses as well as creative menu design and consulting for new ventures. A graduate of the clinical herbalist training program at the Vermont Center of Integrative Herbalism, she has a modest apothecary and private wellness consultation practice where she partners with individuals for health coaching.

Matthew Weiss